ICD-10-CM:
The Questions You Didn't Know to Ask

A Complete Guide for Community Health Centers

Marlegny Mourino
MHSA, AHIMA Approved ICD-10-CM/PCS Trainer, CPC, CMAS, NCMA

Jason Frederick
Amber Braman

Synergy Billing Academy Publishing
M. Jayson Meyer, Publisher

Acknowledgement

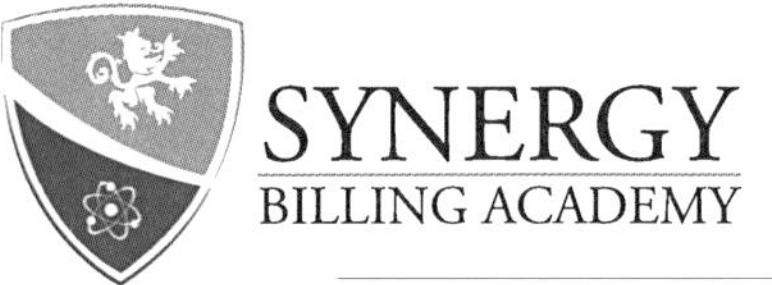

With grateful appreciation, the authors/editors acknowledge the contributions of the Synergy Billing team, especially the ICD-10 Task Force.

Disclaimer

This book and its contents are for educational purposes only. This document is not intended and it does not constitute legal advice. Keep in mind that reimbursement laws, regulations, & policies are constantly changing.

This book was current when it was published. Every reasonable effort has been made to assure the accuracy of the information within these pages. The ultimate responsibility lies with readers to ensure they are using the codes, and following applicable guidelines, correctly. Synergy Billing employees, agents, and staff make no representation, warranty, or guarantee that this compilation of information is error-free, and will bear no responsibility or liability for the results or consequences of the use of this book. This guide is a general summary that explains guidelines and principles in profitable, efficient, healthcare organizations.

TABLE OF CONTENTS

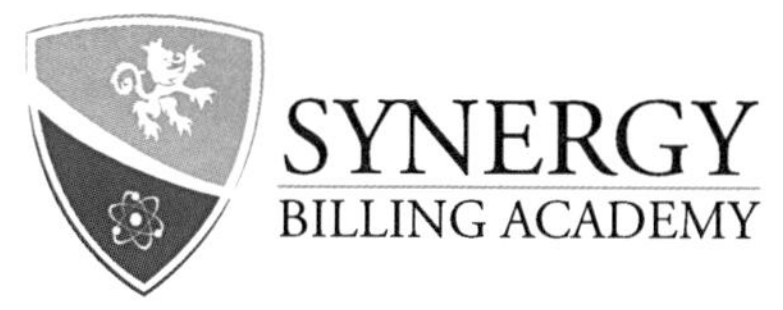

TABLE OF **CONTENTS**

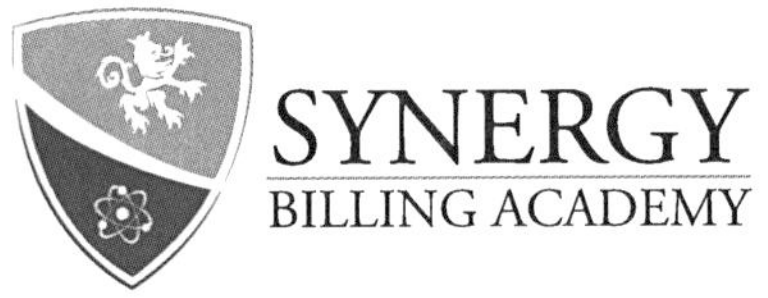

TABLE OF CONTENTS

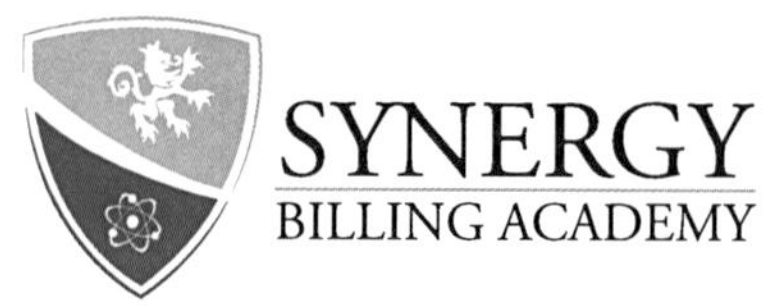

TABLE OF CONTENTS

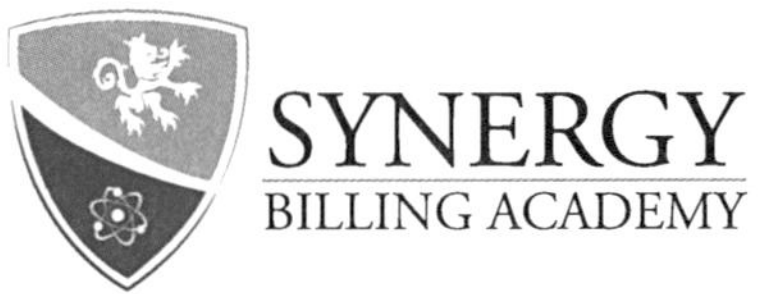

TABLE OF **CONTENTS**

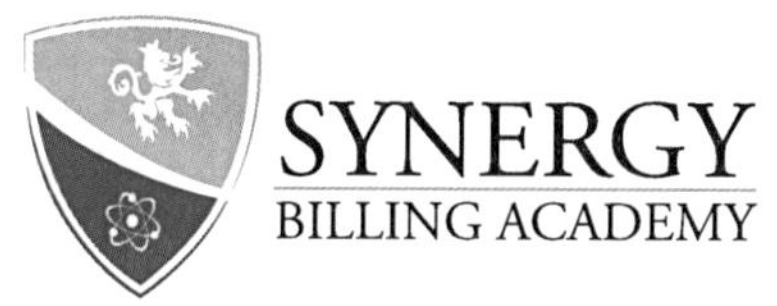

TABLE OF CONTENTS

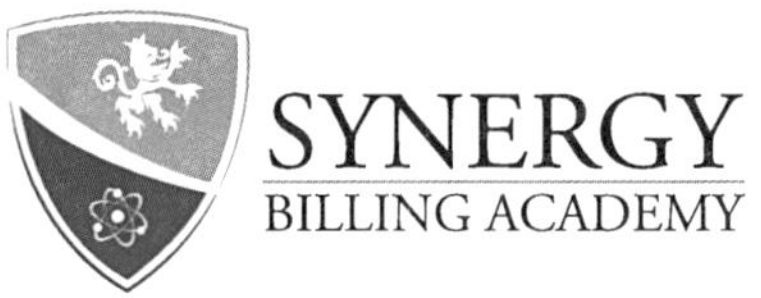

TABLE OF CONTENTS

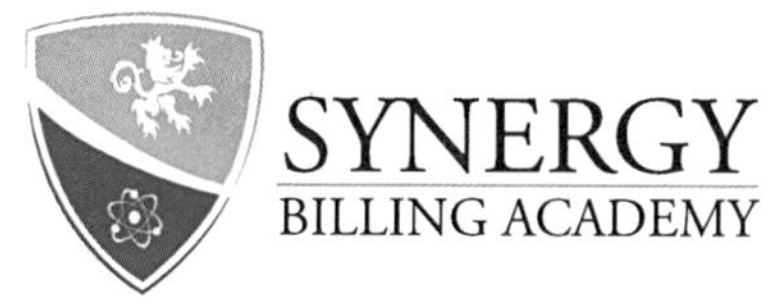

TABLE OF CONTENTS

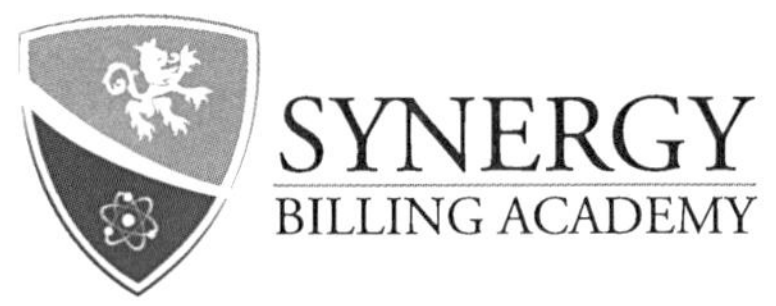

ICD-10-CM International Classification of Diseases 10th Revision Clinical Modification

Introduction to Coding

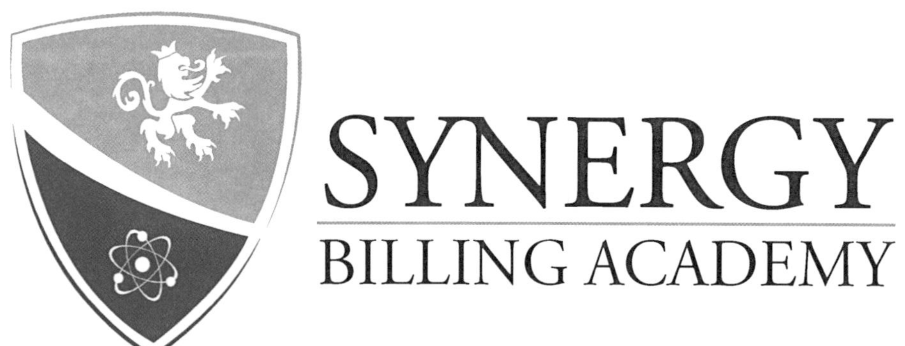

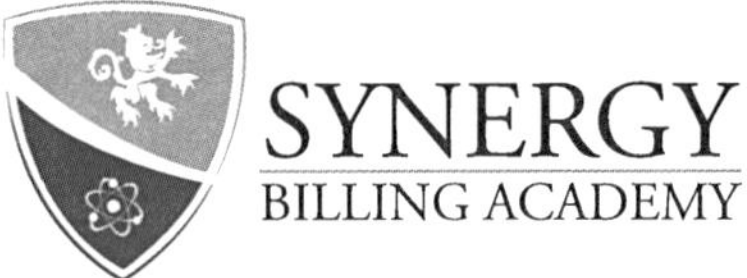

Health Insurance

Many people do not realize that insurance is an actual business—one of the largest businesses in the world. Health insurance is meant to offset the costs of illness and/or injury. By definition, a health insurance plan or a medical insurance plan is a written policy that lists all of the terms of an agreement between an individual and an insurance company.

In other words, this plan protects you from paying the full costs of medical services you receive when injured or sick. Health insurance can be compared to car insurance or even home insurance. With these plans, the individual chooses a plan and agrees to pay a certain rate, or premium, each month; then the company agrees to pay a portion of the covered costs of medical services and treatment.

Billing and Coding: Is Medical Coding the Same as Medical Billing?

No. While the medical coder and medical biller may be the same person or may work closely together to make sure all invoices are paid properly, the medical coder is primarily responsible for abstracting and assigning the appropriate coding on the claims. In order to accomplish this, the coder checks a variety of sources within the patient's medical record, (e.g., the transcription of the doctor's notes, ordered laboratory tests, requested imaging studies, and other sources) to verify the work that was done. Then the coder must assign CPT codes, ICD-9 codes, and HCPCS codes both to report the procedures that were performed and provide the medical biller with the information necessary to process a claim for reimbursement by the appropriate insurance agency.[1]

Medical Billing

The responsibility of the medical biller in a health care facility is to follow medical claims to ensure the practice receives reimbursement for the work its providers perform. Their duties will vary with the size of the facility. The billers assemble all data concerning the bill and translate health care services into billing claims. This can include charge entry, claims transmission, payment posting, insurance follow-up, and patient follow-up. Medical billers regularly communicate with physicians and other health care professionals to clarify diagnoses or obtain additional information. As a result, the medical biller must understand how to read the medical record and, like the coder, be familiar with CPT, HCPCS Level II, and ICD-9-CM codes. A knowledgeable biller can optimize revenue performance for the practice.

Introduction to Coding

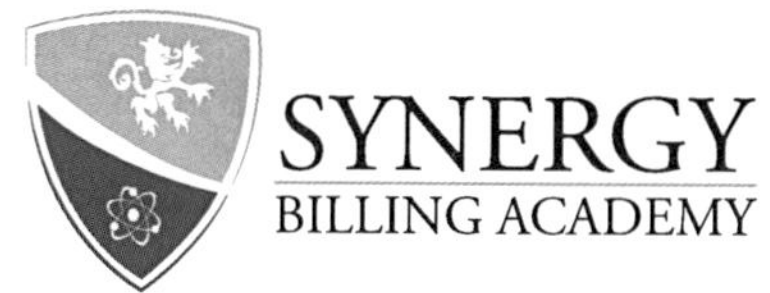

Medical Coding

Medical coding professionals perform a key step in the medical billing process. Every time a patient receives professional health care in a physician's office or outpatient/inpatient hospital facility, the provider must document the services provided. The medical coder extracts the information from the documentation, assigns the appropriate codes, and creates a claim to be paid, whether by a commercial payer, the patient, or the Centers for Medicare and Medicaid Services (CMS).

Coding and Billing Cycle

The medical coder takes the documentation of a patient's encounter with the provider and assigns the correct CPT procedure code(s) and ICD-9-CM diagnosis code(s). They assign the proper modifiers and submit all required documentation with each claim to the billers.The biller uses those codes and the insurance information to review the claims with the help of billing software to ensure that everything is accurate. They also verify the correct billing format so that they can send a clean claim that is free of errors to the appropriate insurance company. Coders and billers are crucial to the office cash flow of any health care provider. They are responsible for correctly billing both the insurance companies and the patients. Coders and billers work together to send out accurate claims so that physicians get paid in a timely manner, and follow up with payers to make sure that these claims are paid in a reasonable time.

Documentation

Documentation is defined as a chronological, detailed recording of relevant facts and observations about the patient and his or her health status that is added to the chart notes and any medical reports.

Have you heard of SOAP? What about CHEDDAR? These are different charting methods. The patient's documentation per encounter must contain certain elements: the history, examination, and medical decision making.

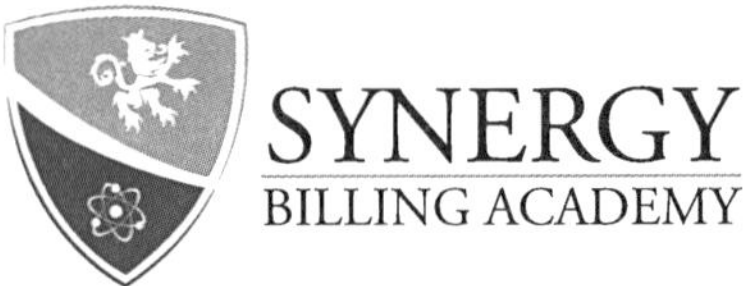

S	**Subjective** statements of symptoms and complaints in the patient's own words	Chief Complaint (CC) *Reason for the encounter*
O	**Objective** findings	Data from physical examination, X-rays, laboratory, and other diagnostic tests *Facts and findings*
A	**Assessment** of subjective and objective findings	Medical decision making *Putting all the facts together to obtain a diagnosis*
P	**Plan** of treatment	Documenting a plan for care to be put into action *Recommendations, instructions, further testing, and medication*

C	**Chief complaint**	What the patient states as the main reason for seeing the doctor; usually a subjective statement
H	**History of present illness**	Includes social history and physical symptoms as well as contributing factors
E	**Examination**	Performed by the physician
D	**Details**	List of complaints and problems
D	**Drugs and dosages**	List of current medications the patient is taking
A	**Assessment**	The diagnostic process and the impression (diagnosis) made by the physician
R	**Return visit information or referral**	Information about return visits or specialists to see for additonal tests

Documentation Elements

The history element entails obtaining and documenting the chief complaint, the history of present illness, and the patient's past, family, and social history. In other words, this procedure involves documenting the reason for the encounter and a description of the development of the current

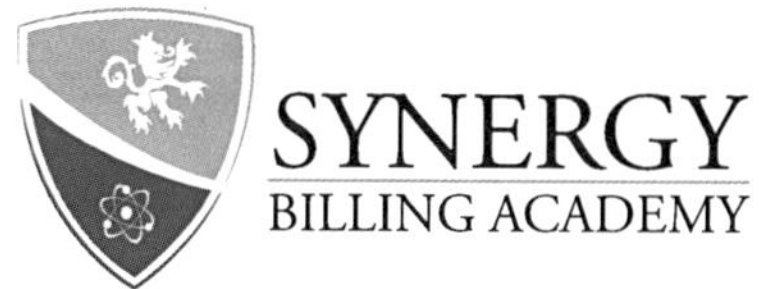

illness (location, severity, quality, duration, timing, and modifying factors).

The physical examination is the objective part of the patient's visit. This is the actual examination by a doctor. The doctor will examine the different body areas and organ systems that are affected. The extent of the examination will depend on the patient's needs and the expert judgment of the physician, although it is based on the patient's chief complaint.

The medical decision-making process depends on what is going on with the patient. The level of medical decision making will vary significantly between different patients, such as one with a chest cold and another with severe chest pain. Assessing medical decision making involves determining how complicated it was for a doctor to diagnose the patient. The difficulty of diagnosis and the available management options are also taken into consideration, as well as the risk of any complications and the amount of data that the doctor has to review.

All of these elements are required in all documentation. Keep in mind that if it is not documented, it did not happen. That is, something may have happened, but you cannot bill for it unless it was documented.

Diagnosis Coding

Diagnosis coding must be accurate because payment for services rendered to a patient is based on the diagnosis. The diagnosis code must correspond to the treatment or services rendered to the patient or payment will be denied. All payments for services are tied into diagnostic coding because of a special requirement called medical necessity.

Depending on the setting, the main reason for the encounter may have different names. In the outpatient setting, the main reason for the encounter is called the first-listed diagnosis or principal diagnosis, whereas for inpatients, it is always called the primary diagnosis.

The main reason for the encounter is related to the chief complaint. Beyond this, there may be other codes, such as secondary codes and others depending on the patient's condition, as they contribute to the primary diagnosis and help clarify other procedures.

How Long Have We Classified Diseases?

The first attempt to classify diseases systematically dates back to François Bossier de Lacroix (1706–1777). The International Conference for the Ninth Revision of the International Classification of Diseases was held from September 30 to October 6, 1975, in Geneva, Switzerland, and the

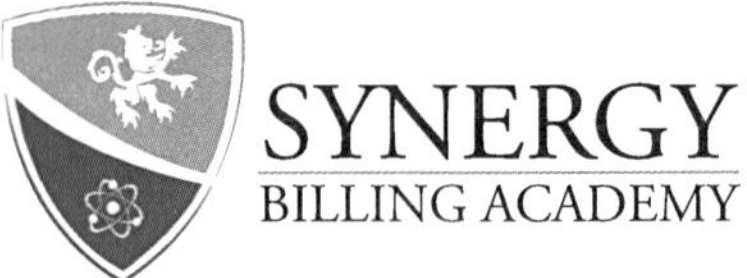

resulting manual was published in 1978. The 10th revision was postponed to 1989 because it had become clear that the established 10-year interval between revisions was too short. Work on the revision process had to start before the current version of the ICD had been in use long enough to be thoroughly evaluated, mainly because the need to consult so many countries and organizations made the revision process a very lengthy one.[2]

U.S. and ICD-9-CM

The ICD-9-CM code set is modeled after the International Classification of Diseases, which is used throughout the world and maintained by the World Health Organization (WHO). In 1978, the World Health Organization published a ninth revision of ICD called ICD-9. The next year, in order to meet statistical data needs in the United States, the U.S. Public Health Service published its modified code set (the CM in the title means clinical modification).[3]

The coding and reporting guidelines were developed and approved by the American Hospital Association (AHA), the American Health Information Management Association (AHIMA), the Centers for Medicare and Medicaid Services (CMS), and the National Center for Health Statistics (NCHS). These parties also maintain the ICD-9-CM. This manual gets updated on October 1 of each year and these new codes must be used as of October 1. ICD-9-CM also updates on April 1, but there is no grace period for these changes.[3]

What Is It?

ICD-9-CM stands for International Classification of Diseases 9th Revision Clinical Modification. ICD-9-CM was designed to classify patients' illnesses and death. This manual is used to:[4]

- Facilitate payment of health services
- Evaluate patients' utilization patterns
- Study health care costs
- Research the quality of health care
- Predict health care trends
- Plan for future health care needs

Diagnoses establish medical necessity, but documentation must always support the diagnosis. The services and diagnoses must correlate; each diagnosis must justify the services provided. Having the correct diagnosis codes permits:[4]

- Accurate reimbursement

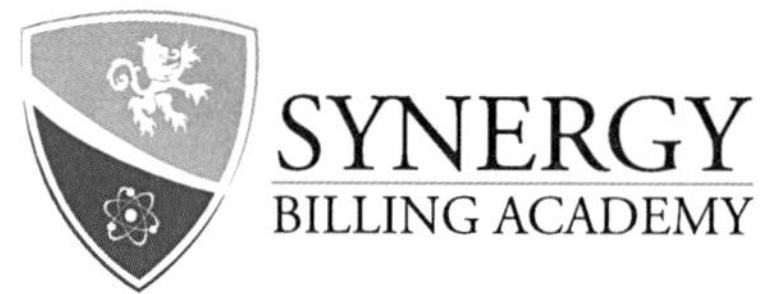

- Fewer rejected claims
- Reduced risk of sanctions/fines from audit

Book Layout

The ICD-9-CM has three volumes:

- Volume 1: Diseases, Tabular List (diagnosis) (17 chapters)
- Volume 2: Diseases, Alphabetic Index to Diseases and Injuries (diagnosis) (3 sections)
- Volume 3: Procedures, Tabular List, and Alphabetic Index (inpatient procedures)

Tabular List – Volume 1 – Division

Volume 1 is the diagnosis list. Right now, there are a total of 17 chapters as well as V Codes and E codes. These chapters are primarily divided based on body systems:[5]

- Chapter 1: Infectious and Parasitic Diseases (001-139)
- Chapter 2: Neoplasms (140-239)
- Chapter 3: Endocrine, Nutritional, and Metabolic Diseases and Immunity Disorders (240-279)
- Chapter 4: Diseases of Blood and Blood-Forming Organs (280-289)
- Chapter 5: Mental, Behavioral, and Neurodevelopmental Disorders (290-319)
- Chapter 6: Diseases of Nervous System and Sense Organs (320-389)
- Chapter 7: Diseases of Circulatory System (390-459)
- Chapter 8: Diseases of Respiratory System (460-519)
- Chapter 9: Diseases of Digestive System (520-579)
- Chapter 10: Diseases of Genitourinary System (580-629)
- Chapter 11: Complications of Pregnancy, Childbirth, and the Puerperium (630-679)
- Chapter 12: Diseases of Skin and Subcutaneous Tissue (680-709)
- Chapter 13: Diseases of Musculoskeletal System and Connective Tissue (710-739)
- Chapter 14: Congenital Anomalies (740-759)
- Chapter 15: Certain Conditions Originating in Perinatal Period (760-779)
- Chapter 16: Symptoms, Signs, and Ill-Defined Conditions (780-799)
- Chapter 17: Injury and Poisoning (800-99)
- V Codes: Factors Influencing Health Status and Contact with Health Services (V01-V91)
- E Codes: External Causes of Injury and Poisoning (E000-E999)

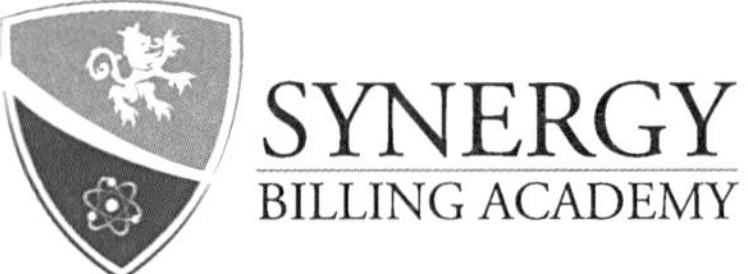

Tabular List – Volume 1

The Tabular List or the numbers list has two major divisions: the classification of diseases and injuries and the supplementary classification.
The Classification of Diseases and Injuries encompasses all 17 chapters based on code range 001.0-999.9.These chapters or main divisions are further divided into:

- Section – A group of three-digit categories that represent a group of conditions or related conditions.
  - Category – A three-digit code that represents a single condition or disease
    - Subcategory – A four-digit code that provides more information or specificity as compared to the category code
      - Subclassification – A five-digit code that adds even more information and specificity to a condition's description

Supplementary Classification is divided into the V Codes, Factors Influencing Health Status, and the E Codes, External Causes of Injury and Poisoning.

Code Format

ICD-9-CM codes contain at least three digits, but a fourth or fifth digit may also be added to provide greater specificity. If additional digits are available, they must be used. Fifth digits may appear at the beginning of the chapter, at the beginning of a section, at the beginning of a three-digit category, or in a fourth-digit subcategory.

Category Code

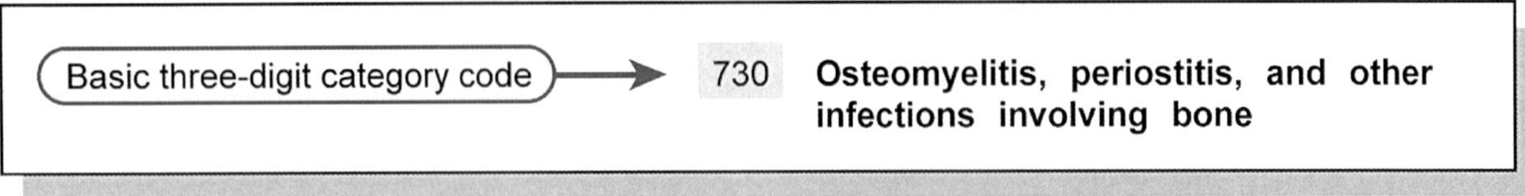

**Modified from Buck CJ: 2013 ICD-9-CM for Hospitals, Volumes 1, 2, & 3, Professional Edition, St. Louis, 2013, Saunders.*

A category represents a single disease or condition (3 digits).

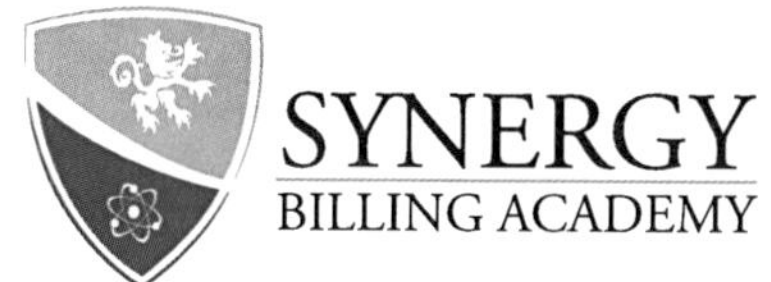
SYNERGY
BILLING ACADEMY

Subcategory Code

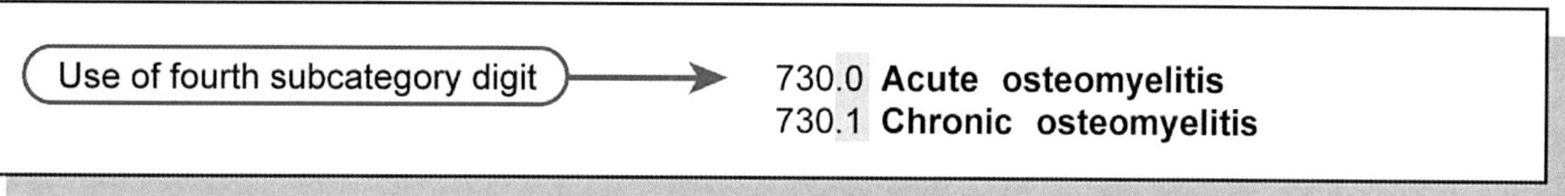
Use of fourth subcategory digit
730.0 Acute osteomyelitis
730.1 Chronic osteomyelitis

**Modified from Buck CJ: 2013 ICD-9-CM for Hospitals, Volumes 1, 2, & 3, Professional Edition, St. Louis, 2013, Saunders.*

A subcategory is more specific, adding a fourth digit.

Subclassification Code

Use of fifth subclassification digit → 730.01 **Acute osteomyelitis, shoulder**

**Modified from Buck CJ: 2013 ICD-9-CM for Hospitals, Volumes 1, 2, & 3, Professional Edition, St. Louis, 2013, Saunders.*

A subclassification is even more specific, adding a fifth digit.

Specificity in ICD-9-CM Codes

Three-digit code	+	Fourth digit	+	Fifth digit	
730	+	.0	+	.01	= 730.01 = acute osteomyelitis of the shoulder
Osteomyelitis	+	Acute	+	Shoulder	

**Modified from Buck CJ: 2013 ICD-9-CM for Hospitals, Volumes 1, 2, & 3, Professional Edition, St. Louis, 2013, Saunders.*

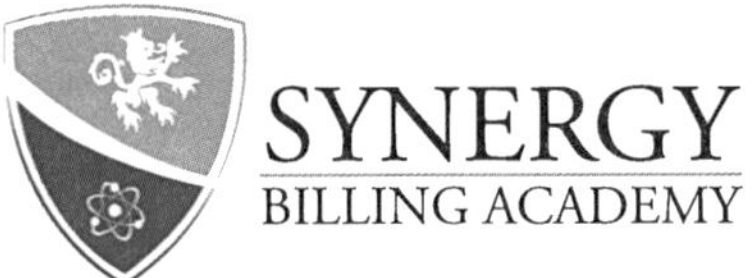

Each digit adds to the specificity (detail). Assign codes to the highest level possible, based on documentation:

- If a 4-digit code exists, do not report the 3-digit code.
- If a 5-digit code exists, do not report the 4-digit code.

V Codes – Volume 1

Code range V01.0–V91.9 is used when a patient not ill but encounters health services, such as going for a vaccination. These codes are also used when a patient requires treatment such as chemotherapy. V Codes are used for factors that influence patient's health status, such as personal history of malignant tumor, organ transplant, or birth status and outcome of delivery.

There is no separate index for V Codes; instead, they appear throughout Volume 2 under certain key terms. The key terms that V Codes are listed under include Impending, History, Examination, Screening, Status, Aftercare, and others.

V Codes are used in four circumstances: When a person who is not currently sick encounters health services for a specific purpose (e.g., vaccination, etc.); when a person with a resolving disease or injury seeks aftercare; when a circumstance influences an individual's health status but the illness is not current; and when it is necessary to indicate the birth status of a newborn.

Examples:

Example 5-3 Supervision of First Pregnancy, Normal

Step 1	Find the heading **pregnancy** in Volume 2.
Step 2	Look for the subheading **supervison.**
Step 3	Look for the second subheading **normal** and a further subheading **first**, which gives you the code V22.0.
Step 4	Find **V22.0** in Volume 1, Tabular List; you will see **"Supervision of Normal Pregnancy."**

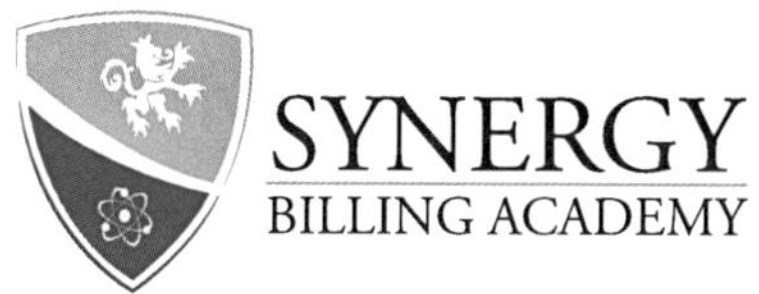

Example 5-4 Routine Annual Physical Examination

Step 1 Look up **examination** and find **annual** as a subterm with the code V70.0.

Step 2 Find **V70** in Volume 1, Tabular List, with the wording **"Routine general medical examination at a health facility."**

Example 5-5 Admission (Encounter) Code

A patient scheduled for gallstone surgery is sent to a cardiologist for evaluation of suspected cardiovascular disease.

Step 1 In Volume 2, look up **admission (encounter) (for) examintion preoperative, cardiovascular V72.81.** Verify it in Volume 1.

Step 2 Code the reason for the surgery as - 574.xx, choleithiasis.

**Modified from Buck CJ: 2013 ICD-9-CM for Hospitals, Volumes 1, 2, & 3, Professional Edition, St. Louis, 2013, Saunders.*

E Codes – Volume 1

These codes are still part of Volume 1 in the ICD-9-CM book; their code range is E000-E999. The E Codes are used as a supplementary classification of external causes of injury and poisoning. E Codes are alphanumeric designations for external causes of injuries, poisonings, and adverse effects. They provide additional information about external causes, such as the nature of the injury/poisoning and where it happened.

Because these codes are used for external causes, they can never be a principal diagnosis. E Codes permit the classification of environmental events, circumstances, and conditions as the cause of illness or injury. An E Code is used in addition to a code from the Tabular List; there is also a separate index for E Codes.

Alphabetic Index: Volume 2

The alphabetic index is the first part of this manual. It is composed of three sections:

- Section I: Index to Diseases and Injuries (A-Z)
  - Hypertension Table
  - Neoplasm Table

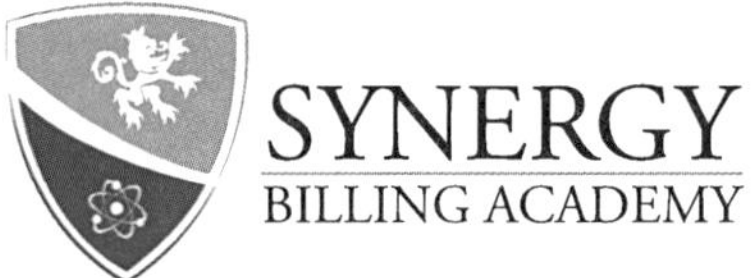

- Section II: Table of Drugs and Chemicals
- Section III: Index to External Causes of Injury (E Codes)

CODING NOTE: NEVER SELECT CODES DIRECTLY FROM THE INDEX

Section I: Index to Diseases

The first section in Volume 2 is the Index to Diseases, in which all of the diseases, disorders, illnesses, signs, and symptoms are listed from A through Z. This is the largest part of Volume 2. The index is where the first few steps in coding happen. When looking at the documentation, after we determine the reason for the encounter, we need to locate the main bold term in the Index and review subterms. Keep in mind that based on the documentation, we may have more than one subterm. When looking at the Index, the subterms will be indented two spaces to the right.[5,6]

A Word of Caution about the Alphabetic Index (Section I, Vol. 2)

To save space, some words in the Alphabetic Index do not appear in the Tabular List and vice versa. Locating the codes in the Alphabetic Index is only the first step; we must locate each term in the Index and then go to the Tabular List and continue to follow directions and instructional notations.

Tables in Section I

Section I includes two tables, the Hypertension Table and the Neoplasms Table. The Hypertension Table has different columns to indicate hypertension and other complications as well as the type of hypertension, such as malignant, benign, or unspecified. The Neoplam Table is also found in Section I. This table lists the neoplasms by anatomical sites, then lists six possible choices in the other columns based on the patient's behavior, such as the malignancy (primary, secondary, ca in situ) and also benign, uncertain behavior, and unspecified.

Section II

Section II comprises the Alphabetic Index to Poisoning and External Causes of Adverse Effects of Drugs and Other Chemical Substances. This table classifies drugs and other chemical substances to identify poisoning classifications. Each of the substances is assigned a code according to poisoning classification (960-989). These codes are used when the documentation states poisoning, overdose, wrong substance given or taken, or intoxication.

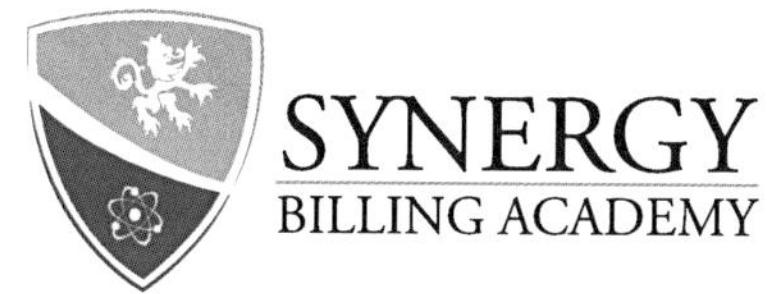

In this table you will find the listing of external causes of adverse effects. The table headings for these adverse effects are accidental poisoning, therapeutic use, suicide attempt, assault, and undetermined.[5, 6]

Section III

Section III is the E Codes index; this is where we can find the code range E000-E999 or the Supplementary Classification of External Causes of Injury and Poisoning. This index is found after the table of drugs and chemicals. The alphabetic index to the E Codes is organized by main terms, which describe the accident, circumstance, event, or specific agent which caused the injury or other adverse effect.[5, 6]

Remember that E Codes are never a principal diagnosis. E Codes permit the classification of environmental events, circumstances, and conditions as the cause of illness or injury. An E Code is used in addition to a code from the Tabular List.

Volume 2, Terms

All main terms in Volume 2 are in bold typeface and all subterms are indented two spaces to right but are not bolded. For example, if you look for "earache," this term is bold because it is the main term. Under it, we can see the subterms "otogenic" and "referred," which are indented two spaces to the right.

ICD-9-CM Conventions

Conventions are abbreviations, punctuation, and notes. These conventions are very important, as they will help you navigate the manual: [5, 6]

- Abbreviations: NEC, NOS
  - NEC is an acronym for "not elsewhere classified." This is used when no more specific code exists. These codes can only be used when the documentation specifies a condition but there is no more specific code for that condition.
  - NOS is an acronym for "not otherwise specified." This is used when the diagnosis has not been specified in the documentation. These codes are equivalent to unspecified; we do not have sufficient documentation to select any other, more specific code.
- Punctuation: [ ] [ ] ( ) : }
  - [ ] Brackets enclose synonyms, alternative wording, or explanatory phrases.

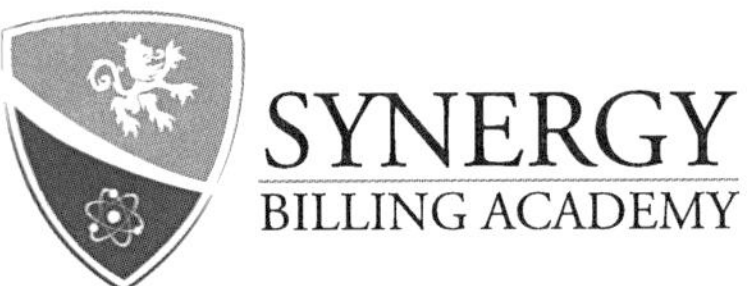

They provide us with additional helpful information. Codes in brackets can affect the main coding. They are only found in the Tabular List (001.0-999.9). Brackets are also used to identify manifestation codes.

   - Etiology refers to the cause of a disease, whereas manifestations are the symptoms. When we can have both in one code, it is called a combination code. In other words, combination codes give you the etiology (cause of disease) and the manifestation (symptoms), using only one code to describe the diagnosis.

- *[ ]* Slanted brackets enclose manifestations of underlying conditions. In cases using this punctuation, you will usually see a note indicating you should "Code first underlying disease." The slanted brackets are used in Volume 2, the Alphabetic Index.
- ( ) Parentheses contain non-essential modifiers: you can choose whether or not to use them. They contain informational, descriptive terms and are found in the Tabular List and the Alphabetic Index. They do not affect code selection but help clarify diagnosis.
   - Example: gonococcal (acute)....
- : Colon: In the Tabular List, a colon completes a statement with one or more modifiers. It is used after an incomplete term that needs one or more of the modifiers that follow in order to allow it to be assigned to a given category.
- } Brace: In the Tabular List, a brace modifies statements to the right of the brace. This is used to enclose a series of terms, each of which modifies the statement appearing to the left of the brace.

- Symbols: § □
   - The lozenge and the section mark are not used in all manuals:
      - □ Lozenge: Indicates codes unique to ICD-9-CM
      - § Section Mark: Indicates that there is a footnote at the bottom of the page
- Notations: Includes, Excludes, Use Additional Code, And/With, and Cross-reference, such as See, See Also, and See Category
   - Includes notes are found in chapters, sections, or categories. They further define or give examples of the content of a category.
   - Excludes notes are used when conditions are coded elsewhere. The terms are excluded from the code and are to be found somewhere else.
   - Use Additional Codes direct you to assign other code(s) as necessary to fully code the patient's condition.
   - The word "And" must be interpreted as "and" as well as "or"
      - Example: 237.0, Neoplasm of uncertain behavior of pituitary gland and/or craniopharyngeal duct

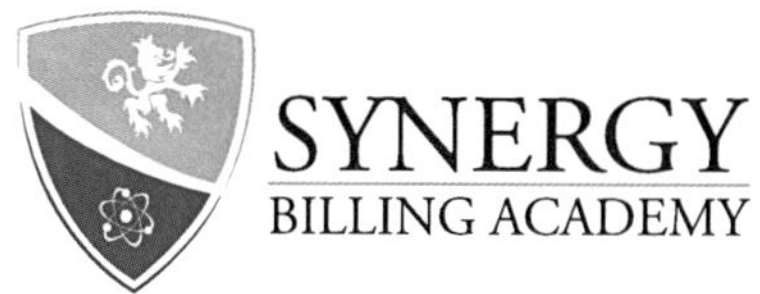

- The word "With" means one condition appears with (in addition to) another condition (associated with or due to). This word is used when two conditions are included in the code.
  - Example: 070.41, Acute hepatitis C with hepatic coma
- Cross-References words direct you to look up other terms. These words include: see, see also, see category
  - "See" directs you to a specific term, suggesting you look elsewhere. This term is used for anatomic sites and for many modifiers and is not normally used in the Alphabetic Index
    - Example: Panotitis—see otitis media
  - "See also" directs you to another term for more information. This means that there is another main term that may also be referenced that could provide us with additional useful information.
    - Example: Perivaginitis (see also vaginitis)
  - "See category" is a cross reference to see other conditions. This note is necessary for proper coding to reference the other term that is given. This note will direct you to Volume 1, Tabular List.
    - Example: Mesencephalitis (see also Encephalitis) 323.9; late effect—see category 326

Volume 2, Notes

Throughout the Alphabetic Index, you will find notes boxes that help you define terms and which give further coding instructions. Mandatory fifth digits also appear as notes—one reason to never code from the Index.

Example: Index: "Melanoma,"

Note: "Except where otherwise indicated…."

Volume 2 Eponyms

Eponyms are used in the medical field to indicate diseases, syndromes, tests, procedures, drugs, and devices named for or after a person. Eponyms are listed both as main terms in their appropriate alphabetic sequence and under the main term "Disease" or "Syndrome."

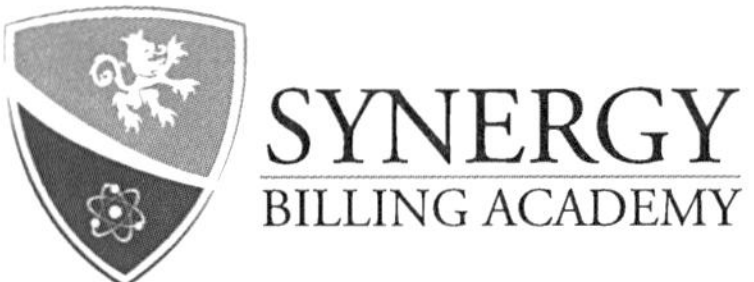

Examples:

- Arnold-Chiari (see also spina bifida)
- Sturge-Weber (encephelotrigeminal angiomatosis)
- Prader-Willi

Volume 3

This volume is only used for inpatient procedures. In this volume, you will find an alphabetic index as well as a tabular listing of all codes. The codes have at least two but no more than four digits.

- 20.41 Simple mastoidectomy

ICD-10 Overview

ICD-10 to CM/PCS

The International Classification of Diseases is a diagnostic tool for epidemiology, health management, and clinical purposes. This mission includes analyzing the general health situation of population groups. It is used to monitor the incidence and prevalence of diseases and other health problems.[2]

It is used to classify diseases and other health problems recorded on many types of health and vital records including death certificates and health records. Many countries use it to help make decisions about reimbursement and resource allocation.[2]

Currently, the United States uses the ninth edition of the ICD code set (ICD-9), published in 1977 and adopted by the U.S. in 1979. It was mandated as the Medicare claims standard in 1989. In 1990, the World Health Organization (WHO) updated its international version of the ICD-10. Other countries began adopting ICD-10 in 1994, but the United States only partially adopted ICD-10 in 1999 for mortality reporting.[7]

The National Center for Health Statistics (NCHS) developed ICD-10-CM following a thorough evaluation by a technical advisory panel and extensive consultation with physician groups, clinical coders, and others to ensure its clinical accuracy and usefulness.[7]

The compliance date for all Health Insurance Portability and Accountability Act (HIPAA)-covered entities to implement ICD-10-CM/PCS was postponed for at least one year from the set date of October 1, 2014, to October 1, 2015. ICD-10-CM/PCS will enhance accurate payment for services rendered and help evaluate medical processes and outcomes. A number of other countries have already moved to ICD-10.

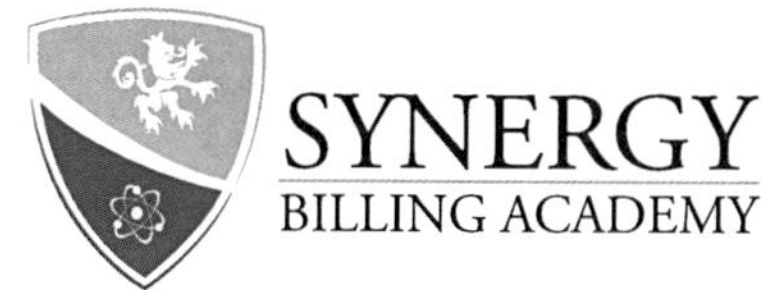

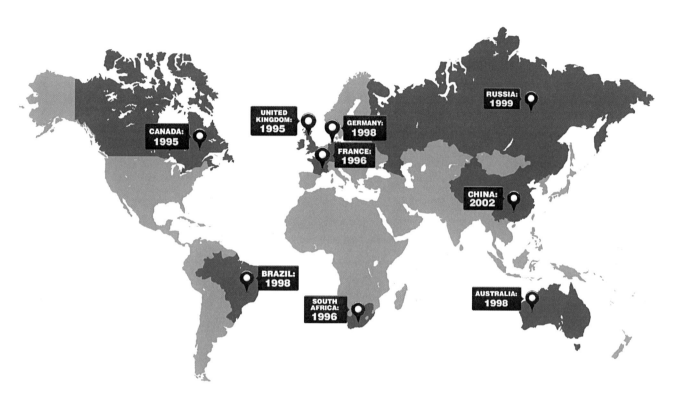

ICD-10 Has Two Parts

Currently, the ICD-9-CM has three volumes: Volume 1, Diseases, Tabular List (diagnosis); Volume 2, Diseases, Alphabetic Index to Diseases and Injuries (diagnosis); and Volume 3, Procedures, Tabular List and Alphabetic Index (inpatient procedures).

Transitioning to ICD-10 will divide the ICD-9 into two books: CM and PCS. ICD-10-CM consists of ICD-9-CM Volumes 1 and 2 and is used for diagnosis coding for inpatient and outpatient settings. ICD-10-PCS consists of ICD-9-CM Volume 3, which is used for procedural coding for inpatient settings.

The "CM" in ICD-10-CM indicates that it is the United States, "clinical modification" of the International Classification of Diseases 10th Revision, which was created by the World Health Organization (WHO). Our modification was developed by the National Center for Health Care Statistics (NCHS) and it contains about 68,000 alphanumeric codes.

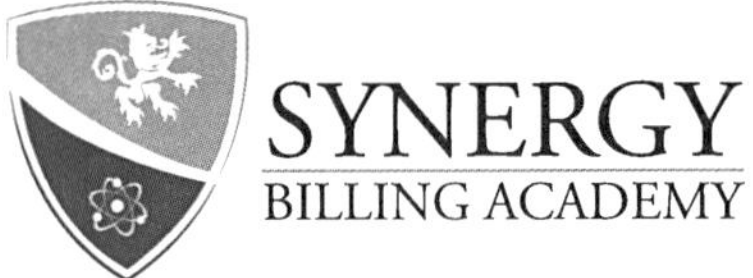

Structural Changes

ICD-10-CM will have 21 chapters instead of the ICD-9-CM's 17. All codes are alphanumeric and they can have up to seven characters. The V Codes and E Codes have been incorporated into the main classification. The diseases of the eyes and ears now have their own chapters instead of being listed in the diseases of the nervous system chapter. Certain diseases were reassigned to other chapters; for example, gout was moved from the endocrine system to the musculoskeletal system. ICD-10-CM groups all injuries by site then type of injury instead of classifying them by injury as ICD-9-CM does. We now also have an "X" character, which is used as a placeholder.[8]

Structural Similarities

The Tabular List is the list of codes, divided into chapters based on body system or condition. The chapters are structured similarly to ICD-9-CM. They are presented in code number order and the codes are looked up the same way, first by looking up diagnostic terms, then by verifying the code number. The codes will be considered invalid if they are missing the appropriate number of characters.

ICD-10-CM also has an Index. This is an alphabetical list of terms and their corresponding codes, structured and formatted the same as ICD-9-CM. The main terms are in alphabetical order with indented subterms. The alphabetical index comprises the Index to Diseases and Injuries, an Index to External Causes, the Table of Neoplasms, and the Table of Drugs and Chemicals.

Conventions in ICD-10-CM have the same meanings they did in ICD-9-CM. The ICD-10-CM also contains a list of Official Guidelines for Coding and Reporting; these need to be followed carefully, as they are the instructions on how to code certain conditions properly. Please keep in mind that adherence to the official coding guidelines in all health care settings is ***required*** under the Health Insurance Portability and Accountability Act (HIPAA).

Why ICD-10-CM

ICD-10-CM provides more specific data than ICD-9-CM. It better records current medical practice, reflecting all the technological advances that have occurred since the implementation of ICD-9-CM. It also allows for better documentation of a condition's severity, risk, complexity, complications, manifestations, and sequelae or late effects, as well as comorbidity, etiology, and external factors and disease classification and stages.[9]

The new structure will also accommodate the addition of new codes. The current coding system (ICD-9-CM) is running out of capacity and cannot accommodate future health care developments.

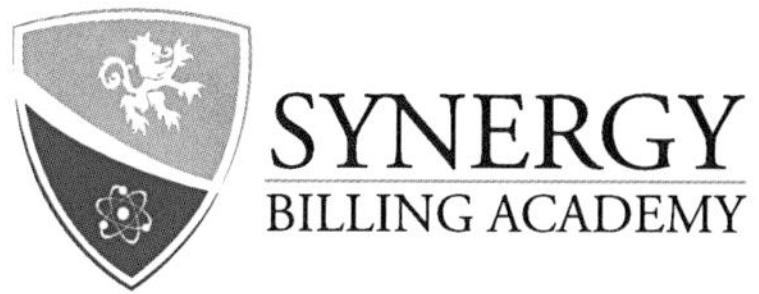

Moreover, new quality measurements will enable ICD-10-CM to reduce coding errors, allow us to better analyze disease patterns, and improve our ability to track and respond to public health outbreaks. It will also make claims submission more efficient and help identify fraud and abuse.

ICD-10-CM Benefits

ICD-10-CM allows better organization and description of each code and offers a greater level of detail than ICD-9-CM. This was accomplished through the expansion of injury codes, the creation and combination of diagnosis/symptom codes to reduce the number of codes needed to describe a condition, the addition of 6th and 7th characters for greater expansion and specificity, revisions to the 4th and 5th digit subclassifications, and the addition of laterality, which will allow for greater specificity regarding the affected side of the body and specific body region.

ICD-10-CM is more flexible, allowing for more expansion than was possible with ICD-9-CM.[9] The greater specificity in code assignment will result in an improved ability to measure health care services and increased sensitivity when refining grouping and reimbursement methodologies, an enhanced ability to conduct public health surveillance, and a decreased need to include supporting documentation with claims.

Index

In ICD-10-CM, the index contains both main terms and subterms. The main terms are in bold font and the subterms are indented two spaces to the right, as in ICD-9-CM.

Aarakog's syndrome Q87.1
Abandonment - *see* Maltreatment
Abasia (-astasia) (hysterical) F44.4
Aberhalden-Kaufmann-Lignac syndrome (cystinosis) E72.04
Andomen, abdominal - *see also* condition
  acute R10.0
  angina K55.1
  muscle deficiency syndrome Q79.4
Abdominalgia - see Pain, abdominal
	Abduction contracture, hip or other joint - *see* Contraction, joint
	Aberrant (congenital) - *see also* Malposition, congenital
	  adrenal gland Q89.1
	  artery (peripheral) Q27.8
	    basilar NEC Q28.1
	    cerebral Q28.3
	    coronary Q24.5
	    digestive system Q27.8
	    eye Q15.8
	    lower limb Q27.8
	    precerebral Q28.1
	    pulmonary Q25.79
	    renal Q27.2
	    retina Q14.1

**ICD-10-CM Index (From Buck CJ: 2013 ICD-10-CM Standard Edition DRAFT (Softbound), St. Louis, 2013, Saunders.)*

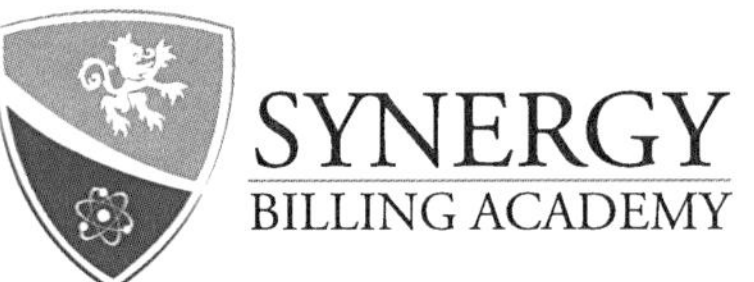

ICD-10-CM Chapters

ICD-10-CM has a total of 21 chapters: [9, 10]

- Chapter 1: Certain Infectious and Parasitic Diseases (A00–B99)
- Chapter 2: Neoplasms (C00–D49)
- Chapter 3: Diseases of the Blood and Blood-Forming Organs and Certain Disorders Involving the Immune Mechanism (D50–D89)
- Chapter 4: Endocrine, Nutritional, and Metabolic Diseases (E00–E89)
- Chapter 5: Mental, Behavioral, and Neurodevelopmental Disorders (F01–F99)
- Chapter 6: Diseases of the Nervous System (G00–G99)
- Chapter 7: Diseases of the Eye and Adnexa (H00-H59)
- Chapter 8: Diseases of the Ear and Mastoid Process (H60–H95)
- Chapter 9: Diseases of the Circulatory System (I00–I99)
- Chapter 10: Diseases of the Respiratory System (J00–J99)
- Chapter 11: Diseases of the Digestive System (K00–K95)
- Chapter 12: Diseases of the Skin and Subcutaneous Tissue (L00–L99)
- Chapter 13: Diseases of the Musculoskeletal System and Connective Tissue (M00–M99)
- Chapter 14: Diseases of the Genitourinary System (N00–N99)
- Chapter 15: Pregnancy, Childbirth, and the Puerperium (O00–O9A)
- Chapter 16: Certain Conditions Originating in the Perinatal Period (P00–P96)
- Chapter 17: Congenital Malformations, Deformations, and Chromosomal Abnormalities (Q00–Q99)
- Chapter 18: Symptoms, Signs, and Abnormal Clinical and Laboratory Findings, Not Elsewhere Classified (R00–R99)
- Chapter 19: Injury, Poisoning, and Certain Other Consequences of External Causes (S00–T88)
- Chapter 20: External Causes of Morbidity (V01–Y99)
- Chapter 21: Factors Influencing Health Status and Contact with Health Services (Z00–Z99)

Tabular List

The Tabular List is where the codes are listed in order. Each section begins with a unique letter and codes are arranged within each letter section in numerical order with the exception of the letter "U."

ICD-10-CM Includes Official Instructional Notations [9, 10]

Includes notes are found in chapters, sections, and categories. They further define or give examples of the content of a category:

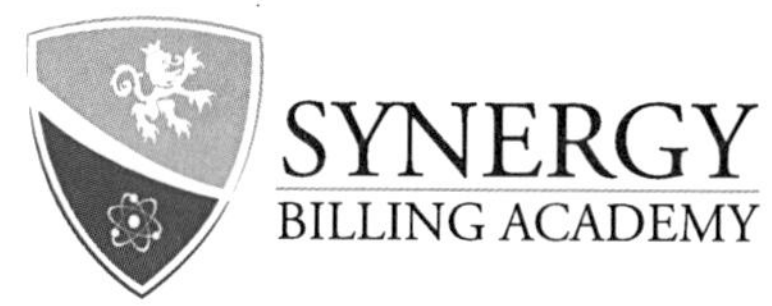

- Excludes1: A type 1 Excludes note is a pure excludes note. It means "Not coded here!" An Excludes1 note indicates that the code excluded should never be used at the same time as the code above the Excludes1 note. An Excludes1 note is used when two conditions cannot occur together, such as a congenital form versus an acquired form of the same condition.
- Excludes2: A type 2 Excludes note represents "Not included here." An Excludes2 note indicates that the condition excluded is not part of the condition represented by the code, but a patient may have both conditions at the same time. When an Excludes2 note appears under a code, it is acceptable to use both the code and the excluded code together if the patient has both conditions.
- Code First/Use Additional Code: A Code First note means that we need to code both the etiology and the manifestation.
  - Etiology refers to the cause of a disease, whereas manifestations are the symptoms. When we can have both in one code, it is called a combination code. In other words, combination codes give you both the etiology (cause of disease) and the manifestation (symptom) in only one code.
- Code Also: A Code Also note means that we are going to need more than one code to fully describe a diagnosis. It's necessary to assign other code(s) to fully code the patient's condition.
- 7th Character and Placeholder X
  - ICD-9-CM has a maximum of 5 characters. With ICD-10-CM, we will have up to 7 characters. This 7th character is required in some categories to provide further specificity about the condition that is being coded. The X is used in some cases as a placeholder for certain codes to allow for future expansion. The placeholder has two uses:
    - As the 5th-digit character for six-character codes. The X will provide for future expansion without disturbing the six-character structure.
    - When a code has fewer than six characters and a seventh character is required. The X is assigned for all characters less than six in order to meet the requirement of coding to the highest level of specificity.
  - Codes with less than six characters that have a 7th character requirement; X is a placeholder.

Outpatient Coding Guidelines[9-10]

The coding guidelines for outpatient diagnoses have been approved for use by hospitals/ providers in coding and reporting hospital-based outpatient services and provider-based office visits.

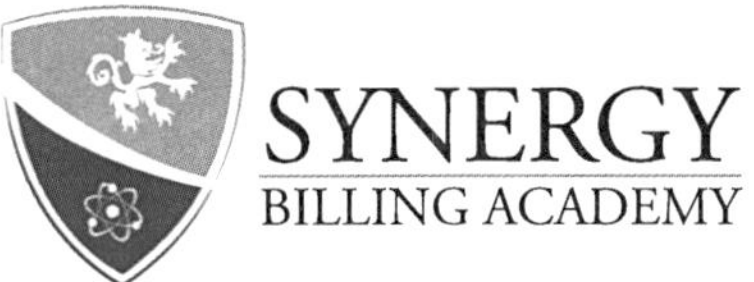

The coding and reporting guidelines were developed and approved by the American Hospital Association (AHA), the American Health Information Management Association (AHIMA), the Centers for Medicare and Medicaid Services (CMS), and the National Center for Health Statistics (NCHS).

First-Listed Diagnosis

Both principal diagnosis and first-listed diagnosis describe the primary reason for encounter. The main difference between the two is the setting in which the patients are being seen. The principal diagnosis is used for inpatient settings and the first-listed diagnosis is used in outpatient settings. For example, documentation states that a patient with inguinal hernia presents with shortness of breath; shortness of breath would be the first-listed diagnosis because this is the reason why the patient was seen and the visit occurred in an outpatient setting.

In determining the first-listed diagnosis, the coding conventions of ICD-10-CM, as well as the general and disease-specific guidelines, take precedence over the outpatient guidelines.

The most critical rule for accurate coding involves beginning the search for the correct code assignment through the Alphabetic Index. Never begin searching initially in the Tabular List, as this will lead to coding errors.

Unconfirmed or Uncertain Diagnosis

Diagnoses often are not established at the time of the initial encounter/visit. It may take two or more visits before the diagnosis is confirmed. In an outpatient setting, it may take several encounters to confirm a diagnosis, but signs/symptoms are reported at each encounter. Do not code diagnoses documented as “probable,” “suspected,” “questionable,” “rule out,” or “working diagnosis,” or other similar terms indicating uncertainty. Rather, code the condition(s) to the highest degree of certainty for that encounter/visit, such as symptoms, signs, abnormal test results, or other reason for the visit.

Codes that describe symptoms and signs, as opposed to diagnoses, are acceptable for reporting purposes when a diagnosis has not been established (confirmed) by the provider. Chapter 18 of ICD-10-CM, Symptoms, Signs, and Abnormal Clinical and Laboratory Findings Not Elsewhere Classified (codes R00-R99), contains many, but not all, codes for symptoms. For example, documentation states that the patient presented with complaint of frequent heartburn. The physician prescribes Prilosec for suspected GERD with patient returning in 10 days. In this case, we would only report frequent heartburn.

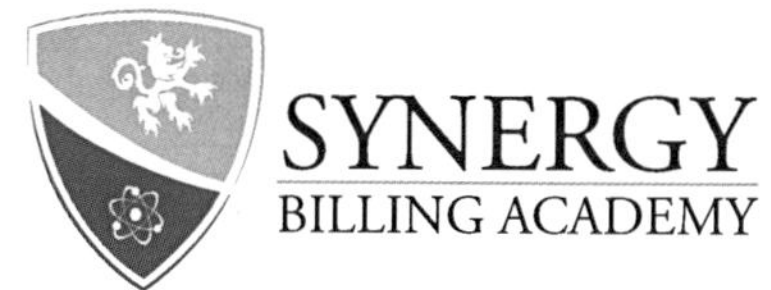

Outpatient Surgery

Code the reason for the surgery first. When a patient presents for outpatient surgery (same-day surgery), code the reason for the surgery as the first-listed diagnosis (reason for the encounter), even if the surgery is not performed due to a contraindication. Follow this with a code to report the reason the procedure was not carried out, such as Z53.09, Procedure not carried out due to other contraindication.

Z Codes

ICD-10-CM provides codes to deal with encounters for circumstances other than a disease or injury. The Factors Influencing Health Status and Contact with Health Services codes (Z00-Z99) are provided to deal with occasions when circumstances other than a disease or injury are recorded as a diagnosis or problem.

Z Codes are informative, reporting circumstances other than disease or injury. They may be listed first or as additional codes depending on the circumstances. For instance, Z23 reports encounters for inoculations and vaccinations and the procedure code will identify the administration.

Coexisting Conditions

Code all documented conditions that coexist at the time of the encounter/visit and require or affect patient care, treatment, or management. Do not code conditions that were previously treated and no longer exist. However, history codes (categories Z80-Z87) may be used as secondary codes if the historical condition or family history has an impact on current care or influences treatment. Example, patient presents with shortness of breath due to asthma. Physician prescribes nebulizer treatments. The patient is morbidly obese, making the examination and treatment more complex. The first-listed diagnosis is asthma and the coexisting condition is obesity.

Chronic Diseases

Chronic diseases that are treated on an ongoing basis may be coded and reported as many times as the patient receives treatment and care for the condition(s). Do not report conditions that were previously treated and no longer exist. In those cases, we would report history codes (Z80-Z87) as secondary diagnosis if the condition impacts the current condition or affects treatment.

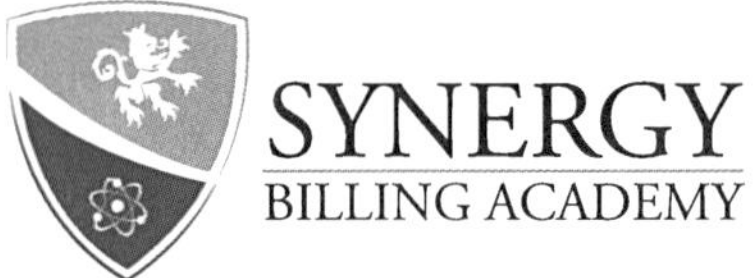

Diagnostic Services

For patients receiving only diagnostic services during an encounter/visit, sequence first the diagnosis, condition, problem, or other reason for encounter/visit shown in the medical record to be chiefly responsible for the outpatient services provided during the encounter/visit. Codes for other diagnoses (e.g., chronic conditions) may be sequenced as additional diagnoses.

For encounters for routine laboratory/radiology testing in the absence of any signs, symptoms, or associated diagnosis, assign Z01.89, Encounter for other specified special examinations. If routine testing is performed during the same encounter as a test to evaluate a sign, symptom, or diagnosis, it is appropriate to assign both the Z Code and the code describing the reason for the non-routine test.

For outpatient encounters for diagnostic tests that have been interpreted by a physician when the final report is available at the time of coding, code any confirmed or definitive diagnosis documented in the interpretation. Do not code related signs and symptoms as additional diagnoses.

When only diagnostic service is provided, report the first reason for service. For example, if a patient presented for a routine periodic gynecological exam, report Z01.419. (no signs, symptoms, or associated diagnosis). As another example, when a patient presents for diagnostic imaging for left, central breast mass, report N63, unspecified breast lump. A later diagnosis of malignant neoplasm would be reported with C50.112.

Preoperative Evaluation

For patients receiving only preoperative evaluations, sequence first a code from subcategory Z01.81, Encounter for pre-procedural examinations, to describe the pre-op consultations. Assign a code for the condition to describe the reason for the surgery as an additional diagnosis. You should also code any findings related to the pre-op evaluation, but the first-listed code will always be the preoperative examination.

Different endings for code Z01.81 will be selected depending on the type of the operation, such as Z01.810, Preoperative cardiovascular examination; Z01.811, Preoperative respiratory examination; Z01.812, Preoperative lab; and Z01.818, Preoperative exam not otherwise specified, examination before chemotherapy.

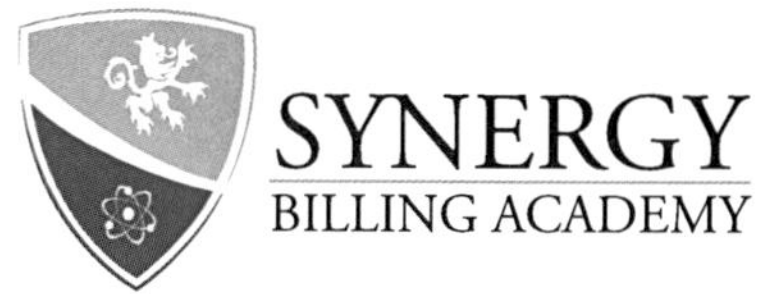

Prenatal Encounters

For routine outpatient prenatal visits when no complications are present, a code from category Z34, Encounter for supervision of normal pregnancy, should be used as the first-listed diagnosis. These codes should not be used in conjunction with Chapter 15 codes. Example: 19-year-old female presents for initial prenatal exam, first pregnancy, Z34.00.

For routine prenatal outpatient visits for patients with high-risk pregnancies, a code from category O09, Supervision of high-risk pregnancy, should be used as the first-listed diagnosis. Secondary Chapter 15 codes may be used in conjunction with these codes if appropriate. Example: 29-year-old first trimester female patient presents for prenatal encounter with varicose veins of legs, O22.01

External Cause Index

The external cause index in ICD-10-CM maps to the E Codes index in the ICD-9-CM manual. This is the Supplementary Classification of External Causes of Injury and Poisoning, found after the table of drugs and chemicals.

This alphabetic index is organized by main terms which describe the accident, circumstance, event, or specific agent which caused the injury or other adverse effect. Remember that these codes may never be used as a principal diagnosis.

These codes permit the classification of environmental events, circumstances, and conditions as the cause of illness or injury. These codes are used in addition to a code from the Tabular List.

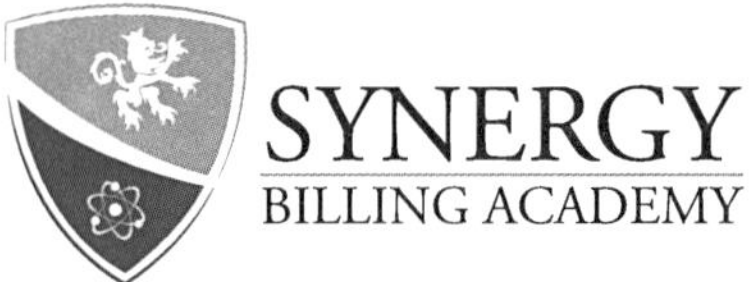

Using the Manual

Alphabetic Index and Tabular List

Example of the use of both the Alphabetic Index and Tabular List

Diagnosis: Pneumoconiosis due to lime dust

Index: Pneumoconiosis (main term)
Dust (subterm)
Lime (subterm) J62.8

Tabular: J62 Pneumoconiosis due to dust containing silica [category code]
J62.8 Pneumoconiosis due to other dust containing silica [subcategory code]

No need for more digits

Code: J62.8 = Pneumoconiosis due to lime dust

Level of Specificity

We must always code to the highest character available. You cannot report only a 5th character if there is a 6th character available. The highest level of specificity has a maximum of 7 characters.

- M48.48XA (A= initial encounter)
- No 6th character for M48.48, but there is a 7th, X = placeholder

Integral Conditions

Integral conditions mean that a condition is part of the diagnosis. In these cases, do not report signs and symptoms separately. For example, a patient presents with fever and shortness of breath due to pneumonia; we would only report the pneumonia, because fever and shortness of breath are symptoms of pneumonia.

Not Integral Conditions

Not integral conditions mean that a condition is not part of the diagnosis. In these cases, we have to report the signs and symptoms separately. For example, a patient presents with pneumonia

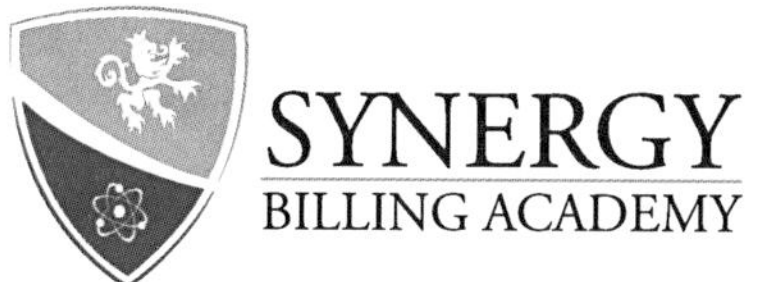

and dehydration. We would report J18.9 for Pneumonia and E86.0 for Dehydration. This is because not all patients with pneumonia have dehydration and dehydration was not stated to be due to the pneumonia.

Etiology and Manifestation

Etiology is the origination; it is the cause or origin of the condition. Manifestation is how the cause shows in the patient; it is an extension of the patient's illness or condition. An example is diabetic retinopathy; in this example, diabetes is the etiology or the cause and retinopathy is the manifestation or the symptom. For this condition, we have a combination code: E10.319, Type 1 diabetic retinopathy. In other cases, such as Staphylococcal aureus cellulitis of face, we would have multiple codes, which in this example are L03.211 for Cellulitis and B95.61 for the Staph.

Acute and Chronic

An acute condition means that symptoms are severe and they appear and change or worsen rapidly. A chronic condition develops and worsens over an extended or long period of time. It is possible for a patient to have a condition that is both acute and chronic. We can have separate codes for this situation or just one. When a patient has a condition that is both acute and chronic, we have to report acute first, then chronic.

Combination Codes

A combination means a grouping of things. In coding, we can have combination codes; this means that diagnoses, manifestations, and complications can be coded using a single code. Combination codes are used to report two diagnoses, a diagnosis with a manifestation, or a diagnosis with an associated complication. An example of this would be K80.00, Acute cholecystitis with cholelithiasis; we have one code for both conditions.

In contrast, when we have to use more than code to report a patient's condition, it is called multiple coding.

Residual and Cause

A late effect is a condition that appears after the acute phase of an earlier condition or after a condition has run its course. There is no time limit for a patient to develop a late effect, because some late effects can occur decades later. In ICD-10-CM, a late effect is referred to as a sequela (plural sequelae). This is the residual of a condition or the leftover from an illness. For example,

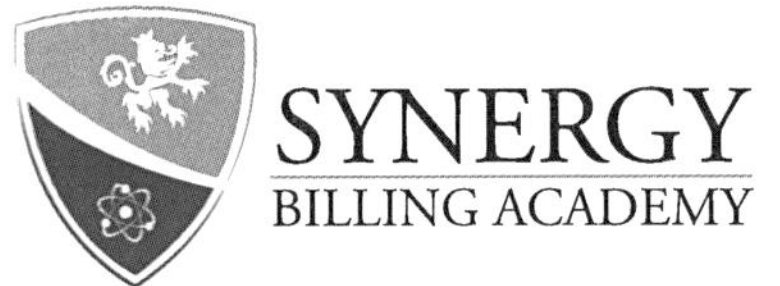

a malunion of a fracture is considered to be a residual, because it is the late effect of a fracture, which was the original cause or injury.

The sequencing of residuals and original cause can be somewhat complicated. When sequencing a sequela or residual, we need to report the residual as first-listed diagnosis, followed by the late effects code. This is because the patient is dealing with the leftover from an earlier condition. If we look at the previous example, we can tell that the patient is being seen for the malunion (the sequela) and not the fracture (the cause).

Laterality

Laterality is a new term used in ICD-10-CM. Laterality is used to indicate which side of the body is affected. In other words, it indicates left versus right.

Use It!
We need to make sure that all claims have the correct codes before they leave the system and go to the clearinghouse or the payer. We need to make sure that the codes capture the essence of every visit and that we have proper documentation to substantiate every code.

There are certain steps in place that we need to follow to be able to accomplish this. We need to know what we are looking for in order to be able to find the accurate code or codes.

Questions to Ask Yourself

While looking at the documentation, there are certain things that we need to know. If we want to code correctly, we need to ask ourselves the following questions before we even begin to code:

- Why was the patient there?
- What are the signs and symptoms?
- Decipher the signs and symptoms
- Was a diagnosis made?
- Are the signs and symptoms related to or due to the diagnosis?
- Is there more than one diagnosis?

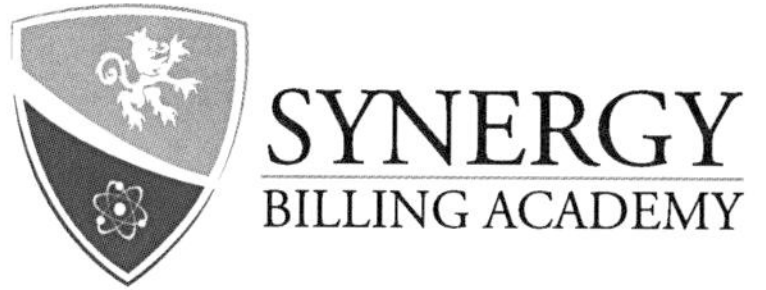

Steps to Coding

Everything goes back to accuracy. In order to make sure we are coding accurately, these are the steps we need to follow: [4]

- Identify the main term.
- Locate the main term in the Alphabetic Index.
- Review the subterms.
- Follow cross-reference instructions like "see" or "see also."
- Verify the code in the Tabular List.
- Refer to instructional notations in the Tabular List.
- Assign codes to the highest level of specificity.
- Code the diagnosis until all elements are completely identified.

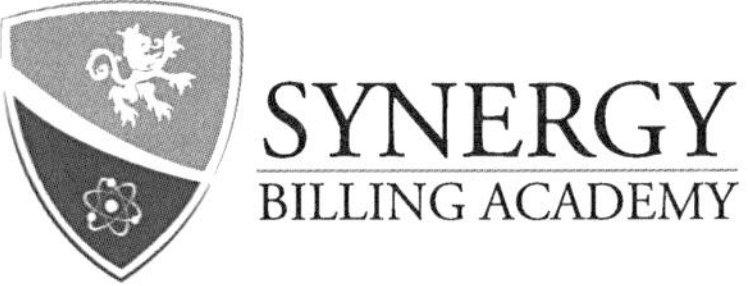

Check Your Understanding

Arrange the steps of coding in order:

1. ____________ Assign codes to the highest level of specificity.

2. ____________ Code the diagnosis until all elements are completely identified.

3. ____________ Follow any cross-reference instructions, such as "see also."

4. ____________ Identify the main terms in the diagnostic statement.

5. ____________ Locate the main terms in the Alphabetic Index (Volume 2).

6. ____________ Refer to any instructional notations in the Tabular List (Volume 1).

7. ____________ Review any subterms under the main term in the Alphabetic Index (Volume 2).

8. ____________ Verify the code(s) selected from the Alphabetic Index (Volume 2) in the Tabular List (Volume 1).

True and False

9. Billing and coding are the same thing.

   a. True
   b. False

10. Clinical documentation of diagnosis is intended to establish medical necessity.

   a. True
   b. False

11. External cause codes can be listed as primary/principal diagnosis.

   a. True
   b. False

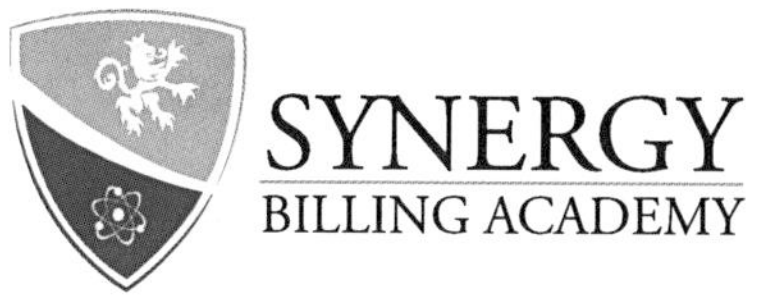

12. We have codes to indicate family and personal history of certain conditions.

    a. True
    b. False

13. ICD was created by WHO.

    a. True
    b. False

14. CM is the ICD version used globally.

    a. True
    b. False

15. We can code signs and symptoms even if the patient has a definite diagnosis.

    a. True
    b. False

16. When signs and symptoms are not integral to a disease, we do not need to add them on the claim.

    a. True
    b. False

Underline the main term and decide what type of code you would use, such as External Cause Code, Health Status Code, or Regular Code:

17. Alcoholic gastritis ________________________

18. Bitten by a duck ________________________

19. Screening for yellow fever ________________________

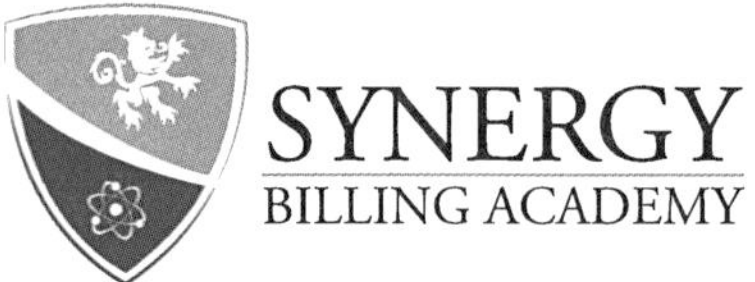

Underline and code the patient's diagnosis following the steps of coding:

20. Established patient is seen for cough, fever, and shortness of breath. Chest X-rays showed pneumonia and the patient was sent home with antibiotics.

21. Follow-up office visit for a 28-year-old male with recent colonoscopy with biopsy and small bowel X-rays. The biopsy and X-rays confirmed that the patient has ulcerative colitis. The patient was started on sulfasalazine.

22. A new 55-year-old male patient presents with jaundice and fatigue. Diagnostic test showed Hepatitis C. He will be treated with interferon therapy.

23. Patient presented for a right inguinal hernia repair. Following an assessment by the nurse, it was discovered that the patient had eaten breakfast; the surgery was canceled and will be rescheduled for next week.

Short Answers

24. Why or when do we have to use health status codes?

____

____

____

25. What is the difference between diagnosis and procedural coding?

____

____

____

ICD-10-CM International Classification of Diseases 10th Revision Clinical Modification

History and Evolution

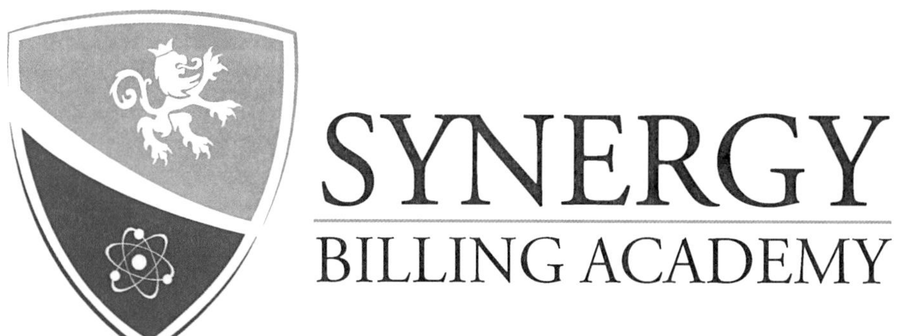

History and Evolution

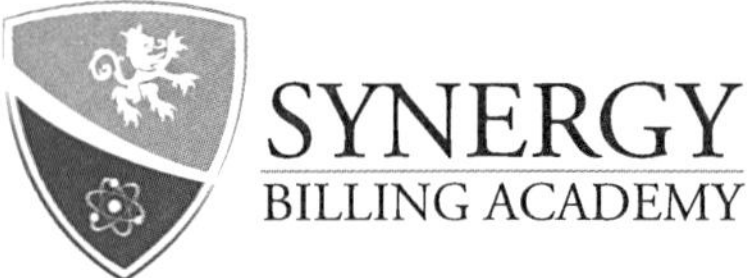

Back In Time[2]

Early History
The first attempt to classify diseases systematically dates back to François Bossier de Lacroix (1706–1777).

1975–1978
The International Conference for the Ninth Revision of the International Classification of Diseases was held from September 30 to October 6, 1975, in Geneva, Switzerland, but the results and manual were not published until 1978.

1989
The 10th revision was postponed from 1985 to 1989, as it had become clear that the established 10-year interval between revisions was too short. The need to consult so many countries and organizations made the revision process a very lengthy one.

ICD-10 to CM/PCS

The International Classification of Diseases is a diagnostic tool used for epidemiology, health management, and clinical purposes. This includes analyzing the general health situation of population groups. It is also used to monitor the incidence and prevalence of diseases and other health problems.[2]

It is used to classify diseases and other health problems recorded on many types of health and vital records including death certificates and health records. It is also used for reimbursement and resource allocation decision-making by countries.[2]

Currently, the United States uses the ninth edition of the ICD code set (ICD-9), published in 1977 and adopted by the U.S. in 1979. It was mandated as the Medicare claims standard in 1989. In 1990, the World Health Organization (WHO) updated its international version of the ICD-10. Other countries began adopting ICD-10 in 1994, but the United States only partially adopted ICD-10 in 1999 for mortality reporting. [7]

The National Center for Health Statistics (NCHS) developed ICD-10-CM following a thorough evaluation by a technical advisory panel and extensive consultation with physician groups, clinical coders, and others to ensure its clinical accuracy and usefulness. [7]

The compliance date for all Health Insurance Portability and Accountability Act (HIPAA)-covered

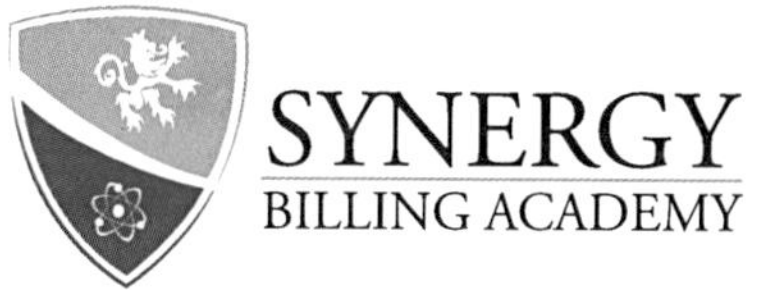

entities to implement ICD-10-CM/PCS was postponed for at least one year from the set date of October 1, 2014. ICD-10-CM/PCS will enhance accurate payment for services rendered and help evaluate medical processes and outcomes.

USA What Happened?

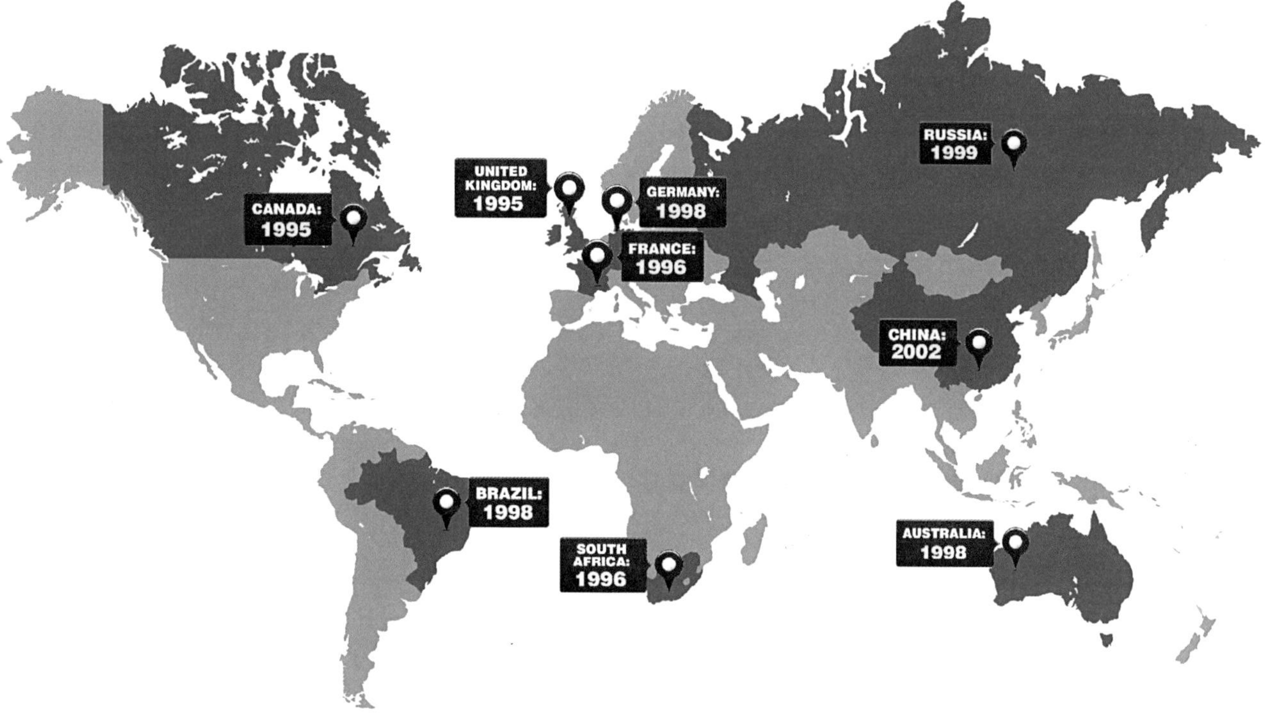

Two Parts

Currently, the ICD-9-CM has three volumes: Volume 1, Diseases, Tabular List (diagnosis); Volume 2, Diseases, Alphabetic Index to Diseases and Injuries (diagnosis); and Volume 3, Procedures, Tabular List and Alphabetic Index (inpatient procedures).

Transitioning to ICD-10 will divide the ICD-9 into two books: CM and PCS. ICD-10-CM consists of ICD-9-CM Volumes 1 and 2, which are used for diagnosis coding for inpatient and outpatient

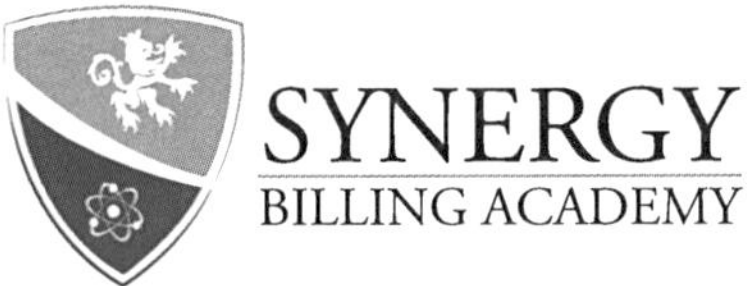

settings. ICD-10-PCS consists of ICD-9-CM Volume 3, which is used for procedural coding for inpatient settings.

ICD-10, or the International Classification of Diseases 10th Revision, was created by the World Health Organization (WHO). The designation "CM" indicates that this is the United States, modification of the code set. Our modification was developed by the National Center for Health Care Statistics (NCHS); it has about 68,000 alphanumeric codes.

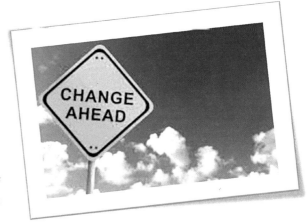

Changes

ICD-10-CM will have 21 chapters instead of ICD-9-CM's 17. All codes are alphanumeric and they can have up to seven characters. The V Codes and E Codes have been incorporated into the main classification. The diseases of the eyes and ears now have their own chapters instead of being listed in the Diseases of the Nervous System chapter. Certain diseases were reassigned to other chapters; for example, gout was moved from the endocrine system to the musculoskeletal system. ICD-10-CM groups all injuries by site then type of injury instead of classifying them by injury as ICD-9-CM does. We now also have an "X," which is used as a placeholder.[8]

Similarities

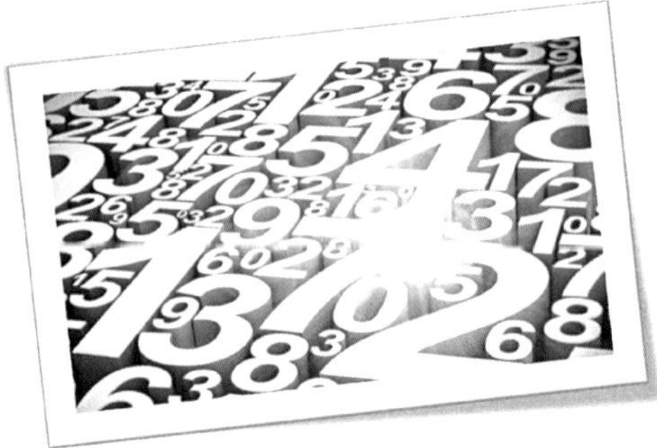

The Tabular List is the list of codes, divided into chapters based on body system or condition. The chapters are structured similarly to ICD-9-CM. They are presented in code number order and the codes are looked up the same way, first by looking up diagnostic terms, then verifying the code number. The codes will be considered invalid if they are missing the appropriate amount of characters.

ICD-10-CM also has an Alphabetic Index. This is an alphabetical list of terms and their

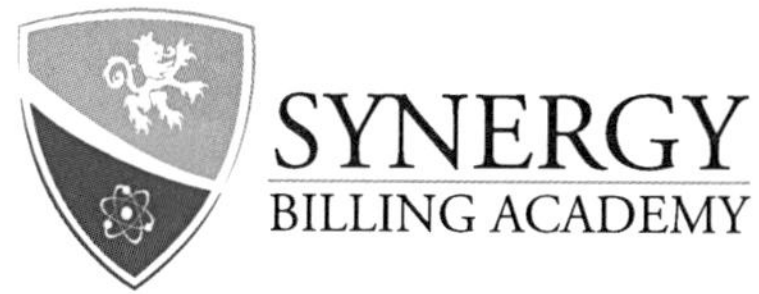

corresponding codes. This is structured and formatted the same as in ICD-9-CM. The main terms are in alphabetical order with indented subterms. This index is composed of the Index to Diseases and Injuries, an Index to External Causes, the Table of Neoplasms, and the Table of Drugs and Chemicals.

Conventions in ICD-10-CM have the same meaning as they did in ICD-9-CM. ICD-10-CM also contains a list of Official Guidelines for Coding and Reporting; these need to be followed carefully, as they are the instructions on how to code certain conditions properly. Please keep in mind that adhering to the official coding guidelines in all health care settings is required under the Health Insurance Portability and Accountability Act (HIPAA).

Why ICD-10-CM

ICD-10-CM provides more specific data than ICD-9-CM. It better reflects current medical practices and accounts for the technological advances that have taken place since the implementation of ICD-9-CM. It also allows for better documentation of a condition's severity, risk, complexity, complications, manifestations, and sequelae or late effects, as well as comorbidity, etiology, external factors, and disease classification and stages. [9]

The new structure will allow the addition of new codes. The current coding system (ICD-9-CM) is running out of capacity and cannot accommodate future developments in the field of health care. Additionally, new quality measurements in ICD-10-CM will help reduce coding errors, give us better analysis of disease patterns, allow us to more accurately track and respond to public health outbreaks, make claims submission more efficient, and help identify fraud and abuse.

ICD-10-CM Benefits

ICD-10-CM allows for better organization and description of each code and a greater level of detail than ICD-9-CM. This was accomplished through the expansion of injury codes, the creation and combination of diagnosis/symptom codes to reduce the number of codes needed to describe a condition, the addition of 6th and 7th characters for greater expansion and specificity, revisions to the 4th and 5th digit subclassifications, and the addition of laterality, which will allow for greater specificity regarding the affected side of the body and specific body region.

ICD-10-CM allows more expansion than was ever possible with ICD-9-CM.[9] The greater specificity in code assignment will result in an improved ability to measure health care services and

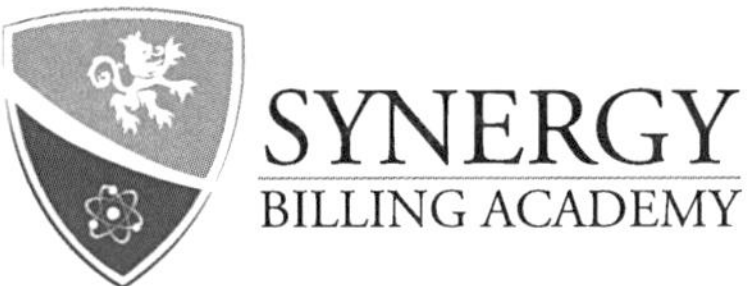

increased sensitivity when refining grouping and reimbursement methodologies, an enhanced ability to conduct public health surveillance, and a decreased need to include supporting documentation with claims.

Chapter Conversion

Chapters	ICD-9-CM	Code Range	ICD-10-CM	Code Range	
Ch. 1	*Infectious and Parasitic Diseases*	001-139	*Certain Infectious and Parasitic Diseases*	A00-B99	
Ch. 2	*Neoplasms*	140-239	*Neoplasms*	C00-D49	*C = Cancer*
Ch. 3	*Endocrine, Nutritional and Metabolic Diseases and Immunity Disorders*	240-279	*Diseases of the Blood and Blood-Forming Organs*	D50-D89	
Ch. 4	*Diseases of the Blood and Blood-Forming Organs*	280-289	*Endocrine, Nutritional, and Metabolic Diseases*	E00-E90	*E = Endocrine*
Ch. 5	*Mental, Behavioral, and Neurodevelopmental Disorders*	290-319	*Mental, Behavioral, and Neurodevelopmental Disorders*	F01-F99	
Ch. 6	*Diseases of Nervous Systems and Sense Organs*	320-389	*Diseases of the Nervous System*	G00-G99	
Ch. 7	*Diseases of the Circulatory System*	390-459	*Diseases of the Eye and Adnexa (new)*	H00-H59	
Ch. 8	*Diseases of the Respiratory System*	460-519	*Diseases of the Ear and Mastoid Process (new)*	H60-H95	*H = Hearing*
Ch. 9	*Diseases of the Digestive System*	520-579	*Diseases of the Circulatory System*	I00-I99	*I = Infarct*
Ch. 10	*Diseases of the Genitourinary System*	580-629	*Diseases of the Respiratory System*	J00-J99	
Ch. 11	*Complications of Pregnancy, Childbirth, and the Puerperium*	630-679	*Diseases of the Digestive System*	K00-K95	
Ch. 12	*Diseases of the Skin and Subcutaneous Tissue*	680-709	*Diseases of the Skin and Subcutaneous Tissue*	L00-L99	
Ch. 13	*Diseases of the Musculoskeletal System and Connective Tissue*	710-739	*Diseases of the Musculoskeletal System and Connective Tissue*	M00-M99	*M = Muscle*
Ch. 14	*Congenital Anomalies*	740-759	*Diseases of the Genitourinary System*	N00-N99	*N = Nephrology*

History and Evolution

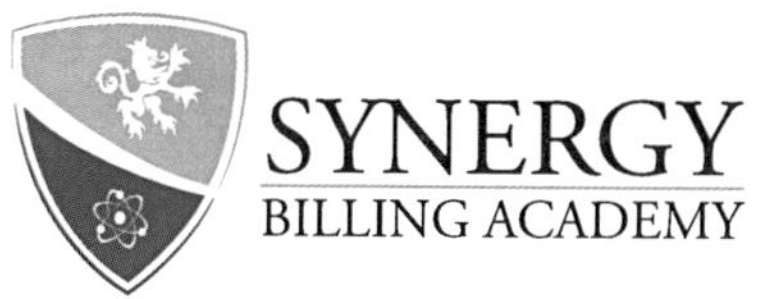

Ch. 15	*Certain Conditions Originating in the Perinatal Period*	760-779	*Pregnancy, Childbirth, and the Puerperium*	O00-O9A	*O = "OB"*
Ch. 16	*Signs, Symptoms, and Ill-Defined Conditions*	780-799	*Certain Conditions Originating in the Perinatal Period*	P00-P96	*P = Perinatal*
Ch. 17	*Injury and Poisoning*	800-999	*Congenital Malformations, Deformations, and Chromosomal Abnormalities*	Q00-Q99	
Ch. 18	*N/A*	-	*Symptoms, Signs, and Abnormal Clinical and Laboratory Findings NEC*	R00-R99	*R = Rule Out*
Ch. 19	*N/A*	-	*Injury, Poisoning, and Certain Other Consequences of External Causes*	S00-T88	*T = Toxicity*
Ch. 20	*N/A*	-	*External Causes of Morbidity (new)*	V01-Y99	*Y = Why did it happen?*
Ch. 21	*N/A*	-	*Factors Influencing Health Status and Contact with Health Services (new)*	Z00-Z99	*Z = Codes*
	Index	-	*Index*		
	Neoplasm Table		*Neoplasm Table*		
	Table of Drugs and Chemicals		*Table of Drugs and Chemicals*		
	Index to External Causes		*Index to External Causes*		
	Classification of Factors Influencing Health Status and Contact with Health Service	V01-V89			
	Supplemental Classification of External Causes of Injury and Poisoning				

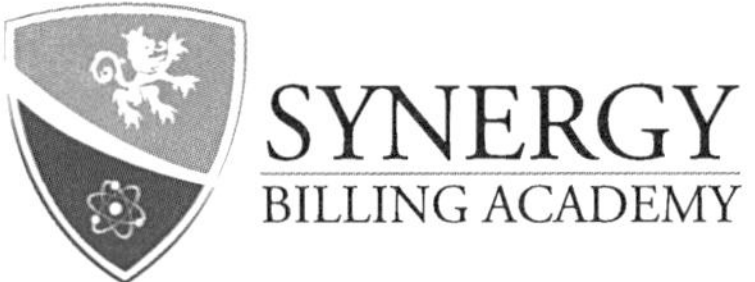

Chapters, Letters, and Meanings

Chapters		Code Range/Letter
Chapter 2	Neoplasms	Code range C00-D49 or C for Cancer
Chapter 4	Endocrine, Nutritional, and Metabolic Diseases	Code range E00-E90 or E for Endocrine
Chapter 7	Diseases of the Ear and Mastoid Process	Code range H60-H95 or H for Hearing
Chapter 9	Diseases of the Circulatory Systems	Code range I00-I99 or I for Infarct
Chapter 13	Diseases of the Musculoskeletal System and Connective Tissue	Code range M00-M99 or M for Muscle
Chapter 14	Diseases of the Genitourinary System	Code range N00-N99 or N for Nephrology
Chapter 15	Pregnancy, Childbirth, and the Puerperium	Code range O00-O9A or O for "OB"
Chapter 16	Certain Conditions Originating in the Perinatal Period	Code range P00-P96 or P for Perinatal
Chapter 18	Symptoms, Signs, and Abnormal Clinical and Laboratory Findings NEC	Code range R00-R99 or R for Rule Out
Chapter 19	Injury, Poisoning, Certain Other Consequences of External Causes	Code range S00-T88 or T for Toxicity
Chapter 20	External Causes of Morbidity	Code range V01-Y99 or Y for "Why did it happen"
Chapter 21	Factors Influencing Health Status and Contact with Health Services	Code range Z00-Z99 or Z for V Codes

GEMs

General Equivalency Mappings (GEMs) were created by the Centers for Medicare and Medicaid Services (CMS) to help with the analysis and conversion of codes to ICD-10-CM, but they are not meant for crosswalks. We are going from about 14,000 to 69,000 codes and from 17 to 21 chapters. Nonetheless, some ICD-9-CM codes do not have an equivalent ICD-10-CM code.

History and Evolution

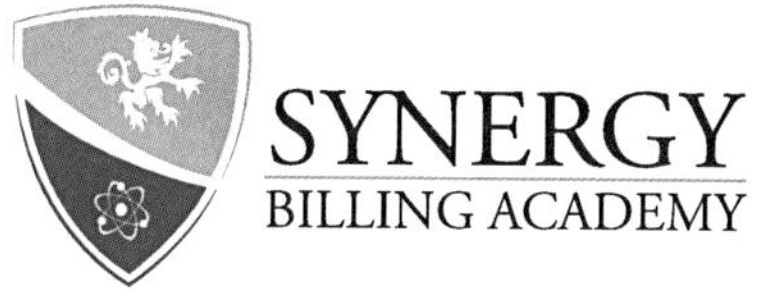

<u>Three things could happen when using these files</u>:

- You could end up with an exact match in code but the description might be slightly different.
- With forward mapping (ICD-9 to ICD-10), you could end up with multiple ICD-10-CM codes corresponding to one ICD-9-CM code.
- With backward mapping (ICD-10 to ICD-9), you could end up with multiple ICD-9-CM codes corresponding to one ICD-10-CM code.

General Equivalency Mappings

896.2 Traumatic Amputation of Foot (complete) (partial), bilateral without mention of complications

OR

S98011: Complete traumatic amputations of right foot at ankle level
AND
S98012: Complete traumatic amputations of left foot at ankle level

S98011: Complete traumatic amputations of right foot at ankle level
AND
S98022: Partial traumatic amputations of left foot at ankle level

S98021: Partial traumatic amputations of right foot at ankle level
AND
S98012: Complete traumatic amputations of left foot at ankle level

S98021: Partial traumatic amputations of right foot at ankle level
AND
S98022: Partial traumatic amputations of left foot at ankle level

History and Evolution

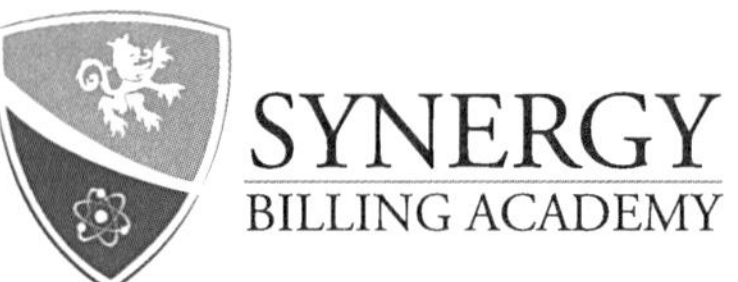

1 Code to 26 Options

Was

ICD-9-CM

728.85 - Spasm of Muscle

Now

ICD-10-CM

M62.40	CONTRACTURE OF MUSCLE UNSPECIFIED SITE
M62.411	CONTRACTURE OF MUSCLE RIGHT SHOULDER
M62.412	CONTRACTURE OF MUSCLE LEFT SHOULDER
M62.419	CONTRACTURE OF MUSCLE UNSPECIFIED SHOULDER
M62.421	CONTRACTURE OF MUSCLE RIGHT UPPER ARM
M62.422	CONTRACTURE OF MUSCLE LEFT UPPER ARM
M62.429	CONTRACTURE OF MUSCLE UNSPECIFIED UPPER ARM
M62.431	CONTRACTURE OF MUSCLE RIGHT FOREARM
M62.432	CONTRACTURE OF MUSCLE LEFT FOREARM
M62.439	CONTRACTURE OF MUSCLE UNSPECIFIED FOREARM
M62.44I	CONTRACTURE OF MUSCLE RIGHT HAND
M62.442	CONTRACTURE OF MUSCLE LEFT HAND
M62.449	CONTRACTURE OF MUSCLE UNSPECIFIED HAND
M62.451	CONTRACTURE OF MUSCLE RIGHT THIGH
M62.452	CONTRACTURE OF MUSCLE LEFT THIGH
M62.459	CONTRACTURE OF MUSCLE UNSPECIFIED THIGH
M62.461	CONTRACTURE OF MUSCLE RIGHT LOWER LEG
M62.462	CONTRACTURE OF MUSCLE LEFT LOWER LEG
M62.469	CONTRACTURE OF MUSCLE UNSPECIFIED LEG
M62.471	CONTRACTURE OF MUSCLE RIGHT ANKLE AND FOOT
M62.472	CONTRACTURE OF MUSCLE LEFT ANKLE AND FOOT
M62.479	CONTRACTURE OF MUSCLE UNSPECIFIED ANKLE AND FOOT
M62.48	CONTRACTURE OF MUSCLE OTHER SITE
M62.49	CONTRACTURE OF MUSCLE MULTIPLE SITES
M62.831	MUSCLE SPASM OF CALF
M62.838	OTHER MUSCLE SPASM

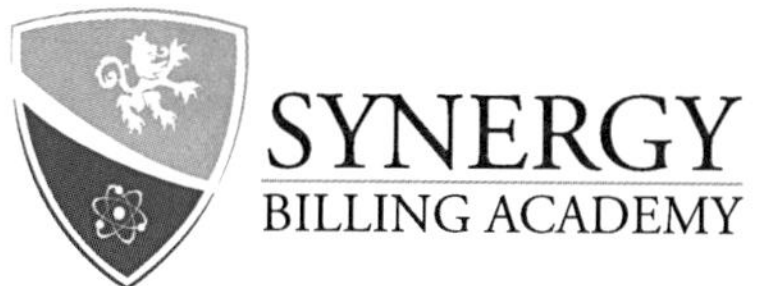

Conventions [9,10]

Conventions are abbreviations, punctuation, and notes. These conventions are very important, as they will help you navigate the manual. [5, 6] The coding conventions were developed and approved by the American Hospital Association (AHA), the American Health Information Management Association (AHIMA), the Centers for Medicare and Medicaid Services (CMS), and the National Center for Health Statistics (NCHS). The guidelines are divided into four sections just like in ICD-9-CM:

Section I: Structure and Conventions

Abbreviations = NEC and NOS

- NEC is an acronym for "not elsewhere classified." This is used when no more specific code exists. These codes can only be used when the documentation specifies a condition but there is no more specific code for that condition.

- NOS is an acronym for "not otherwise specified." This is used when the diagnosis is not specified in the documentation. These codes are equivalent to unspecified. They are used when we do not have sufficient documentation to select any other, more specific code.

Punctuation = () []

- [ ] Brackets enclose synonyms, alternative wording, or explanatory phrases. They provide us with additional helpful information. Codes in brackets can affect how we code. They are only found in the Tabular List. Brackets are also used to identify etiology and manifestation codes.

  - Etiology refers to the cause of a disease, whereas manifestations are the symptoms. When we can have both in one code, it is called a combination code. In other words, combination codes give you the etiology (cause of disease) and the manifestation (symptom) using only one code to describe the diagnosis.

- *[ ]* Slanted brackets enclose manifestations of underlying conditions. They are typically accompanied by a note that states, "Code first underlying disease." The slanted brackets are used in Volume 2, the Alphabetic Index.

- ( ) Parentheses contain non-essential modifiers, which you can choose whether or not

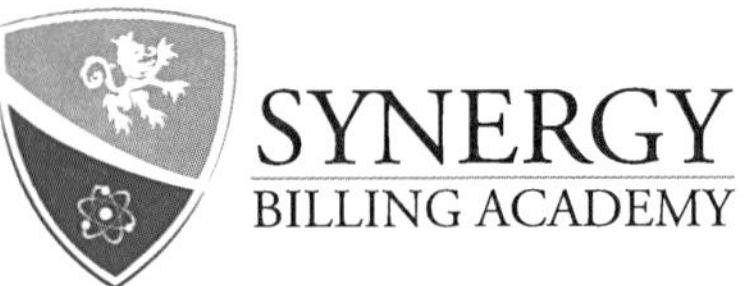

to use.They contain informational, descriptive terms and are found in the Tabular List and Alphabetic Index. They do not affect code selection but do help clarify the diagnosis.

– Example: gonococcal (acute)....

- : In the Tabular List, a colon completes a statement with one or more modifiers. It is used after an incomplete term that needs one or more of the modifiers that follow in order to assign it to a given category.

- } In the Tabular List, a brace modifies statements to the right of the brace. This is used to enclose a series of terms, each of which modifies the statement appearing to the left of the brace.

Notes: Excludes, includes, code first, use additional, cross-references (see and see also)

- Excludes1: A type 1 Excludes note is a pure excludes note. It means "Not coded here!" An Excludes1 note indicates that the code excluded should never be used at the same time as the code above the Excludes1 note. An Excludes1 is used when two conditions cannot occur together, such as a congenital form versus an acquired form of the same condition.

- Excludes2: A type 2 Excludes note means "Not included here". An Excludes2 note indicates that the condition excluded is not part of the condition represented by the code, but a patient may have both conditions at the same time. When an Excludes2 note appears under a code, it is acceptable to use both the code and the excluded code together if the patient has both conditions.

- Code First/Use Additional Code: A Code First note means that we need to code for the etiology and manifestation(s).

  – Etiology refers to the cause of disease, whereas manifestations are the symptoms. When we can have both in one code, it is called a combination code. In other words, combination codes give you the etiology (cause of disease) and the manifestation (symptom), using only one code to describe the diagnosis.

- Code Also: A Code Also note means that we will need more than one code to fully express the diagnosis. We must assign other code(s) to fully code the patient's condition.

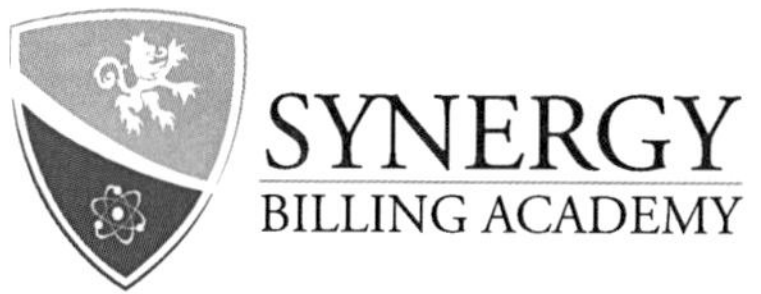

- See: The See note indicates that another term should be referenced. It is necessary to go to the main term referenced with the see note to obtain the correct code.

- See Also: The See Also note indicates that there is another main term that we might also need to reference. It is not necessary to cross-reference this new term.

- See Condition: The See Condition note indicates that this is not the main term, but rather a term that describes the immediate condition but not the actual condition of the patient.

- 7th Character and Placeholder X: ICD-9-CM allows a maximum of 5 characters. With ICD-10-CM, we will have up to 7 characters. This 7th character is required in some categories to provide further specificity about the condition that is being coded. The X is used in some cases as a placeholder for certain codes to allow for future expansion.

  The placeholder has two uses:

  - As the 5th-digit character for 6-character codes. The X will allow for future expansion without disturbing the 6-character structure.
  - When a code has fewer than 6 characters but a 7th character is required. The X is assigned for all characters less than 6 in order to meet the requirement of coding to the highest level of specificity.

Section IV: Outpatient Coding and Reporting

First-Listed Diagnosis

Both the principal diagnosis and the first-listed diagnosis describe the primary reason for an encounter. The main difference between these terms is the setting in which the patients are being seen. The principal diagnosis is used for inpatient settings and the first-listed diagnosis is used in outpatient settings. For example: Documentation states that a patient with inguinal hernia presents with shortness of breath; in this case, shortness of breath would be the first-listed diagnosis because this is the reason the patient was seen.

In the outpatient setting, the term first-listed diagnosis is used in the place of principal diagnosis. In determining the first-listed diagnosis, the coding conventions of ICD-10-CM, as well as the general and disease-specific guidelines take precedence over the outpatient guidelines.

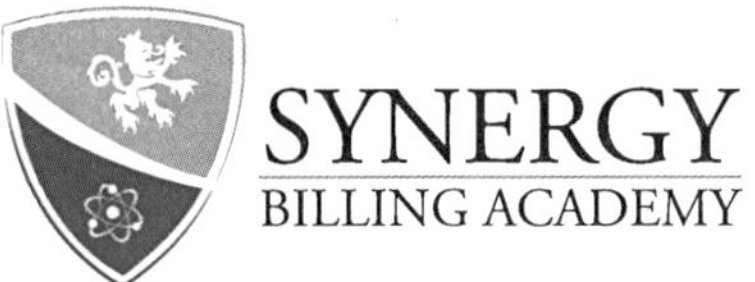

The most critical rule involves beginning the search for the correct code(s) through the Alphabetic Index. Never begin searching initially in the Tabular List, as this will lead to coding errors.

Unconfirmed or Uncertain Diagnosis

Diagnoses often are not established at the time of the initial encounter/visit. It may take two or more visits before the diagnosis is confirmed, but signs/symptoms are reported at each visit. Do not code diagnoses documented as "probable," "suspected," "questionable," "rule out," "working diagnosis," or other similar terms indicating uncertainty. Rather, code the condition(s) to the highest degree of certainty for that encounter/visit, such as symptoms, signs, abnormal test results, or other reason for the visit.

Codes that describe symptoms and signs, as opposed to diagnoses, are acceptable for reporting purposes when a diagnosis has not been established (confirmed) by the provider. Chapter 18 of ICD-10-CM, Symptoms, Signs, and Abnormal Clinical and Laboratory Findings Not Elsewhere Classified (codes R00-R99), contains many, but not all, codes for symptoms. For example: Documentation states that the patient presented with complaint of frequent heartburn. The physician prescribes Prilosec for suspected GERD with patient returning in 10 days. In this case, we would only report frequent heartburn.

Outpatient Surgery

Code the reason for the surgery first. When a patient presents for outpatient surgery (same-day surgery), code the reason for the surgery as the first-listed diagnosis (reason for the encounter), even if the surgery is not performed due to a contraindication. Follow this with a code to report the reason the procedure was not carried out, such as Z53.09, Procedure not carried out due to other contraindication.

Z Codes

ICD-10-CM provides codes to deal with encounters for circumstances other than a disease or injury. The Factors Influencing Health Status and Contact with Health Services codes (Z00-Z99) are provided to deal with occasions when circumstances other than a disease or injury are recorded as a diagnosis or problems.

Z Codes are informative; they report circumstances other than disease or injury. They may be used first or listed as additional codes depending on the circumstances. For instance, Z23 reports encounters for inoculations and vaccinations, while the procedure code will identify the administration.

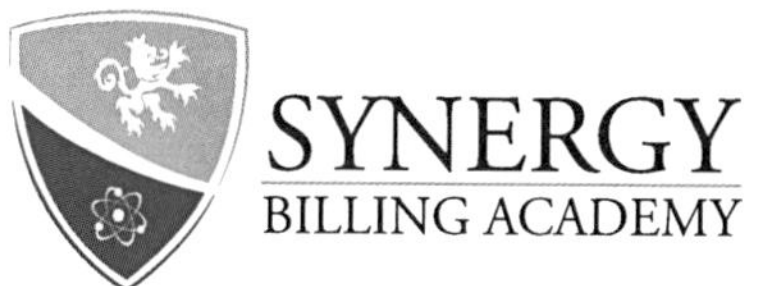

Coexisting Conditions

Code all documented conditions that coexist at the time of the encounter/visit and require or affect patient care, treatment, or management. Do not code conditions that were previously treated and no longer exist. However, history codes (categories Z80-Z87) may be used as secondary codes if the historical condition or family history has an impact on current care or influences treatment.

For example, patient presents with shortness of breath due to asthma. Physician prescribes nebulizer treatments. The patient is morbidly obese, making the examination and treatment more complex. The first-listed diagnosis is asthma and the coexisting condition is obesity.

Chronic Diseases

Chronic diseases that are treated on an ongoing basis may be coded and reported as many times as the patient receives treatment and care for the condition(s). Do not report conditions that were previously treated and no longer exist. In those cases, we would report history codes (Z80-Z87) as secondary diagnoses if the condition impacts the current condition or affects treatment.

Diagnostic Services

For patients receiving only diagnostic services during an encounter/visit, sequence first the diagnosis, condition, problem, or other reason for encounter/visit shown in the medical record to be chiefly responsible for the outpatient services provided during the encounter/visit. Codes for other diagnoses (e.g., chronic conditions) may be sequenced as additional diagnoses.

For encounters for routine laboratory/radiology testing in the absence of any signs, symptoms, or associated diagnosis, assign Z01.89, Encounter for other specified special examinations. If routine testing is performed during the same encounter as a test to evaluate a sign, symptom, or diagnosis, it is appropriate to assign both the Z Code and the code describing the reason for the non-routine test.

For outpatient encounters for diagnostic tests that have been interpreted by a physician, if the final report is available at the time of coding, code any confirmed or definitive diagnosis or diagnoses documented in the interpretation. Do not code related signs and symptoms as additional diagnoses.

If only diagnostic service was provided, report the first reason for service. For example, the patient presented for a routine periodic gynecological exam; report Z01.419, No signs, symptoms, or

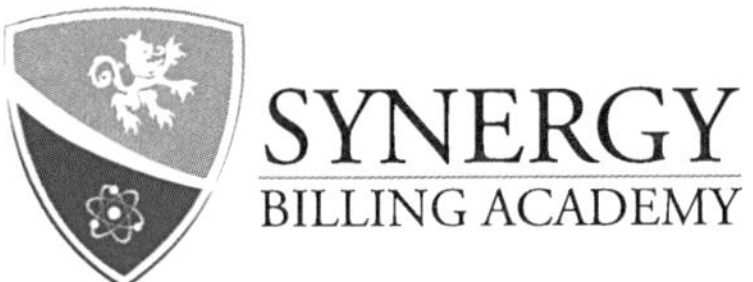

associated diagnosis. Another example would be when a patient presents for diagnostic imaging for left, central breast mass: report N63, unspecified breast lump. A later diagnosis might be malignant neoplasm, which would be reported with C50.112.

Preoperative Evaluation

For patients receiving only preoperative evaluations, sequence first a code from subcategory Z01.81, Encounter for pre-procedural examinations, to describe the pre-op consultations. Assign a code for the condition to describe the reason for the surgery as an additional diagnosis. You may also code any findings related to the pre-op evaluation, but the first-listed code should be the preoperative examination.

Depending on the type of operation, code Z01.81 may have different endings, such as Z01.810, Preoperative cardiovascular examination; Z01.811, Preoperative respiratory examination; Z01.812, Preoperative lab; or Z01.818, Preoperative exam not otherwise specified, examination before chemotherapy.

Prenatal Encounters

For routine outpatient prenatal visits when no complications are present, a code from category Z34, Encounter for supervision of normal pregnancy, should be used as the first-listed diagnosis. These codes should not be used in conjunction with Chapter 15 codes. Example: 19-year-old female presents for initial prenatal exam, first pregnancy, Z34.00.

For routine prenatal outpatient visits for patients with high-risk pregnancies, a code from category O09, Supervision of high-risk pregnancy, should be used as the first-listed diagnosis. Secondary Chapter 15 codes may be used in conjunction with these codes if appropriate. Example: 29-year-old first trimester female patient presents for prenatal encounter with varicose veins of legs, O22.01.

External Cause Index

The external cause index in ICD-10-CM maps to the E Codes index in the ICD-9-CM manual. This is the Supplementary Classification of External Causes of Injury and Poisoning, found after the table of drugs and chemicals.

The alphabetic index is organized by main terms, which describe the accident, circumstance, event, or specific agent that caused the injury or other adverse effect. Remember that these codes are never used as the principal diagnosis.

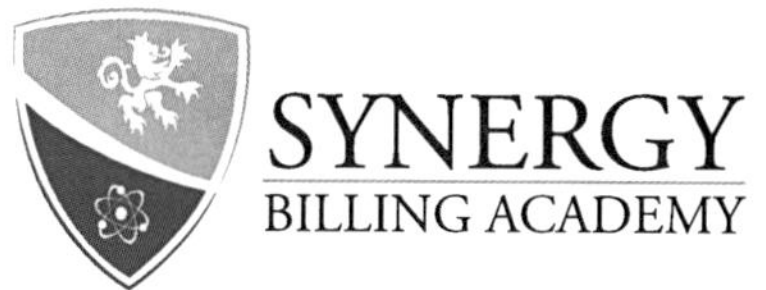

These codes permit the classification of environmental events, circumstances, and conditions as the cause of illness or injury. These codes are used in addition to a code from the Tabular List.

Level of Specificity

We must always report to the highest character available. You cannot report only to the 5th character if there is a 6th character available. The highest level of specificity has a maximum of 7 characters.

- M48.48XA (A= initial encounter)
- No 6th character for M48.48, but there is a 7th, X = placeholder

Integral Conditions

Integral conditions mean that a condition is part of the diagnosis. In these cases, do not report signs and symptoms separately. For example, for a patient with fever and shortness of breath due to pneumonia, we would only report the pneumonia, because fever and shortness of breath are symptoms of pneumonia.

Not Integral Conditions

Not integral conditions mean that a condition is not part of the diagnosis. In these cases, we have to report the signs and symptoms separately. For example, a patient presents with pneumonia and dehydration. We would report J18.9 for Pneumonia and E86.0 for Dehydration. This is because not all patients with pneumonia have dehydration and dehydration was not stated to be due to the pneumonia.

Etiology and Manifestations

Etiology is the origination; it is the cause or origin of the disease or condition. Manifestations are how the cause shows in the patient; it is an extension of the patient's illness or condition. An example is diabetic retinopathy; diabetes is the etiology or the cause and retinopathy is the manifestation or the symptom. For this condition, we have a combination code: E10.319, Type 1 diabetic retinopathy. In other cases such as Staphylococcal aureus cellulitis of face, we would have multiple codes; in this case, they are L03.211 for Cellulitis and B95.61 for the Staph infection.

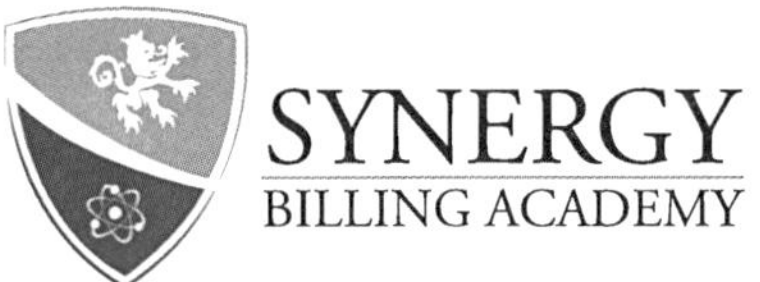

Acute and Chronic

An acute condition means that symptoms are severe; they appear and change or worsen rapidly. A chronic condition develops and worsens over an extended or long period of time. It is possible for a patient to have a condition that is both acute and chronic. We might have have separate codes for this or just one. When a patient has a condition that is both acute and chronic, we have to report acute first, then chronic.

Combination Codes

A combination means a grouping of things. In coding, we can have combination codes; this means that diagnoses, manifestations, and complications can be coded using one code. Combination codes are used to report two diagnoses, a diagnosis with a manifestation, or a diagnosis with an associated complication. An example of this would be K80.00, Acute cholecystitis with cholelithiasis; we have one code for both conditions.

In contrast, when we have to use more than code to report a patient's condition, it is called multiple coding.

Residual and Cause

A late effect is a condition that appears after the acute phase of an earlier condition or after a condition has run its course. There is no time limit for a patient to develop a late effect, as some late effects can occur decades later. In ICD-10-CM, a late effect is referred to as a sequela (plural sequelae). This is the residual of a condition or the leftover from an illness. For example, a malunion of a fracture is considered to be residual because it is the late effect of the fracture, which was the original the cause.

The sequencing of residuals and their causes can be somewhat complicated. When sequencing a sequela or residual, we need to report the residual as the first-listed diagnosis, followed by the late effects code. This is because the patient is dealing with the "leftovers" of a disease or condition. If we look at the previous example, we can tell that the patient is being seen for the malunion (the sequela) and not the fracture (the cause).

Structure and Format [11]

The expanded number of characters in the ICD-10-CM diagnosis codes provides greater specificity to identify disease etiology, anatomical site, and severity. The ICD-10-CM code structure is as follows:

History and Evolution

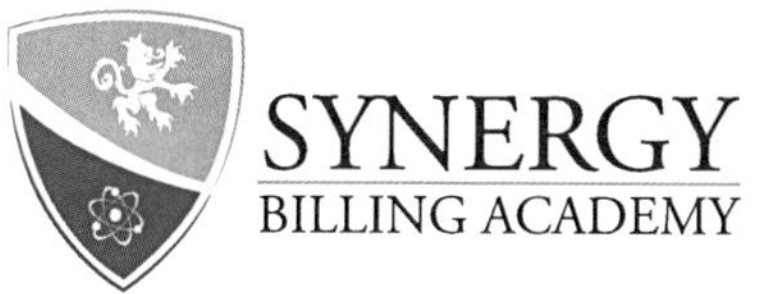

- Characters 1–3: Category
- Characters 4–6: Etiology, anatomical site, severity, or other clinical detail
- Character 7: Extension

The increased specificity of the ICD-10-CM codes is more flexible, allowing emerging diseases to be quickly incorporated. The higher level of detail in the codes provides the ability to more precisely code the diagnosis. It reflects advances in medicine and medical technology, making the code set more relevant to today's understanding of diagnoses. ICD-10-CM provides an improved ability to measure health care services.

ICD-10-CM codes are to be reported at the highest level of detail possible within the code structure.

Representation of Codes ICD-9-CM to ICD-10-CM

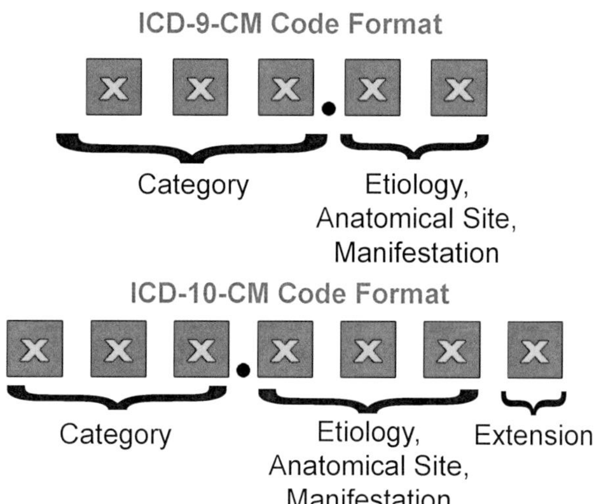

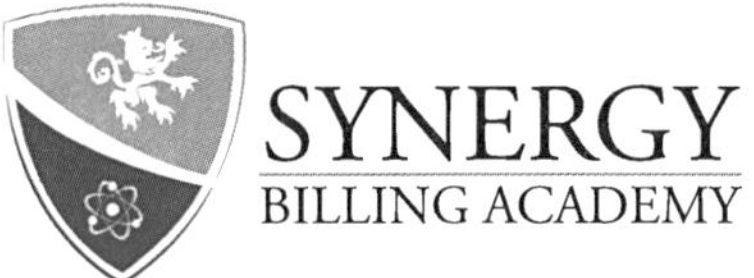

New V Codes[4]

The listing of codes for factors influencing health status and contact with health services are a bit different in ICD-10-CM than in ICD-9-CM. Factors Influencing Health Status and Contact with Health Services (Z00-Z99) are as follows:

Range	Description
Z00-Z13	Persons encountering health services for examinations
Z14-Z15	Genetic carrier and generic susceptibility to disease
Z16	Resistance to antimicrobial drugs
Z17	Estrogen receptor status
Z18	Retained foreign body fragment
Z20-Z28	Persons with potential health hazards related to communicable diseases
Z30-Z39	Persons encountering health services in circumstances related to reproduction
Z40-Z53	Encounters for other specific health care with potential health
Z55-Z65	Persons with potential health hazards related to socioeconomic and psychosocial circumstances
Z66	Do not resuscitate status
Z67	Blood type
Z68	Body mass index (BMI)
Z69-Z76	Persons encountering health services in other circumstances
Z77-Z99	Persons with potential health hazards related to family and personal history and certain conditions influencing health status

New E Codes[4]

The new E Codes are the External Causes of Morbidity (V00-Y99). An external cause code may be used with any code in the range of A00.0–T88.9 or Z00–Z99; they comprise classifications that are health conditions due to an external cause. They are mostly used with injuries and are also valid for use with infections or diseases due to an external source, or other health conditions such as a heart attack that occurs during strenuous physical activity.

History and Evolution

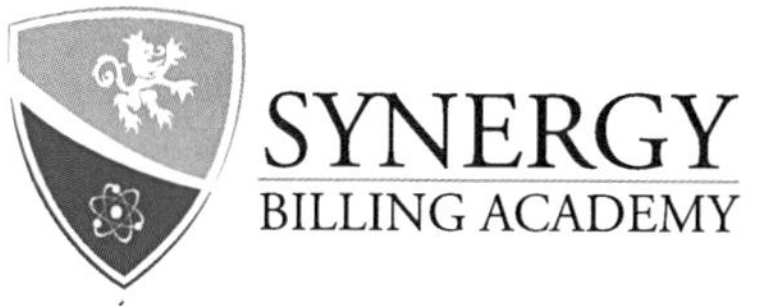

The E Codes chapter covers the letters V, W, X, and Y and represents a significant expansion from ICD-9-CM. Make sure to assign the external cause code with the appropriate seventh character (initial encounter, subsequent encounter, or sequela) for each encounter for which the injury or condition is being treated.

It will be necessary to make behavioral changes to how you prepare documentation. We have more characters overall.

You need to ask yourself the following questions:

How many elements are you currently documenting?

- Are you currently documenting the side of the body that is affected?
- Are you documenting severity?
- Are you documenting external causes?
- Are you documenting the episode of care?
- Are you documenting the underlying condition?
- Are you documenting degrees and stages? Phases and weeks?

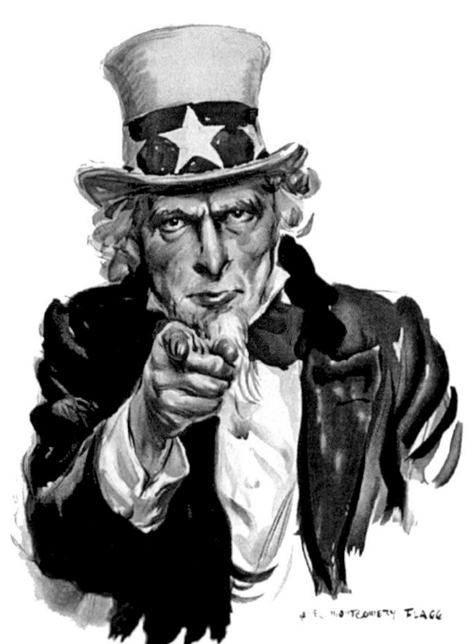

I WANT YOU
TO TELL ME
WHAT ICD-10 IS

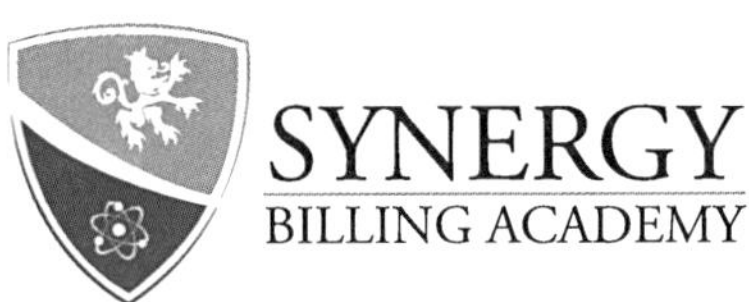

Are you ready for ICD-10?

See how it will affect your office.

Physicians

The code set will increase tremendously needing increase documentation in the following areas: laterality, stages of healing, weeks in pregnancy, episodes of cares, etc.

Managers

All policies and procedures will need to be reevaluated as well as the contracts with software vendors and all insurance companies.

Nurses

Since there will be more codes and this will call for increased documentation, every form used by nurses will need to be revised and updated. Policies could also change which will require updates

Front Desk

All patient forms need to be revised to meet HIPAA regulations. The practice management software will also be in need of updates.

Labs

The increase in the number of codes will require payers to have new requirements on how labs are ordered, as well as how they are reported.

Coding

Due to the increased number in codes, new code books will be required along with extensive knowledge of medical terminology and Anatomy of the human body.

Billing

Billing guidelines and payer reimbursement will be revised for all payers and policies and procedures training on this new code set will be required.

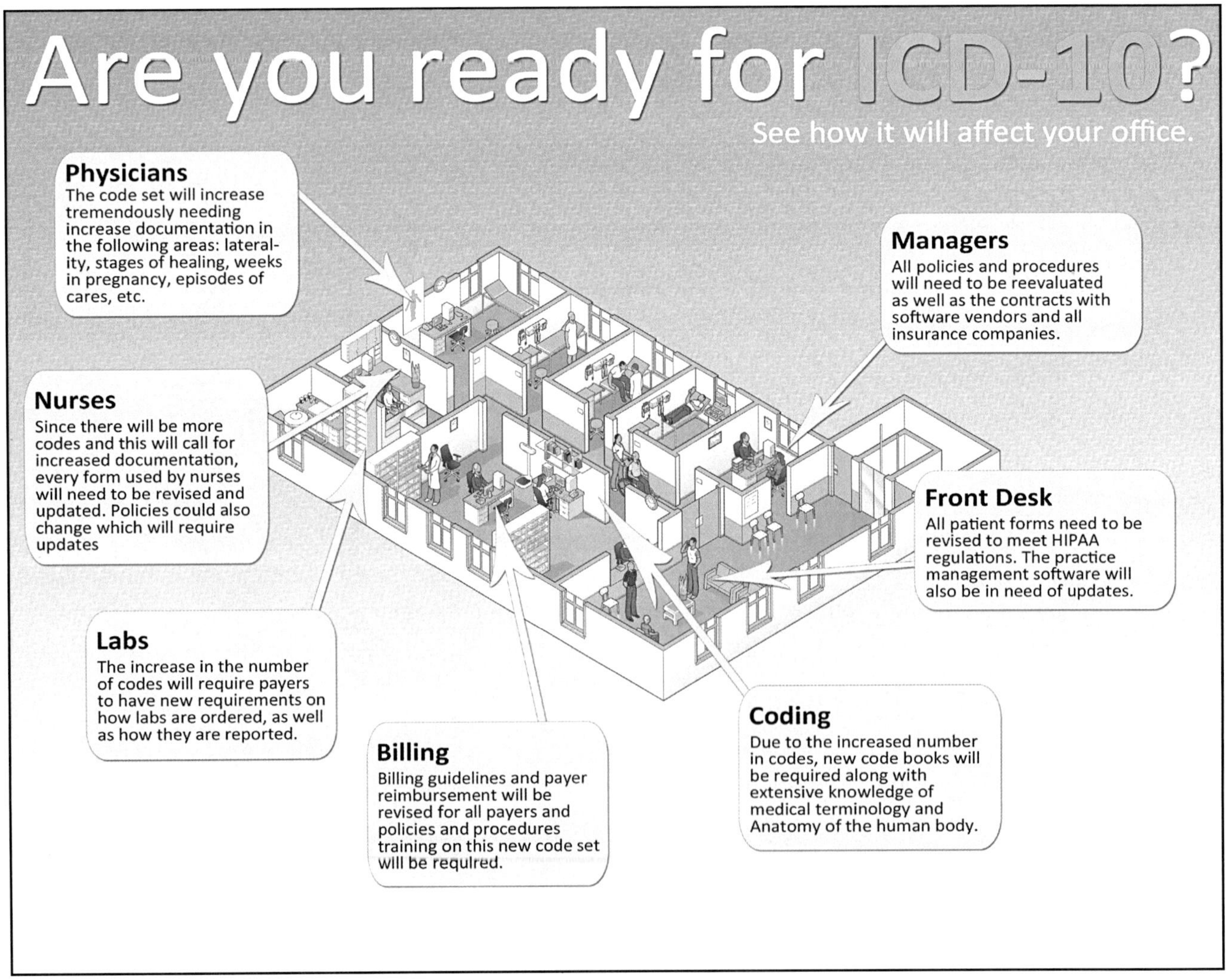

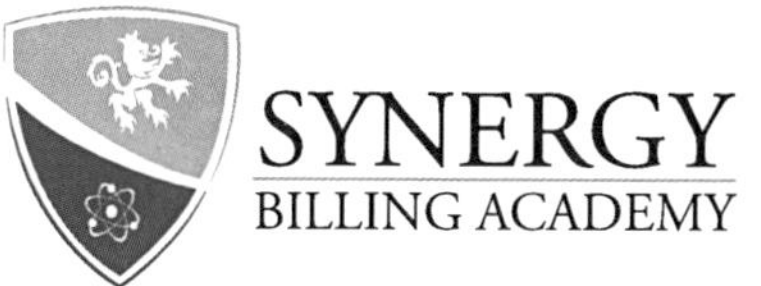

Specialties [12]

These specialties have been greatly affected by ICD-10-CM:

- Pediatrics and Primary Care
  - A larger volume of codes is applicable because these physicians treat the whole body.
- Cardiology
  - Both code and definition changes have occurred.
    - Acute phase of myocardial infarctionis now four weeks instead of eight.
- Nephrology
  - Hypertensive chronic kidney disease is now reported with two codes.
- Orthopedics
  - Laterality has been added to codes and injury codes have been expanded.

Code Increase [13]

Specialties	Number of ICD-9 Codes	Number of ICD-10 Codes	Additional Codes
Gastroenterologists	596 ICD-9 codes	706 ICD-10 codes	+110 Additional codes
Pulmonologists	255 ICD-9 codes	336 ICD-10 codes	+81 Additional codes
Urologists	389 ICD-9 codes	591 ICD-10 codes	+202 Additional codes
Endocrinologists	335 ICD-9 codes	675 ICD-10 codes	+340 Additional codes
Neurologists	459 ICD-9 codes	591 ICD-10 codes	+132 Additional codes
Pediatricians	702 ICD-9 codes	591 ICD-10 codes	-111 Fewer codes
Infectious disease	1,270 ICD-9 codes	1,056 ICD-10 codes	-214 Fewer codes

Process Changes

The two major areas that will be impacted by this transition involve changes in clinical documentation and the patient workflow. This is because the clinical documentation will increase tremendously. Insufficient documentation may lead to inquiries and potentially take-backs by CMS or other payers. Meanwhile, the number of patients being seen will be affected because of the time that must be spent documenting the facts of each visit.

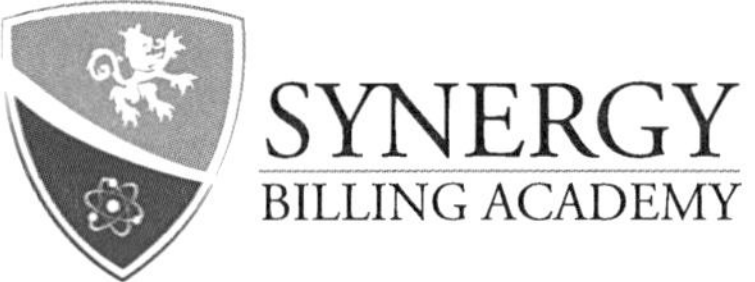

Daily Workflow [14]

- Workflow disruption before, during, and after the transition should be taken into consideration:
  - Training will require time loss for key members of the team.
  - Initial challenges with coding quality and accuracy may result in an increase in claims being denied or paid inappropriately.
    - It will take time to rework and resubmit those claims.
  - Physician productivity may be similarly impacted because of new documentation requirements to support ICD-10-CM coding.
    - The call for more accurate documentation will take more time away from the physicians.
    - Documentation needs to be specific, detailed, and complete.
    - Physician documentation will need to meet the higher standard. If the clinical documentation does not improve, accurate coding and proper payment will not be possible.
    - It is estimated that physician productivity will decrease by 10% to 20% because of the significant increase in documentation. This could have a huge impact on revenue.

Specificity

- One of the new features in the ICD-10-CM manual is the greater level of clinical detail. This is the reason why we went from about 14,000 codes to about 68,000.
  - Expansion of injury, diabetes, alcohol and substance abuse, and postoperative complication codes
  - Inclusion of trimesters in obstetrics codes
  - Changes in time frames from pregnancy to heart attack
  - New combination codes
- An example of increased specificity is:
  - S72.044G, Non-displaced fracture of base of neck of right temur, subsequent encounter for closed fracture with delayed healing
    - The fractured bone
      - Femur
    - What part of the bone
      - Base of neck
    - Type of fracture
      - Non-displaced

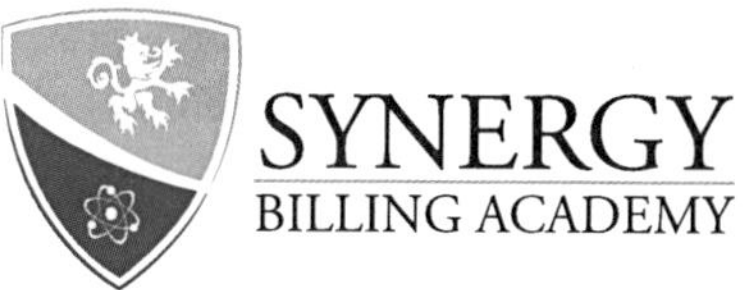

- The extent of the fracture
  - Closed
- Stage of healing
  - Delayed healing
- Laterality
  - Right
- Number of encounter(s)
  - Subsequent

Because of the additional characters, coders will have to change their habits and behavior.

Right vs. Left

Laterality is a new term used in this classification system. Laterality is used throughout the entire manual to indicate the side of the body that has been affected. In other words, it indicates left versus right. The final character of the codes in the ICD-10-CM indicate laterality.

An unspecified side code is also provided for times when the site is not identified in the medical record. Note that if no bilateral code is provided and the condition is bilateral, you will have to use one code for the left side and one code for the right side.

- Dacryops (excess tears)
  - In ICD-9-CM, there is only one code available: [5]
    - 375.11
  - In ICD-10-CM, there are four codes: [10]
    - H04.111, dacryops of right lacrimal gland
    - H04.112, dacryops of left lacrimal gland
    - H04.113, dacryops of bilateral lacrimal glands
    - H04.119, dacryops of unspecified lacrimal gland

Specific Site [4]

For some conditions, we must not only specify left or right, but also upper or lower, as indicated in the following example.

- Blepharochalasis (inflammation of the eyelid).
  - In ICD-9-CM, there is only one code available: [5]
    - 374.46

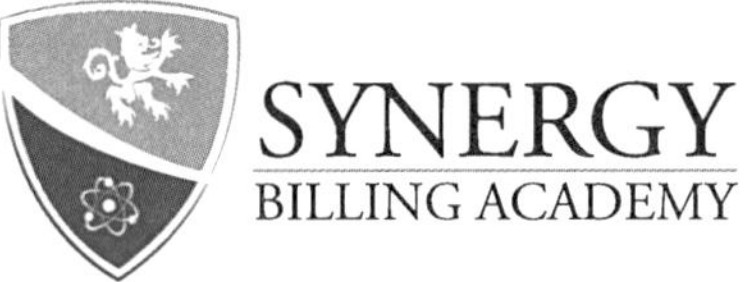

- The ICD-10-CM codes not only specify right and left eye, they also denote upper and lower eyelid: [10]
  - H02.30, blepharochalasis unspecified eye, unspecified eyelid
  - H02.31, blepharochalasis right upper eyelid
  - H02.32, blepharochalasis right lower eyelid
  - H02.33, blepharochalasis right eye, unspecified eyelid
  - H02.34, blepharochalasis left upper eyelid
  - H02.35, blepharochalasis left lower eyelid
  - H02.36, blepharochalasis left eye, unspecified eyelid

As you can see, there is an increase from one code to seven, because there was also an addition of the specific site of the inflammation.

7th Character [5]

- ICD-9-CM has a maximum of 5 characters. With ICD-10-CM, we will have up to 7 characters.
  - 1 Character: Alpha
  - 2–7 Characters: Alpha or Numeric
- The 7th character is required in some categories to provide further specificity about the condition that is being coded.
  - This 7th character will be either a letter or a number.
- The 7th character describes the encounter
  - **Initial encounter:** As long as a patient is receiving active treatment for a condition
    - Surgical treatment, emergency department encounter, or evaluation and treatment by a new physician
  - **Subsequent encounter:** After a patient has received active treatment for a condition and is receiving routine care for the condition during the healing or recovery phase
    - Cast change or removal, removal of external or internal fixation device, medication adjustment, or other aftercare and follow-up visits following treatment of the injury or condition
  - **Sequela:** Complications or conditions that arise as a direct result of a condition
    - Scar formation after a burn or any other late effect

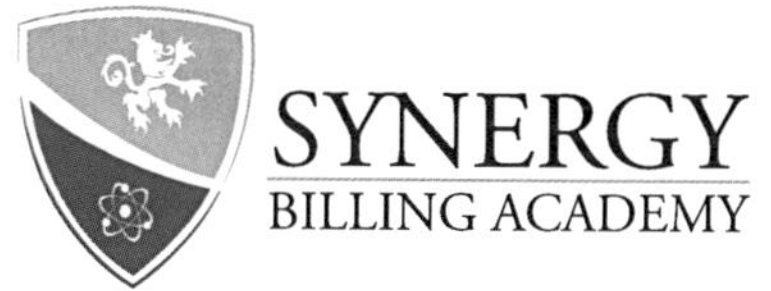

Character	Injury
A	Initial Encounter / Closed Fracture
B	Intial Encounter / Open Fracture
D	Subsequent Encounter / Fracture, Routine Healing
G	Subsequent Encounter / Fracture, Delayed Healing
K	Subsequent Encounter / Fracture, Nonunion
P	Subsequent Encounter / Fracture, Malunion
S	Sequela

Injury Classification [16]

In ICD-10-CM, injuries are grouped by body part rather than by categories of injury, so that all injuries of a specific site are grouped together, instead of grouping all fractures or all open wounds; for example, categories in ICD-9-CM grouped by injury, such as fractures, dislocations, and sprains and strains, are grouped in ICD-10-CM by site, such as injuries to the head, injuries to the neck, and injuries to the thorax.

Example:

- Injury Changes
  - ICD-9-CM – Type of Injury [5]
    - Fractures (800-829)
    - Dislocations (830-839)
    - Sprains and strains(840-848)
  - ICD-10-CM – Site Affected [10]
    - Injuries to the head (S00-S09)
    - Injuries to the neck (S10 S19)
    - injuries to the thorax (S20-S29)

Example: [16]

- Larry was seen in the ER for shoulder pain. X-rays indicated there was a displaced fracture of the right clavicle, shaft.

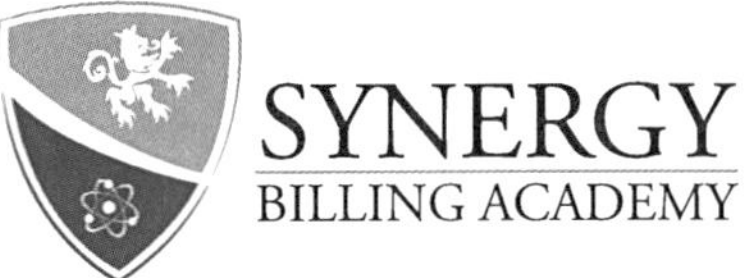

   - Code: S42.021A, Displaced fracture of shaft of right clavicle, initial encounter. "A" would be assigned for the initial encounter.
- Larry returns three months later with complaints of continuing pain; X-rays are taken and indicate a nonunion.
   - Code: S42.021K, Displaced fracture of the shaft of right clavicle, subsequent encounter for fracture with nonunion
- Larry returns six months later for a follow-up appointment
   - Code: S42.021S, Displaced fracture of the shaft of the right clavicle, sequela.

Gustilo Anderson

ICD-10-CM uses the Gustilo Anderson system to identify the severity of soft tissue damage for open fractures. Only three categories of codes in ICD-10-CM require the Gustilo Anderson classifications: [15]

- S52, fracture of forearm
- S72, fracture of femur
- S82, fracture of lower leg, including ankle

For documentation of an open fracture without specifying the amount of soft tissue damage, you should default to type I open fracture.

Example:

- Encounter for occupational therapy for open nondisplaced fracture neck of right radius, with extensive soft tissue injury with routine healing.
   - Code: S52.134F

For open fractures, the 7th characters from the Gustilo classification are B, C, E, F, H, J, M, N, Q, or R. They can be used with codes in categories S52, S72, and S82.

Gustilo Classification

Character	Description
B	Initial encounter for open fracture type I or II Initial encounter for open fracture NOS

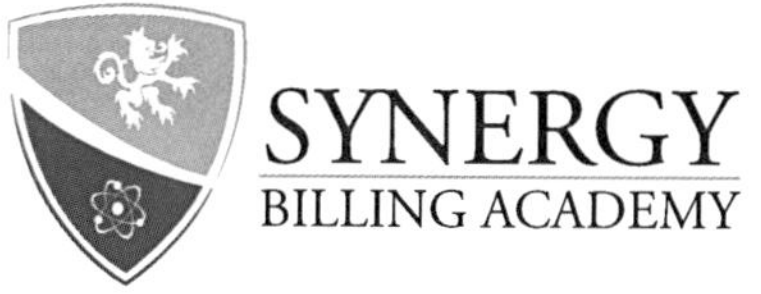

C	Initial encounter for open fracture type III A, III B, or III C
E	Subsequent encounter for open fracture type I or II with routine healing
F	Subsequent encounter for open fracture type III A, III B, or IIIC with routine healing
H	Subsequent encounter for open fracture type I or II with delayed healing
J	Subsequent encounter for open fracture IIIA, IIIB, or IIIC with delayed healing
M	Subsequent encounter for open fracture type I or II with nonunion
N	Subsequent encounter for open fracture type IIIA, IIIB, or IIIC with nonunion
Q	Subsequent encounter for open fracture type I or II with malunion
R	Subsequent encounter for open fracture type IIIA, IIIB, or IIIC with malunion

Placeholder "X" [16]

- The X is used in some cases as a placeholder for certain codes to allow for future expansion.
- When the placeholder character applies, it must be used in order for the code to be considered valid.
- "X" is not case-sensitive.
  - T46.1x5A or T46.1X5A, Adverse effect of calcium channel blockers, initial encounter
  - T15.02xD or T15.02XD, Foreign body in cornea, left eye, subsequent encounter
- Without the placeholder, the code is incomplete and will be rejected by the payer.
  - S06.0X0A, concussion without loss of consciousness, initial encounter
  - O64.1XX1, obstructed labor due to breech presentation, fetus 1
  - W92.XXXD, exposure to excessive heat of man-made origin, subsequent encounter

SOAP Note: Select The Variables [17]

<u>Subjective</u>

- Mrs. Finley presents today after having a new cabinet fall on her last week, suffering a concussion as well as some cervicalgia. She was cooking dinner at the home she shares with her husband. She did not seek treatment at that time. She states that the

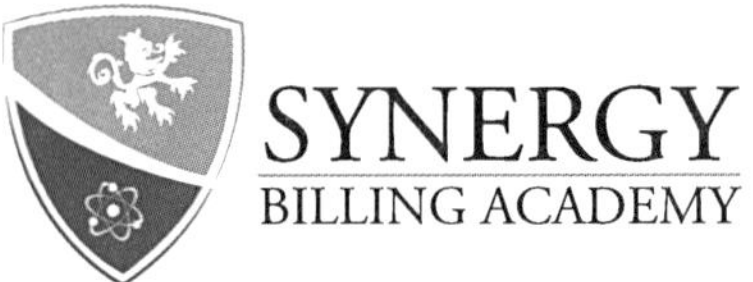

people who installed the cabinet in her kitchen missed the stud by about two inches. Her husband, who was home with her at the time, told her she was "out cold" for about two minutes. The patient continues to have cephalgias since the accident, primarily occipital, extending into the bilateral occipital and parietal regions. The headaches come on suddenly, last for long periods of time, and occur every day. They are not relieved by Advil. She denies any vision changes, any taste changes, any smell changes. The patient has a marked amount of tenderness across the superior trapezius.

Objective

- Her weight is 188 pounds, which is up 5 pounds from last time; blood pressure 144/82, pulse rate 70, respirations are 18. She has full strength in her upper extremities. DTRs (Deep Tendon Reflexes) in the biceps and triceps are adequate. Grip strength is adequate. Heart rate is regular and lungs are clear.

Assessment

1. Status post-concussion with acute persistent headaches
2. Cervicalgia
3. Cervical somatic dysfunction

Plan

- The plan at this time is to send her for physical therapy, three times a week for four weeks, for cervical soft tissue muscle massage, as well as upper dorsal. We will recheck her in one month, sooner if needed.

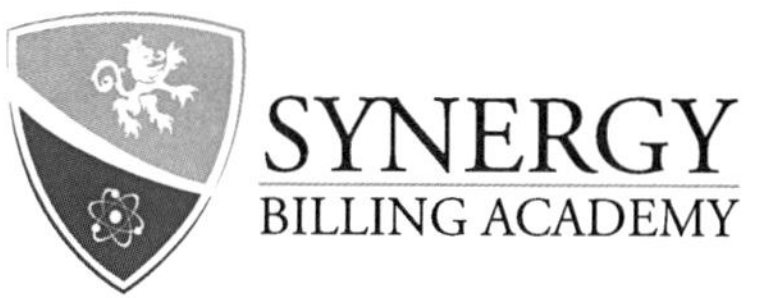

S: Mrs. Finley presents today after having a new cabinet fall on her last week, suffering a concussion, as well as some cervicalgia. She was cooking dinner at the home she shares with her husband. She did not seek treatment at that time. She states that the people who installed the cabinet in her kitchen missed the stud by about two inches. Her husband, who was home with her at the time, told her she was "out cold" for about two minutes. The patient continues to have cephalgia since the accident, primarily occipital, extending up into the bilateral occipital and parietal regions. The headaches come on suddenly, last for long periods of time, and occur every day. They are not relieved by Advil. She denies any vision changes, any taste changes, any smell changes. The patient has a marked amount of tenderness across the superior trapezius.

O: Her weight is 188, which is up 5 pounds from last time; blood pressure 144/82, pulse rate 70, respirations are 18. She has full strength in her upper extremities. DTRs in the biceps and triceps are adequate. Grip strength is adequate. Heart rate is regular and lungs are clear.

A:
1. Status post-concussion with acute persistent headaches
2. Cervicalgia
3. Cervical somatic dysfunction

P: The plan at this time is to send her for physical therapy, three times a week for four weeks, for cervical soft tissue muscle massage, as well as upper dorsal. We'll recheck her in one month, sooner if needed. [17]

Acute vs. Chronic Documentation of the patient's condition must include acute or chronic to assign the most appropriate ICD-10-CM code.

Relief or No Relief: Intractable vs. not intractable notes are an inherent part of the ICD-10-CM code for headaches and documentation needs to be clear to assign the appropriate code.

External Cause: The falling cabinet is what caused the injuries. Description of the cause is required.

Activity: In ICD-10-CM, the activity of the patient needs to be documented. An activity code is only used once, at the initial encounter.

7th Character: Injury codes require a 7th character extender that identifies the encounter. Documentation must be clear so that the correct extender can be applied.

Location: Documentation needs to include the location of the patient at the time of the injury or other condition. In ICD-10-CM, the details include the actual room of the house the patient was in when the injury occurred.

Applied Specificity: Concussion: For a concussion, documentation needs to include if the patient suffered loss of consciousness.

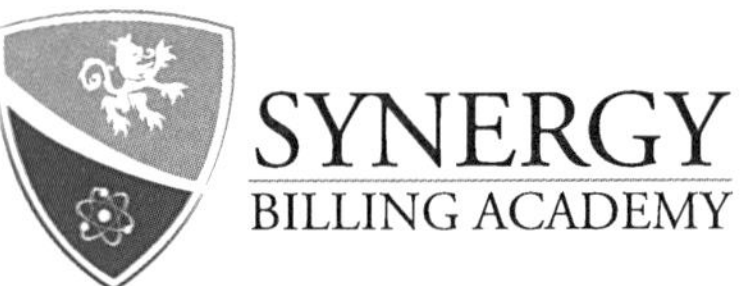

Components [17]

Applied Specificity: Concussion – For a concussion, documentation needs to include if the patient suffered loss of consciousness.	S: Her husband, who was home with her the time, told her she was "out cold" for about two minutes.	S06.0X1A	• Concussion with loss of consciousness of 30 minutes or less
7th Character: Injury codes require a 7th character extender that identifies the encounter. Documentation must be clear so that the correct extender can be applied.	S: She did not seek treatment.		• Initial encounter
Acute vs. Chronic: Documentation of the patient's condition must include acute or chronic to assign the most appropriate ICD-10-CM code. **Relief or No Relief:** Intractable vs. not intractable notes are an inherent part of the ICD-10-CM code for headaches and documentation needs to be clear to assign the appropriate code.	A: Status post concussion with acute persistent headaches. S: The headaches come on suddenly, last for long periods of time, and occur every day. They are not relieved by Advil.	G44.311	• Acute post traumatic headache • Intractable
Patient Diagnosis	A: Cervicalgia A: Cervical somatic dysfunction	M54.2 M99.01	• Cervicalgia • Segmental and somatic dysfunction of cervical region
External Cause: The falling cabinet is what caused the injuries. Description of the cause is required.	S: After having a cabinet fall on her last week.	W20.8XXA	• Struck by falling object (accidentally)
7th Character: Injury codes require a 7th character extender that identifies the encounter. Documentation must be clear so that the correct extender can be applied.	S: She did not seek treatment		• Initial encounter
Activity: In ICD-10-CM, the activity of the patient needs to be documented. An activity code is only used once at the initial encounter.	S: In her kitchen	Y93.G3	• Cooking and baking
Location: Documentation needs to include the location of the patient at the time of injury or other condition. In ICD-10-CM, the details include the actual room of the house the patient was in when the injury occurred.		Y92.010	• Place of occurrence, house, single family, kitchen

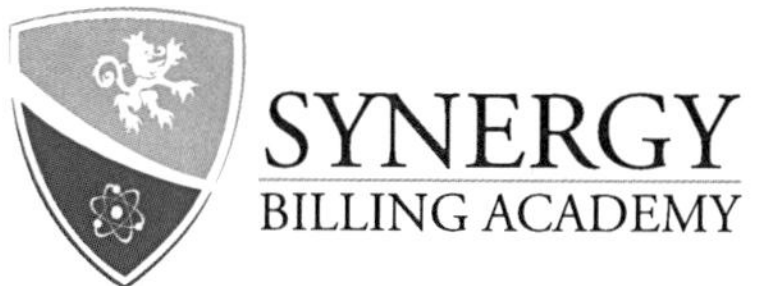

The Codes [17]

ICD-9		ICD-10	
850.11	Concussion with loss of consciousness of 30 minutes or less	S06.0x1A	Concussion with loss of consciousness of 30 minutes or less, *initial encounter*
339.21	Acute post-traumatic headache	G44.311	Acute post-traumatic headache, *intractable*
723.1	Cervicalgia	M54.2	Cervicalgia
739.1	Non-allopathic lesions of the cervical region	M99.01	Segmental and somatic dysfunction of cervical region
E916	Struck accidentally by falling object	W20.8xxA	Struck by falling object (accidentally), *initial encounter*
E015.2	Activities involving cooking and baking	Y93.G3	Activity, cooking and baking
E015.2	Place of occurrence, home	Y92.010	Place of occurrence, home, *single family, kitchen*

Burns, Degrees, and Percentages [9,18]

- There are certain things that we need to know about our burn patients. What kind of burn is it? What caused the burn? Where is the burn located? What degree? What percentage? What type of encounter (initial or subsequent)? Is there information about the incident and where it happened? ICD-10-CM is very specific. Here are a few examples of places for burns to the head:
  - Cheek, Chin, Ear, Eye(s) only, Forehead, Lip, Neck, Nose, Scalp
- Each area is further divided into degrees:
  - First degree (erythema)
  - Second degree (blistering)
  - Third degree (full-thickness involvement)
- If the patient suffered multiple burns in the same local site (three-character category level, T20-T28), but of different degrees, report the code for the subcategory identifying the highest degree recorded in the diagnosis.
- If the patient suffered first- and second-degree burns to his right forearm, report only the code for the second-degree burn (T22.211A, burn of second degree of right forearm, initial encounter)..

History and Evolution

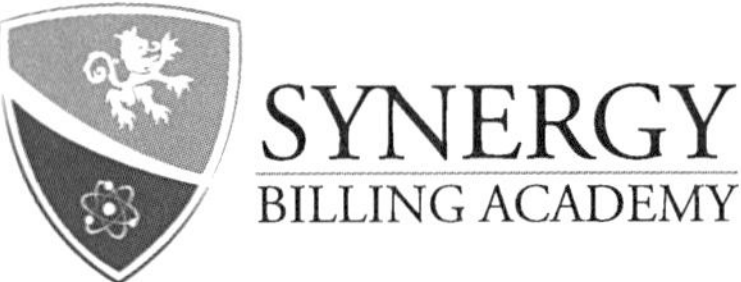

- If the patient suffered burns at different sites, such as the left forearm and left upper arm, we would report separate codes for each burn because they are different sites, even if they are the same degree.
- The ICD-10-CM codes follow the "rule of nines" to estimate body surface involved:
  - Head and neck, 9%
  - Each arm, 9%
  - Each leg, 18%
  - Anterior trunk, 18%
  - Posterior trunk, 18%
  - Genitalia, 1%
    - T31.30, Burns involving 30–39% of body surface with 0–9% third-degree burns
    - T31.31, Burns involving 30–39% of body surface with 10–19% third-degree burns
    - T31.32, burns involving 30–39% of body surface with 20–29% third-degree burns
    - T31.33, burns involving 30–39% of body surface with 30–39% third-degree burns
- External Causes
  - X00-X19, X75-X77, X96-X98, and Y92 identify the source, place, and intent of the burn.
  - X12.XXXA, Contact with other hot fluids, initial encounter
  - Y92.017, Garden or yard in single-family (private) house as the place of occurrence of the external cause

History and Evolution

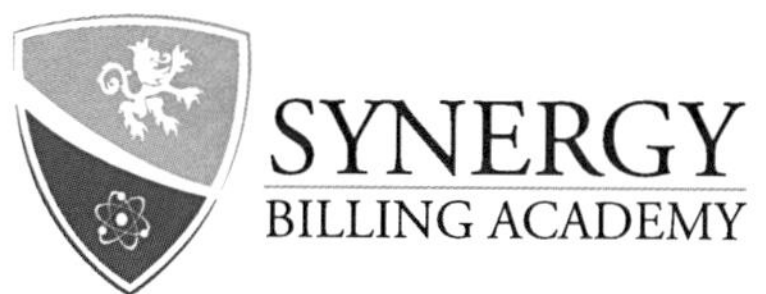

Example:
Burns

942.23
2nd degree burn of abdomen

T2122xA
2nd degree burn of abdominal wall, initial episode

T2122xD
2nd degree burn of abdominal wall, subsequent episode

T2162xA
2nd degree corrosion of abdominal wall, initial episode

T2162xA
2nd degree corrosion of abdominal wall, subsequent episode

- ICD-9-CM codes do not distinguish between thermal and chemical burns.
- ICD-10-CM codes have separate codes for thermal versus chemical burns.
- Documentation is key!

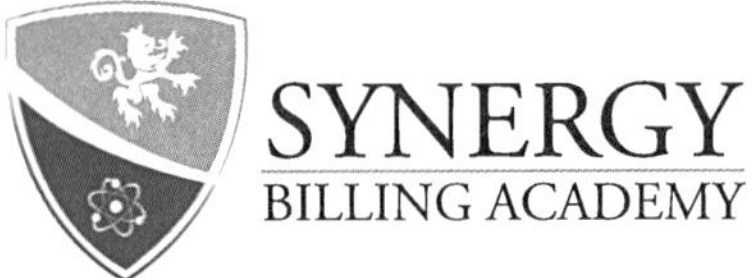

Manifestations, Complications, and Severities Documentation [19]

The 4th and 5th characters for diabetes have been expanded to reflect manifestations and complications of the disease, instead of having to use additional codes for them.

When documenting diabetes, we must include the type, the body system affected, and any complications or manifestations. Also, because type 2 diabetes usually does not require insulin or medications, we need to indicate the use of insulin for type 2 diabetes management when applicable.

ICD-10-CM	Defintion	ICD-9-CM
I25.110	Atherosclerotic heart disease of native coronary artery with unstable angina pectoris	411.1 & 414.01
E11.311	Type 2 diabetes mellitus with unspecified diabetic retinopathy with macular edema	250.50, 362.01, & 362.07
K50.012	Crohn's disease of small intestine with intestinal obstruction	555.0 & 560.9

Asthma, even though it is a very common chronic inflammatory disease, has undergone a tremendous amount of documentation changes in ICD-10-CM. With asthma, we are required to document its frequency and severity. We need to indicate the asthma's severity: if it is mild intermittent, mild persistent, or severe persistent. We also need to indicate if it is a chronic condition versus acute, as well as exacerbation and status asthmaticus.

- Example
  - J45.41: Moderate persistent asthma with (acute) exacerbation

The following table shows the difference between the severities:

Classification	Severity of Symtoms	Nighttime Symptoms	Forced Expiratory Volume
Mild Intermittent	Sx<2x/wk, otherwise asymptomatic	Sx<= 2x/mo	> 80%

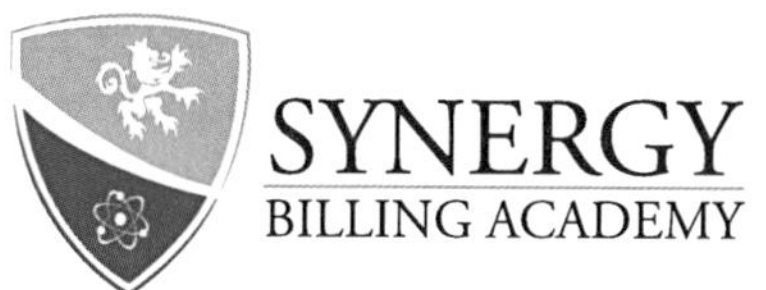

Mild Persistent	Sx > 2x/wk, < 1x/day	Sx > -2x/mo	> 80%, variability from 20% to 30%
Moderate Persistent	Daily Sx, daily use of beta 2 agonist	Sx > 1x/wk	60% to 80%
Severe Persistent	Continual Sx, limited physical activity	Frequent	< 60%
*A patient qualifying for two different stages should be classified in the more severe stage.			

- Mild intermittent asthma is diagnosed when symptoms happen about twice a week or less frequently during the day and when the patient has the symptoms at night twice a month or less.
- Mild persistent asthma is diagnosed when, during the day, symptoms happen more than twice a week but no more than once in a single day, and when the patient has the symptoms at night more than twice a month.
- Moderate persistent asthma is when symptoms occur every day during the day and the nighttime symptoms happen more than once a week.
- Severe persistent asthma is when symptoms occur throughout the day on most days and the nighttime symptoms happen often.

The neoplasm table has also been expanded in ICD-10-CM. For example, malignant neoplasm of the breast not only has 54 choices but also requires the specification of male and female breast, the site of the neoplasm of the breast, and the laterality. Also, if known, we need to add the corresponding code for estrogen receptor status. Thus, the documentation for neoplasm will need the: [19]

- Type:
  - Malignant (Primary, Secondary, Ca in situ)
  - Benign
  - Uncertain
  - Unspecified behavior
- Location(s) (site specific)
- Secondary sites, if malignant
- Laterality, in some cases

Example:

C50.411, Malignant neoplasm of upper-outer quadrant of the left female breast and Z17.1, Estrogen receptor status negative status [ER-]

History and Evolution

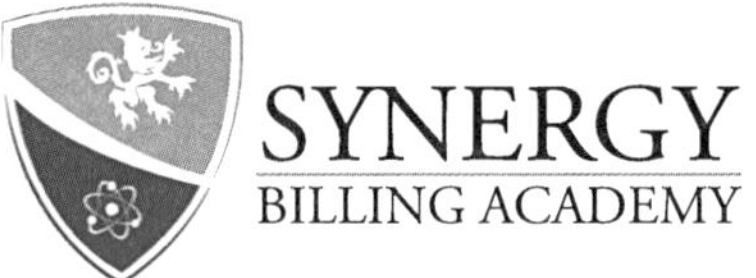

Currently in ICD-9-CM, when classifying hypertension, we have to identify the type: malignant, benign, or unspecified. In ICD-10-CM, we no longer have a hypertension table, and what was category 401 is now I10 (Essential hypertension).

This code includes high blood pressure and hypertension, whether it is arterial, benign, essential, malignant, primary, or systemic. There are excludes notes that indicate the following:

- Excludes1:
  - Hypertensive disease complicating pregnancy, childbirth, and the puerperium (O10-O11, O13-O16)

- Excludes2:
  - Essential (primary) hypertension involving vessels of brain (I60-I69)
  - Essential (primary) hypertension involving vessels of eye (H35.0)

Software Changes

- The ICD-10-CM transition and implementation will be a very large undertaking for IT staff. Without the proper software updates, reimbursement will drop, affecting the clinic's revenue.

- Further configuration will need to be done to ensure that providers are able to select the proper diagnosis codes, converting their current ICD-9-CM code selections to the ICD-10-CM equivalents.

- Configuring systems to be ready for ICD-10-CM will be time consuming. The IT staff and software vendor support teams need to update all of the electronic medical record (EMR) templates for the physicians to be able to accurately document the patient's visits.

  - These templates have to be more specific about the reasons why patients were seen at the time of visit, along with enabling physicians to record a detailed treatment plan for that patient for a correct level of billing.

- If these things are not in place, there will be a decrease in overall provider productivity and an increase in billing turnaround time.

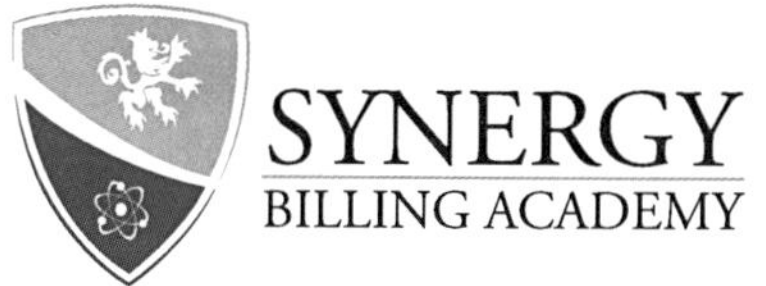

Bottom Line [20]

- ICD-10-CM implementation is an investment in time, but ICD-10-CM will help physicians:
  - Increase compensation and reimbursement
    - ICD-9-CM codes were not developed with reimbursement in mind. ICD-10-CM will offer a more decisive system to determine payments. The specificity of data will help determine accurate and fair physician compensation and reimbursement for services.
  - Prove medical necessity
    - ICD-10-CM codes are much more specific and provide choices that will allow the reality of the patient's condition to be condensed into a code based on the documentation. ICD-10-CM will reflect how sick the patients really are to a third-party payer and even to auditors.
  - Ensure a strong reputation
    - Documentation is the basis used by ICD-10-CM codes to more accurately reflect the quality of care provided by physicians. Documentation will tell a more complete story of the gravity of the patient's illness, the complexity of the services, and utilization of resources.
  - Reduce the stress of audits
    - ICD-10-CM codes will allow the documentation to give a more accurate clinical picture. In doing so, it will reduce the chances of misinterpretation by third parties, auditors, and attorneys. The new required documentation will help save time or even prevent an audit in the first place.
  - Document better clinical information
    - ICD-10-CM requires a deeper level of clinical detail in the medical record. This information will be used to reduce errors and provide guarantees of appropriate reimbursement. It offers significant opportunities for data mining and research.

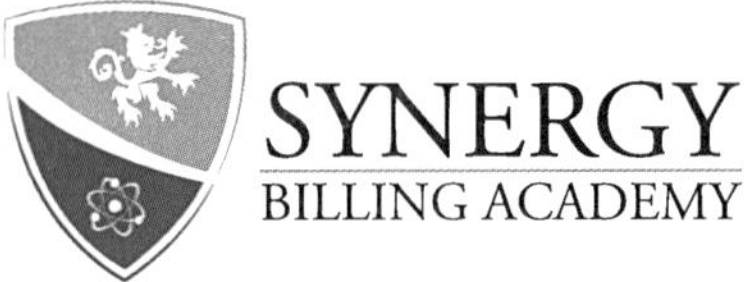

Review Questions – Check Your Understanding

1. ICD-10-CM stands for International Classification of Deaths 10th Revision Clinical Modification.

   a. True
   b. False

2. The National Center of Health Statistics, along with three other cooperating parties, developed the conventions and guidelines for ICD-10-CM.

   a. True
   b. False

3. We now have fewer chapters in ICD-10-CM than we did in ICD-9-CM.

   a. True
   b. False

4. V Codes and E Codes were incorporated into the main classification.

   a. True
   b. False

5. Diseases of the eyes and ears do not have their own chapters.

   a. True
   b. False

6. GEMs were created as a 100% crosswalk from ICD-9-CM to ICD-10-CM.

   a. True
   b. False

7. Laterality indicates the site of the body that has been affected.

   a. True
   b. False

8. It is optional for providers to use the seventh character with ICD-10-CM.

   a. True
   b. False

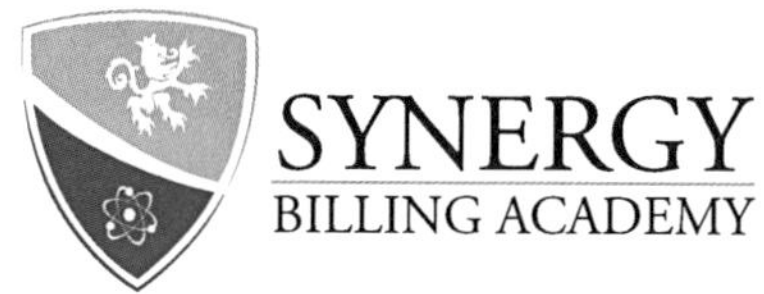

9. The letter "Y" is used as a placeholder.

   a. True
   b. False

10. Documentation always needs to be detailed, specific, and complete.

   a. True
   b. False

11. ICD-10-CM contains codes that specify laterality.

   a. True
   b. False

12. ICD-10-CM uses inclusion terms in the same way that ICD-9-CM uses them.

   a. True
   b. False

13. Which of the following abbreviations is used in ICD-10-CM?

   a. NOC
   b. NES
   c. NEC

14. What indicates synonyms, alternative wording, or explanatory phrases?

   a. Parentheses
   b. Brackets
   c. Dash

15. Which of the following is a convention found in the ICD-10-CM manual?

   a. Symbols
   b. The abbreviation NEC
   c. External cause

ICD-10-CM International Classification of Diseases 10th Revision Clinical Modification

Primary Care Providers

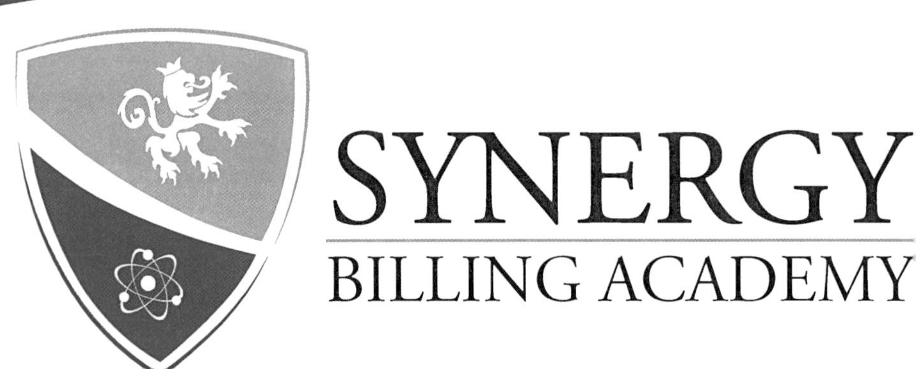

Primary Care Providers

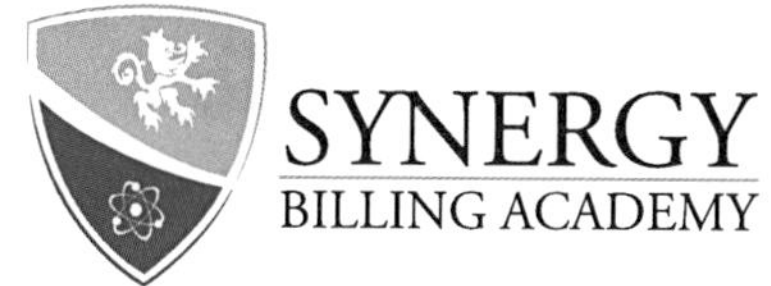

Background and Practice

Family Physicians and Family Medicine

Family medicine (FM), formerly known as Family Practice (FP), is a medical specialty devoted to comprehensive health care for people of all ages. The specialist is called a family physician, family doctor, or, formerly, family practitioner. This discipline is often referred to as general practice and a practitioner as a General Practice Doctor or GP. This name emphasizes the holistic nature of this specialty, as well as its roots in the family. It is a division of primary care that provides continuing and comprehensive health care for the individual and family across all ages, genders, diseases, and parts of the body. It is based on knowledge of the patient in the context of the family and the community, emphasizing disease prevention and health promotion. According to the World Organization of Family Doctors (WONCA), the aim of family medicine is to provide personal, comprehensive, and continuing care for the individual in the context of the family and the community. [21]

Pediatrics

Pediatrics (also spelled paediatrics or pædiatrics) is the branch of medicine that deals with the medical care of infants, children, and adolescents; the age limit usually ranges from birth up to 18 (in some places, pediatrics continues until completion of secondary education, or until age 21 in the United States). The word pediatrics and its cognates mean "healer of children;" the term derives from two Greek words: παῖς (pais, "child") and ἰατρός (iatros, "doctor, healer"). [22]

Internal Medicine

Internal medicine is the medical specialty dealing with the prevention, diagnosis, and treatment of adult diseases. Physicians specializing in internal medicine are called internists, or physicians. They are especially skilled in the management of patients who have undifferentiated or multi-system disease processes. Internists care for patients and may play a major role in teaching and research. They often have subspecialty interests in diseases affecting particular organs or organ systems. [23]

Claims and Coding Manuals

In 2003, it was mandated that all HIPAA-covered entities use diagnostic codes. In other words, even primary care providers are required to use ICD-9-CM codes to report a patient's diagnosis and the reason for his or her visit.

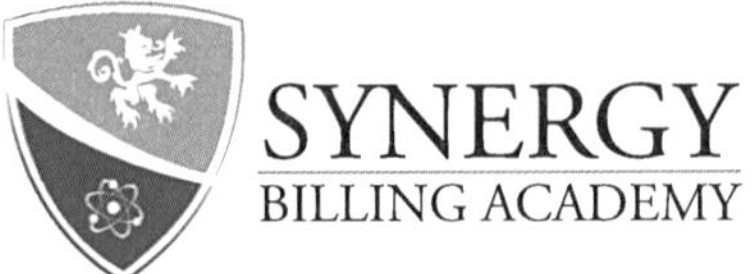

On October 1, 2015, the ICD-10-CM (International Classification of Diseases 10th Revision Clinical Modification) will replace ICD-9-CM, which is what all providers have been using to add the diagnosis or reason for visit to their patients' claims. ICD-10-CM is an improvement over ICD-9-CM because ICD-9-CM codes do not have sufficient coverage due to a lack of specificity.

Please keep in mind that ICD-10-CM will not have any effects on Current Procedural Terminology (CPT) codes.

ICD-10- CM Diseases and Disorders [9,10,24]

Transitioning to ICD-10-CM will completely change the codes used in family medicine, internal medicine, and pediatrics. Each and every one of the codes and their descriptions will be more specific to the patient's condition. Overall, ICD-9-CM codes are vague and not very descriptive, whereas ICD-10-CM codes are more descriptive. Family medicine, internal medicine, and pediatrics relate to several parts of ICD-10-CM. Below is a list of where these conditions will be classified:

Chapters	Description
Chapter 1	Certain Infectious and Parasitic Diseases (A00-B99)
Chapter 4	Endocrine, Nutritional, and Metabolic Diseases (E00-E89)
Chapter 5	Mental, Behavioral, and Neurodevelopmental Disorders (F01-F99)
Chapter 7	Diseases of the Eye and Adnexa (H00-H59)
Chapter 8	Diseases of the Ear and Mastoid Process (H60-H95)
Chapter 9	Diseases of the Circulatory System (I00-I99)
Chapter 10	Diseases of the Respiratory System (J00-J99)
Chapter 11	Diseases of the Digestive System (K00-K95)
Chapter 13	Diseases of the Musculoskeletal System (M00-M99)
Chapter 14	Diseases of the Genitourinary System (N00-N99)
Chapter 15	Pregnancy, Childbirth, and the Puerperium (O00-O9a)
Chapter 16	Certain Conditions Originating in the Perinatal Period (P00-P96)
Chapter 17	Congenital Malformations, Deformations, and Chromosomal Abnormalities (Q00-Q99)
Chapter 18	Symptoms, Signs and Abnormal Clinical, and Laboratory Findings, Not Elsewhere Classified (R00-R99)

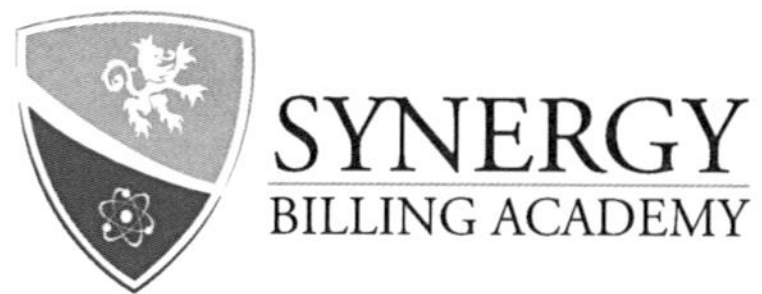

Chapter 19	Injury, Poisoning, and Certain Other Consequences of External Causes (S00-T88)
Chapter 20	External Causes of Morbidity (V00-Y99)
Chapter 21	Factors Influencing Health Status and Contact with Health Services (Z00-Z99)

Many medical specialties have experienced a significant amount of changes in ICD-10-CM. Family medicine, internal medicine, and pediatrics are among those affected. In the transition to ICD-10-CM, all of the chapters that make up family medicine, internal medicine, and pediatrics include a variety of changes related to diagnosis codes. Here we will provide a detailed list of all the changes in the organization of diseases and disorders, organized per chapter.

ICD-9-CM and ICD-10-CM – Chapter 1

Chapter 1 in ICD-10-CM has been indexed similarly to ICD-9-CM, but keep in mind that some of the category and subcategory titles have been changed. For example, in ICD-9-CM, 008 is for Intestinal infections due to other organisms, whereas in ICD-10-CM, A08 is for Viral and other specified intestinal infections; in ICD-9-CM, 024 is for Glanders and 025 for Melioidosis, whereas in ICD-10-CM, A24 is used for both Glanders and Melioidosis. Another example is ICD-9-CM, which codes 036.4 for Meningococcal carditis; in ICD-10-CM, A39.5 is used for Meningococcal heart disease.

This chapter includes diseases that are generally recognized as communicable or transmissible. In this chapter we also have a new section: infections with a predominantly sexual mode of transmission. Some conditions in this chapter have been rearranged and we now have separate subchapters where conditions have been grouped together.

Terminology was also revised all throughout the chapter in reference to specific infectious and parasitic diseases. An example of this is the term sepsis. Sepsis was used in ICD-9-CM, but in ICD-10-CM, it has been replaced with the term septicemia.

In this chapter, we have more combination codes, as the codes have been expanded to reflect manifestations and complications of diseases by using the fourth and fifth characters. Instead of using multiple codes to identify the patient's condition, we can now use one code instead.

ICD-9-CM and ICD-10-CM – Chapter 4

ICD-10-CM contains a major change in the diabetes mellitus classification. When in ICD-9-CM we

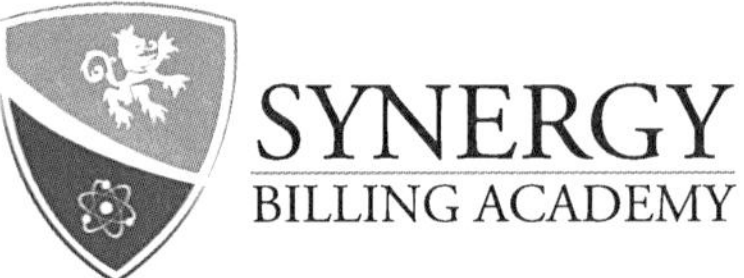

had the single category of 250, in ICD-10-CM, we now have a total of five categories for diabetes mellitus. These codes were expanded to reflect manifestations and complications of the disease by using the fourth or fifth characters instead of multiple coding and using an additional code to identify the manifestation. Moreover, ICD-10-CM does not classify diabetes as controlled or uncontrolled but instead inadequately controlled, out of control, and poorly controlled. Diabetes mellitus is classified by type with hyperglycemia. These are five categories for diabetes mellitus:

- E08: Diabetes mellitus due to underlying condition
- E09: Drug or chemical induced diabetes mellitus
- E10: Type 1 diabetes mellitus
- E11: Type 2 diabetes mellitus
- E13: Other specified diabetes mellitus

Another change within this chapter is the addition of new subchapters. An example of a new subchapter is diabetes mellitus and malnutrition; before, these were found with diseases of other endocrine glands and nutritional deficiencies.

ICD-9-CM and ICD-10-CM – Chapter 5

Mental and behavioral disorders now contain more subchapters, categories, and subcategories, as well as more codes than in ICD-9-CM. Some of the disorders are classified differently, allowing for greater clinical detail. These changes are because many parts of this chapter previously had outdated terminology. For example, in ICD-9-CM subcategory 296.0 is called Bipolar I disorder, single manic episode, but in ICD-10-CM the equivalent is category F30, Manic episode.

In this chapter, we can find conditions classified as disorders of psychological development, but it actually excludes their symptoms, signs, and abnormal findings. The symptoms, signs, and abnormal findings are found in Chapter 18, code range is R00-R99. In the past 20 years there have been many discoveries relating to the effects of nicotine; because of this, ICD-10-CM now contains a separate category, F17, for nicotine dependence and has added subcategories to help identify the specific tobacco product and any nicotine-induced disorders.

We now have unique codes for alcohol and drug abuse, as well as abuse and dependence. Also, in order to note that the patient has a history of alcohol and drug abuse, we can identify it as in remission; ICD-10-CM does not have a separate history code section for this. We can now specify the level of alcohol in the patient's blood using code Y90.-, which is assigned as an additional code when the documentation indicates it.

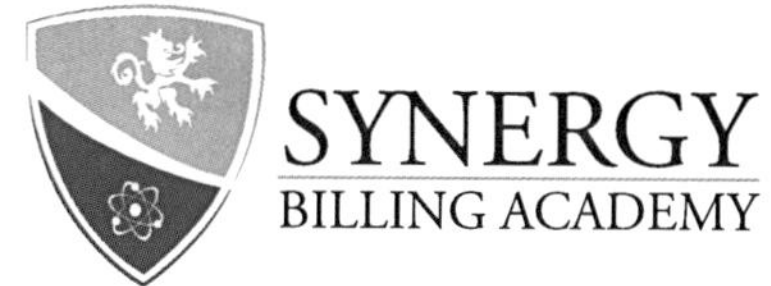

ICD-9-CM to ICD-10-CM – Chapter 7

Diseases of the eye and the adnexa were originally combined with diseases of the nervous system and sense organs in ICD-9-CM. Now diseases of the eye and adnexa have their own chapter, which is an entirely new chapter in ICD-10-CM. In this new chapter, the structure was based on the site of the diseases just as in ICD-9-CM, but now the order is somewhat different. Because of the new terminology in use today, some categories been changed to reflect these differences. For example, ICD-9-CM uses senile cataract while ICD-10-CM uses the descriptor age-related cataract. Keep in mind that by adding a new chapter for diseases of the eye and adnexa, we now have more instructions on which conditions are excluded from this chapter.

Many changes in this chapter are due to the addition of laterality. Laterality was added in order to indicate which side of the body was affected and is being treated. In other words, we now have codes for right, left, bilateral, and unspecified. In some cases, we even have to indicate upper and lower in addition to the side, such as upper eyelid versus lower eyelid.

- H16.011, Central corneal ulcer, right eye
- H16.012, Central corneal ulcer, left eye
- H16.013, Central corneal ulcer, bilateral
- H16.019, Central corneal ulcer, unspecified eye

ICD-9-CM to ICD-10-CM – Chapter 8

Diseases of ear and mastoid process were originally combined with diseases of the nervous system and sense organs in ICD-9-CM. Now diseases of the ear and the mastoid process have their own chapter, which is an entirely new chapter in ICD-10-CM. In this new chapter, the diseases of the ear and mastoid process are arranged into blocks. This new arrangement will make it easier when identifying the types of conditions that occur in the external ear, middle ear and mastoid process, and inner ear. Other disorders of the ear and codes for intraoperative and postprocedural complications are now grouped at the end of the chapter instead of being scattered throughout different categories.

Even though this chapter is similar to the section for diseases of the ear and mastoid process in ICD-9-CM, the category and subcategory titles have been revised in a number of places. Other changes include greater specificity, which was added at the fourth, fifth, and sixth character levels; the addition of laterality; the addition of more notes to be able to "code first the underlying disease;" and the division of some categories to better reflect new medical terminology updates and to enable better documentation. For example, ICD-9-CM code 381 is Nonsuppurative otitis

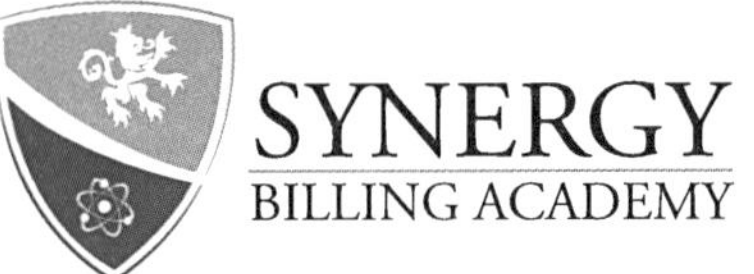

media and Eustachian tube disorders, but in ICD-10-CM, this category was split into two: H65 for Nonsuppurative otitis media and H68 for Eustachian salpingitis and obstruction.

Keep in mind that by adding a new chapter for diseases of the ear and mastoid process, we now have more instructions and guidelines on the usage of the codes and classification of the conditions. For example, ICD-9-CM contains a note excluding otitis media with perforation of tympanic membrane from subcategory 384.2, but in ICD-10-CM, the note directly under its equivalent, H72, Perforation of tympanic membrane, states "code first any associated otitis media."

Another new guideline is found under the categories for nonsuppurative otitis media (H65) and suppurative and unspecified otitis media (H66). The note instructs coders to use an additional code to identify: exposure to environmental tobacco smoke (Z77.22), exposure to tobacco smoke in the perinatal period (P96.81), history of tobacco use (Z87.891), occupational exposure to environmental tobacco smoke (Z57.31), tobacco dependence (F17.-), or tobacco use (Z72.0).

ICD-9-CM to ICD-10-CM – Chapter 9

In the diseases of the circulatory system, the terminology has changed to reflect current terminology and medical practice for cardiovascular conditions. Because of the addition of chapters, what was Chapter 7 in ICD-9-CM is now Chapter 9 in ICD-10-CM. In ICD-10-CM, there have also been changes to the order in which some conditions are listed.

ICD-10-CM contains a major change in hypertension and its classification. In ICD-9-CM, hypertension was classified as benign, malignant, or unspecified; in ICD-10-CM, we no longer have those classifications. Now we have one code for all of them, which is I10 for a description of essential (primary) hypertension. This code includes high blood pressure and hypertension (arterial) (benign) (essential) (malignant) (primary) (systemic), but hypertensive disease complicating pregnancy, childbirth, and the puerperium are found in a different section (O10-O11, O13-O16). If the patient has essential hypertension involving the vessels of the brain or vessels of the eyes, we would use I10 along with code range I60-I69 or H35.0-.

Some diseases were actually taken from other chapters and added to Chapter 9. For example, we now have Binswanger's diseases, chronic and mesenteric lymphadenitis, and gangrene, which came from ICD-9-CM Chapter 9, which is now Chapter 11. Moreover, changes in terminology were necessary and some conditions were renamed. An example of this is in intermediate coronary syndrome, which is now unstable angina in ICD-10-CM.

The category for late effects of cerebrovascular disease has also been retitled as "Sequelae

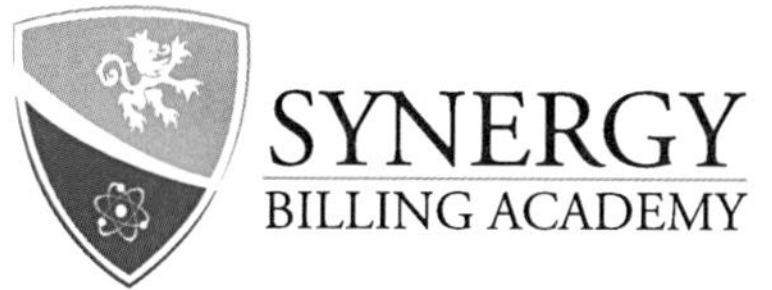

of cerebrovascular diseases," and it was restructured by expanding all subcategory codes. The expansion involved specifying laterality, changing subcategory titles, making terminology changes, adding sixth characters, and providing greater specificity in general. Late effects of cerebrovascular disease are differentiated by type of stroke (e.g., hemorrhage, infarction).

ICD-9-CM to ICD-10-CM – Chapter 10

Even though some diseases in Chapter 10 were rearranged, the diseases of the respiratory system in ICD-10-CM were ordered much like in the equivalent Chapter 8 in ICD-9-CM. The modifications in this chapter were made to specific categories to help bring the terminology up to date with current medical practice. This chapter has also received enhancements to the classification, providing greater specificity than what was available in ICD-9-CM. Some examples are as follows:

- ICD-10-CM has individual codes for acute recurrent sinusitis for each sinus whereas ICD-9-CM does not have a specific code for acute recurrent sinusitis.
- ICD-10-CM subcategory J10.8, Influenza due to other identified influenza virus with other manifestations, has been expanded to reflect manifestations of the influenza.
- ICD-10-CM category J20, Acute bronchitis, has been expanded to reflect the manifestations of the acute bronchitis.

A note at the beginning of the chapter states that when a respiratory condition is described as occurring in more than one site and is not specifically indexed, it should be classified to the lower anatomic site (for example, tracheobronchitis to bronchitis in J40).

An additional instructional guideline also appears at the beginning of this chapter, which instructs the coding professional to use an additional code, where applicable, to identify: exposure to environmental tobacco smoke (Z77.22), exposure to tobacco smoke in the perinatal period (P96.81), history of tobacco use (Z87.891), occupational exposure to environmental tobacco smoke (Z57.31), tobacco dependence (F17.-), or tobacco use (Z72.0).

Moreover, codes were added to this chapter that had been in other chapters in ICD-9-CM. An example of this is streptococcal sore throat. Additionally, lobar pneumonia has a unique code in a category for pneumonia, unspecified organism, instead of being classified to the code for pneumococcal pneumonia as before. For documentation purposes, we need to indicate when known or applicable any infectious agents, any viruses, any associated lung abscess, any underlying disease, or any tobacco use or exposure.

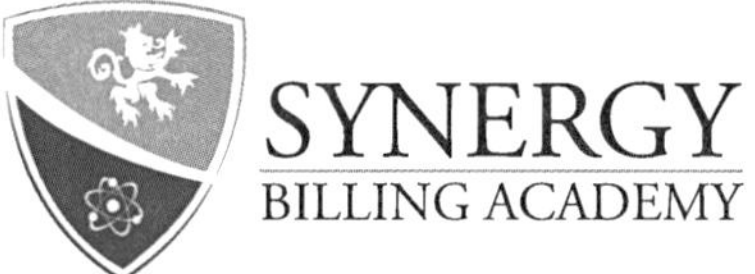

Asthma, even though it is a very common chronic inflammatory disease, has undergone a significant series of changes in ICD-10-CM. With asthma, we are required to document its frequency and severity of it. We need to indicate if the severity is mild intermittent, mild persistent, or severe persistent. We also need to indicate if it is a chronic condition versus acute, as well as exacerbation and status asthmaticus. Intrinsic asthma (nonallergic) and extrinsic (allergic) are both classified to J45.909, Unspecified asthma, uncomplicated.

ICD-9-CM and ICD-10-CM – Chapter 11

In ICD-10-CM, Chapter 11 is the chapter designated for diseases of the digestive system. In this chapter, a number of new subchapters have been added. In ICD-10-CM, diseases of the liver have their own subchapter or block, whereas these conditions were grouped with other diseases of the digestive system in ICD-9-CM. Terminology changes and revisions to specific digestive conditions have been made and some subcategory headings have been changed.

For example, in ICD-9-CM, angiodysplasia of intestines is in a subcategory for "other specified disorders of intestines," but in ICD-10-CM, this is in a subcategory for "vascular disorders of intestines." We also have notes indicating that we need to include additional codes for associated conditions and external causes; other expanded notes indicate that an underlying condition should be coded first.

ICD-9-CM to ICD-10-CM – Chapter 13

Chapter 13, diseases of the musculoskeletal system, contains many more subchapters, categories, and codes. In ICD-9-CM, this chapter has four subchapters, grouping many conditions together. Now, nearly every code has been expanded to include very specific sites as well as laterality. Many codes were moved from other chapters and added to this one. For example, Category 274 for Gout and Code 268.2 for Osteomalacia unspecified in ICD-9-CM are found in Chapter 3, which is the Endocrine, Nutritional and Metabolic Diseases, and Immunity Disorders chapter; these codes are now in ICD-10-CM Chapter 13. Another example is Code 524.4 for Malocclusion unspecified, which in ICD-9-CM is found in Chapter 9, Diseases of the Digestive System; in ICD-10-CM it has been added to Chapter 13.

In this chapter, we also have new guidelines with definitions regarding infections and how the codes should be assigned. In this chapter, we can find any kind of bone, joint, or muscle condition that might be the result of a healed injury, as well as recurrent bone, joint, or muscle conditions. The use of the seventh character is required in some instances to specify the initial encounter for a fracture, a subsequent encounter for a fracture with routine healing, a subsequent encounter for a fracture with delayed healing, a subsequent encounter for a fracture with nonunion, a

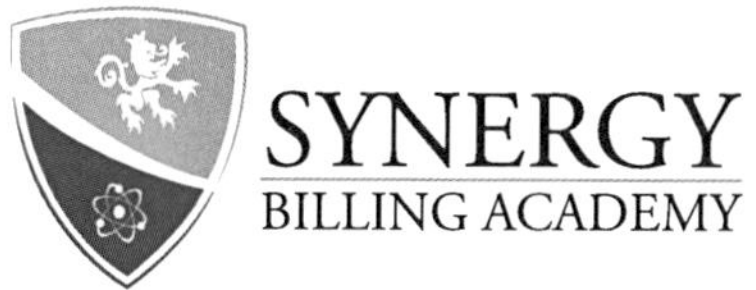

subsequent encounter for a fracture with malunion, or for sequelae.

In ICD-10-CM, pathologic fractures can be classified in different categories: pathologic fractures that are due to neoplastic disease, pathologic fractures that are due to osteoporosis, and pathologic fractures that are due to other specified disease. Another classification that we are able to make is the difference between the types of origin, such as spontaneous versus fragility. Spontaneous rupture occurs when normal force is applied to tissues that are inferred to have less than normal strength, whereas fragility fractures are sustained with trauma no more than a fall from a standing height or less occurring under circumstances that would not cause a fracture in a normal healthy bone. These types of fractures need to be specified in the doctor's documentation; the coder is not able to make the judgment without the specific and clear documentation.

ICD-9-CM and ICD-10-CM – Chapter 14

ICD-10-CM is replacing ICD-9-CM because the terminology in ICD-9-CM is outdated, among other reasons. In Chapter 14, diseases of the genitourinary system, changes were necessary in specific sections. For example, because of new discoveries about male erectile dysfunction since the last revision of ICD-9-CM, ICD-10-CM now includes a whole category for this condition, N52, as well as subcategories to identify the different causes of the dysfunction; in ICD-9-CM, we only have a single code, 607.84, Impotence of organic origin. Another change is that now we also have to document the patient's gender to be able to code to the highest level of specificity.

Throughout this chapter, there are new includes notes that help to clarify the types of disorders that are classified to the various categories.

A similar change has occurred to the instruction for menopausal and other perimenopausal disorders. In ICD-9-CM, there is no guideline under category 627 to help coding professionals select a code for these disorders. However, ICD-10-CM includes a note stating that menopausal and other perimenopausal disorders due to naturally occurring (age-related) menopause and perimenopause are classified to category N95.

Several blocks and category title changes have been made in this particular chapter. An example of this is subsection 617-629 in ICD-9-CM, which is Other disorders of female genital tract, whereas the corresponding section in ICD-10-CM, N80-N98, is Noninflammatory disorders of the female genital tract.

Codes have also moved to this chapter from other chapters. An example of this is code 099.40, which was previously in Chapter 1; it is now found in this chapter as the new ICD-10-CM code N34.1.

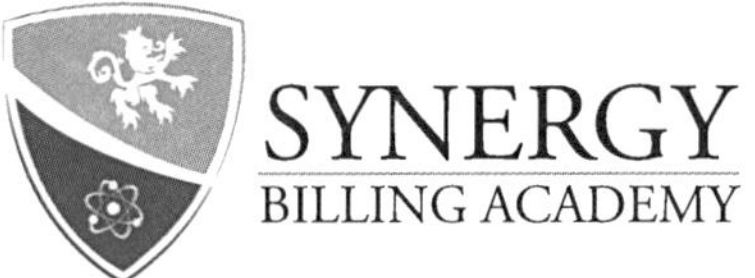

ICD-9-CM and ICD-10-CM – Chapter 15

The codes in Chapter 15, Pregnancy, Childbirth, and the Puerperium, are only to be used on the mother's record; this is the same guideline as in ICD-9-CM. These codes are to never be used on a newborn record. Some title changes were required in this chapter. For instance, ICD-9-CM code 654 for Abnormality of organs and soft tissues of pelvis is now called O34, Maternal care for abnormality of pelvic organs. Another example of a title change involves ICD-9-CM code 664 for Trauma to perineum and vulva during delivery; this is now called O70, Perineal laceration during delivery. In ICD-9-CM, the codes for elective (legal or therapeutic) abortion are classified with the abortion codes. Now, elective abortion (without complication) has been moved to code Z33.2 (Encounter for elective termination of pregnancy) and elective abortion with complication is now O04.

For certain conditions, we need to specify the fetus that is being affected. For a single pregnancy, the 7th character will be "0," which will also be used for multiple gestations where the fetus is unspecified. 7th characters of 1 through 9 are used for cases of multiple gestations to identify the fetus for which the code applies. Below are the 7th characters for fetus identification:

Seventh Character for Fetus	
0	Not applicable or unspecified
1	Fetus 1
2	Fetus 2
3	Fetus 3
4	Fetus 4
5	Fetus 5
9	Other Fetus

The trimester is now the measurement of classification in Chapter 15. In ICD-9-CM, we used the episode of care, such as delivered, antepartum, intrapartum, and postpartum. We also have to keep in mind that not all codes include the ability to select the trimesters. The trimesters are counted from the first day of the last menstrual period and are classified as follows:

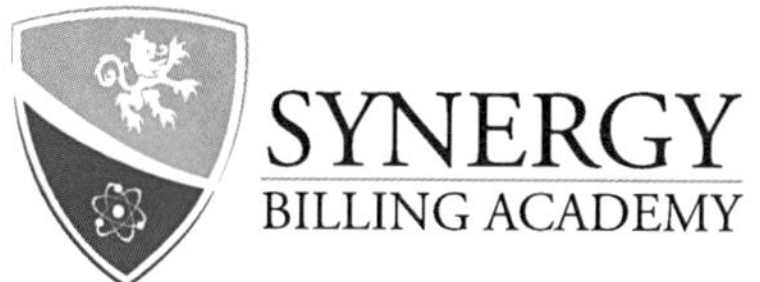

Trimesters	
1st	Less than 14 weeks 0 days
2nd	14 weeks 0 days to less than 28 weeks 0 days
3rd	28 weeks 0 days until delivery

We must also specify the week of gestation in the documentation. We are now required to code it using category code Z3A. In Chapter 15, we have a combination code that incorporates obstructed labor with the reason for the obstruction into one code. Some definition changes in this chapter are worth noting, such as: abortion versus fetal death is now set at 20 weeks instead of 22; early versus late vomiting is now 20 weeks instead of 22; and preterm labor still happens before completing a full 37 weeks of gestation.

One of the blocks in Chapter 21, Factors Influencing Health Status and Contact with Health Services is Z30-Z39, Persons encountering health services in circumstances related to reproduction. Several categories relate to the pregnant female. They are:

Code	Description
Z32	Encounter for pregnancy test and childbirth and childcare instruction
Z33	Pregnant state
Z34	Encounter for supervision of normal pregnancy
Z36	Encounter for antenatal screening of mother
Z3A	Weeks of gestation
Z37	Outcome of delivery
Z39	Encounter for maternal postpartum care and examination

Outcome of delivery codes (Z37.0-Z37.9) are intended for use as an additional code to identify the outcome of delivery on the mother's record. These codes are not for use on the newborn record. These codes exclude stillbirth (P95).

ICD-9-CM and ICD-10-CM – Chapter 16

Codes from this chapter are for use on newborn records only, never on maternal records. The codes in this chapter, Certain Conditions Originating in the Perinatal Period, include conditions that have their origin in the fetal or perinatal period (before birth through the first 28 days after

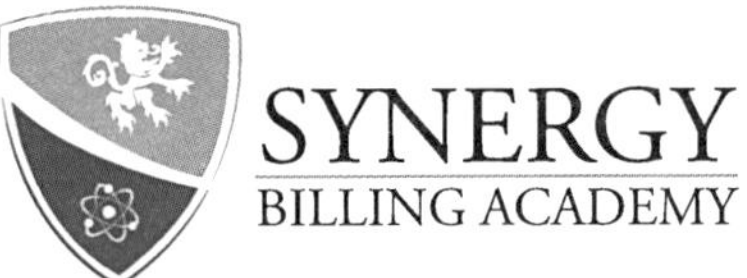

birth) even if morbidity occurs later. Subchapters were added for certain conditions originating in the perinatal period or the time after 22 weeks of pregnancy to about one month after birth. Because of updated terminology, some revisions to the classification of this chapter occurred.

Examples of these changes are in the first blocks in ICD-10-CM, regarding newborns affected by maternal factors and by complications of pregnancy, labor, and delivery. For example, the phrase "suspected to be" is included in the code title as a nonessential modifier to indicate that the codes are for use when the listed maternal condition is specified as the cause of confirmed or suspected newborn morbidity or potential morbidity.

Another example is in ICD-9-CM subsection 760-763, titled "Maternal causes of perinatal morbidity and mortality;" in ICD-10-CM, this is now titled "Newborn affected by maternal factors and by complications of pregnancy, labor, and delivery" and the code range is P00-P04. Also, the subclassification for 2,500 grams and over for birth weight is no longer an option for category P05, Disorders of newborn related to slow growth and fetal malnutrition.

The codes in block P00-P04 (Newborn affected by maternal factors and by complication of pregnancy, labor, and delivery) are for use when the listed maternal conditions are specified as the cause of confirmed morbidity or potential morbidity that have their origin in the perinatal period, which is before birth through the first 28 days after birth. These codes can be used for newborns who are suspected of having an abnormal condition resulting from exposure from the mother or the birth process, but without signs or symptoms, and which, after examination and observation, is found not to exist. The codes may also be used even if treatment is begun for a suspected condition that is ruled out.

When using codes from this chapter, we need to pay close attention to instructional notes appearing all throughout the chapter and in several of the classifications. For deliveries, we need to make sure that we use category Z38, Liveborn infants according to place of birth and type of delivery.

ICD-9-CM and ICD-10-CM – Chapter 17

ICD-10-CM Chapter 17, Congenital Malformations, Deformations, and Chromosomal Abnormalities, is the equivalent of ICD-9-CM Chapter 14. This chapter also went through some changes; it is now in a better format than the chapter in ICD-9-CM. The conditions in this chapter have been grouped into subchapters or blocks, making it easier to identify the type of conditions classified to Chapter 17.

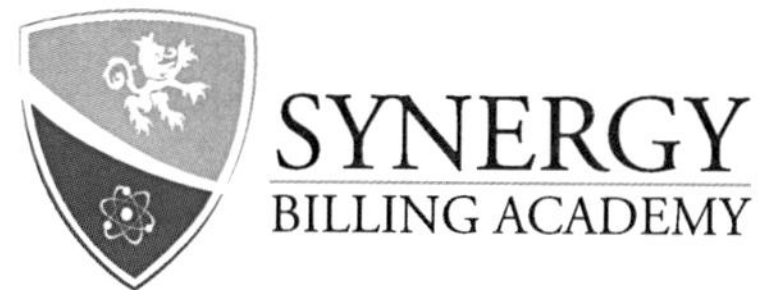

We can use the codes from Chapter 17 when a malformation/deformation or chromosomal abnormality is actually documented by the physician. When no unique code is available, assign additional code(s) for any manifestations. When a malformation/deformation or chromosomal abnormality does not have a unique code assignment, assign additional code(s) for any manifestations that may be present.

Modifications were also made to specific categories to bring the terminology in this chapter up to date with current medical practice. Another improvement is the increased specificity of classifications.

When the code assignment specifically identifies the malformation/deformation or chromosomal abnormality, manifestations that are inherent components of the anomaly should not be coded separately. Additional codes should be assigned for manifestations that are not inherent components. These codes are to be used throughout the life of the patient. Although present at birth, malformation/deformation or chromosomal abnormality may not be identified until later in life. Whenever the condition is diagnosed by the physician, it is appropriate to assign a code from codes Q00-Q99.

ICD-9-CM to ICD-10-CM – Chapter 18

Chapter 18, Symptoms, Signs, and Abnormal Clinical and Laboratory Findings, Not Elsewhere Classified, has also experienced some organizational changes. General symptoms and signs codes follow those related specifically to a body system or other relevant grouping in ICD-10-CM. Hematuria, or blood the in the urine, underwent an extensive classification change. Now, different types of hematuria are coded in this chapter unless they are included in an underlying condition such as acute cystitis with hematuria. In those instances, the code will be found in Chapter 14, Diseases of the Genitourinary System.

ICD-10-CM Chapter 18 is the equivalent of Chapter 16 in ICD-9-CM. Some codes have been moved from a different chapter to this one and some titles have been modified. An example of this is seen with ICD-9-CM Chapter 7 code 427.89, Other specified dysrhythmias; this is now in Chapter 18 in ICD-10-CM and its code is R00.1, Bradycardia, unspecified. Another example is ICD-9-CM code 511.0 for Pleurisy without mention of effusion or current tuberculosis, which moved from Chapter 8 to become ICD-10-CM code R09.1, Pleurisy.

The conditions, signs, and symptoms included in this chapter consist of:

- Cases for which no more specific diagnosis can be made even after all the facts

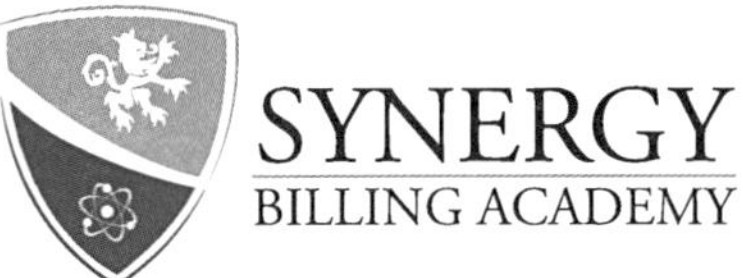

bearing on the case have been investigated.
- Signs or symptoms existing at the time of the initial encounter that proved to be transient and whose causes could not be determined.
- Provisional diagnosis in a patient who failed to return for further investigation or care.
- Cases referred elsewhere for investigation or treatment before the diagnosis was made.
- Cases in which a more precise diagnosis was not available for any other reason.
- Certain symptoms, for which supplementary information is provided, that represent important problems in medical care in their own right.

ICD-9-CM to ICD-10-CM – Chapter 19

Chapter 19 also went through an extensive modification to its classifications. Chapter 19 is the chapter where injury, poisoning, and certain other consequences of external causes have been classified. This chapter has a total of two letters, "S" for injuries that are related to a body region and "T" for injuries to unspecified regions as well as poisoning and external causes. Here you will find the classification for injuries, which is different from ICD-9-CM. In ICD-9-CM, injuries were grouped by the type of injury, such as fracture, strain, sprain, etc. In ICD-10-CM, injuries are now grouped by body part then by type of injury. An example of the classification is as follows:

Body Part	Code Section
Head	(S00 - S09)
Neck	(S10 - S19)
Thorax	(S20 - S29)

The listings of conditions are then followed by type of injury, such as:

- Superficial injury
- Open wound
- Fracture
- Dislocation and sprain
- Injury of nerves
- Injury of blood vessels
- Injury of muscle and tendon
- Crushing injury
- Traumatic amputation
- Other and unspecified injuries

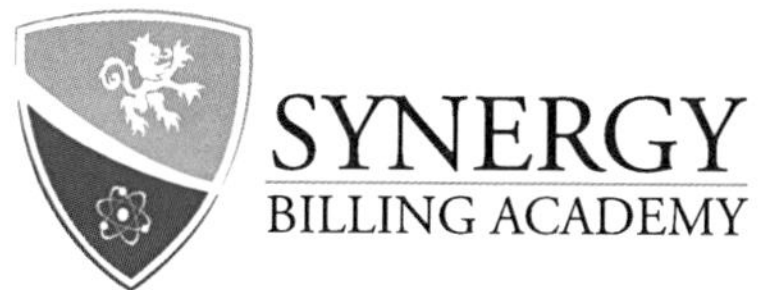

When it comes to fractures, many elements need to be taken into consideration. If a fracture is not indicated as open or closed, we would code it as closed. Also, if a fracture is not indicated as displaced or nondisplaced, we would code it as displaced. Some other elements that need to be included in the documentation are the type of fracture, the specific anatomical site, displaced vs. nondisplaced, laterality, routine vs. delayed healing, nonunion, malunion, and the type of encounter (initial, subsequent, sequela). Depending on the fracture, the following shows what the seventh character will be:

7th Character	Description
A	Initial closed
B	Initial open
D	Subsequent routine
G	Subsequent delayed
K	Subsequent nonunion
P	Subsequent malunion
S	Sequela

Initial encounter is used when the patient is receiving active treatment for the condition, such as surgical treatment, an emergency department encounter, or an evaluation and treatment by a new physician. A subsequent encounter is used after a patient has received active treatment for the condition and is now receiving routine care during the healing or recovery phase, such as a cast change or removal, a removal of an external or internal fixation device, a medication adjustment, or other aftercare and follow-up visits following injury treatment. Sequela is used when complications or conditions arise as a direct result of a condition, such as a scar formation after burn.

We must understand the difference between poisoning, adverse effect, and underdosing, as all of these terms are used in this chapter.

Term	Definition
Poisoning	Overdose of substances; wrong substance given or taken in error
Adverse effect	“Hypersensitivity,” “reaction,” or correct substance properly administered
Underdosing	Taking less of medication than is prescribed or instructed by manufacturer, either inadvertently or deliberately

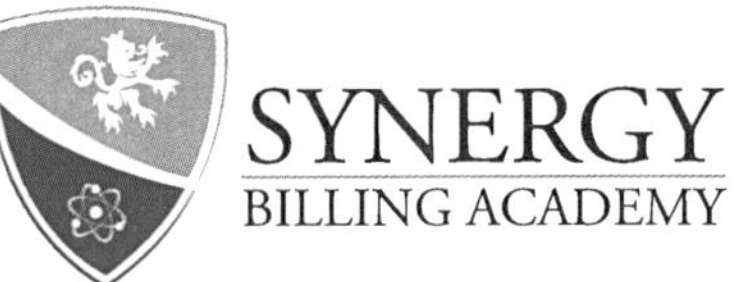

Some fracture categories provide for 7th characters to designate the specific type of open fracture (these designations are based on the Gustilo Anderson open fracture classification):

Character	Description
A	Initial encounter for closed fracture
B	Initial encounter for open fracture type I or II Initial encounter for open fracture NOS
C	Initial encounter for open fracture type IIIA, IIIB, or IIIC
D	Subsequent encounter for closed fracture with routine healing
E	Subsequent encounter for open fracture type I or II with routine healing
F	Subsequent encounter for open fracture type IIIA, IIIB, or IIIC with routine healing
G	Subsequent encounter for closed fracture with delayed healing
H	Subsequent encounter for open fracture type I or II with delayed healing Subsequent encounter for open fracture type IIIA, IIIB, or IIIC with delayed healing
K	Subsequent encounter for closed fracture with nonunion
M	Subsequent encounter for open fracture type I or II with nonunion
N	Subsequent encounter for open fracture type IIIA, IIIB, or IIIC with nonunion
P	Subsequent encounter for closed fracture with malunion
Q	Subsequent encounter for open fracture type I or II with malunion
R	Subsequent encounter for open fracture type IIIA, IIIB, or IIIC with malunion
S	Sequela(e)

ICD-9-CM to ICD-10-CM – Chapter 20

Chapter 20 is where we can find the codes for external causes of morbidity or illness. This chapter, External Causes of Morbidity, and Chapter 19, Injury, Poisoning, and Certain Other Consequences of External Causes, contain what we originally knew as E Codes in ICD-9-CM. Codes in this chapter capture the cause of the injury or health condition, the intent (unintentional or accidental vs. intentional, such as suicide or assault), the place where the event occurred, the activity of the patient at the time of the event, and the person's status (e.g., civilian, military).

Revisions to the whole chapter were necessary due to changes in terminology. Conditions included as subcategory codes in ICD-9-CM have been given a specific category code in ICD-

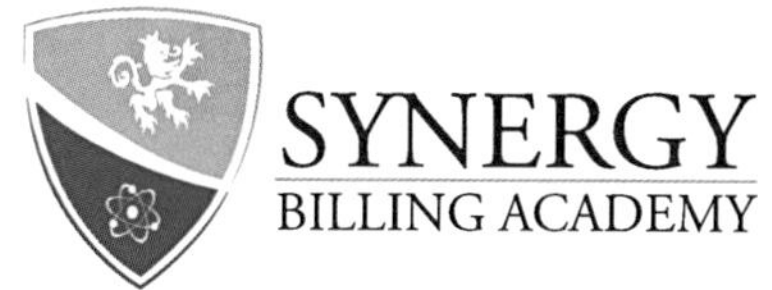

10-CM, allowing expansion of the codes at the fourth-, fifth-, and sixth-character levels. In ICD-9-CM, we would use E884.0 to indicate the patient fell from playground equipment; with ICD-10-CM, we can be more specific than listing simply W09, Fall on and from playground equipment; we can say exactly which equipment, such as:

- W09.0, Fall on or from playground slide
- W09.1, Fall from playground swing
- W09.2, Fall on or from jungle gym
- W09.8, Fall on or from other playground equipment

ICD-9-CM to ICD-10-CM – Chapter 21

Chapter 21 is a brand-new chapter. This chapter is for factors influencing health status and contact with health services. In ICD-9-CM, these were the V Codes; now, in ICD-10-CM, they are Z Codes, which is a huge difference from before. Some codes were moved from other chapters in ICD-9-CM to Chapter 21. An example of this is elective, legal, or therapeutic abortions, which have been moved from ICD-9-CM Chapter 11, Complications of Pregnancy, Childbirth, and the Puerperium, to ICD-10-CM Chapter 21.

These codes are used when a person who may or may not be sick encounters health services for some specific purpose, such as to receive limited care or service for a current condition, to donate an organ or tissue, to receive prophylactic vaccination, or to discuss a problem. These codes are used when some circumstance or problem is present which influences a person's health status but is not a current illness or injury.

This chapter also has category titles that were rephrased to reflect current medical practice and terminology. It also has a decrease in specificity: codes were actually removed for easier classification. An example of decreased specificity in ICD-10-CM is code Z23, Encounter for immunization. This code is not further classified. In ICD-9-CM, category codes V03, V04, V05, and V06 are used to identify the types of immunizations.

Several codes have been expanded, such as personal and family history. Codes have been added for concepts that do not exist in ICD-9-CM. Category Z67 identifies the patient's blood type. Category Z68, Body Mass Index (BMI) is divided into adult and pediatric codes.

The adult BMI codes are for use for persons 21 years of age or older. Pediatric BMI codes are for use for persons 2–20 years of age. The percentiles listed with the codes are based on the growth charts published by the Centers for Disease Control and Prevention (CDC).

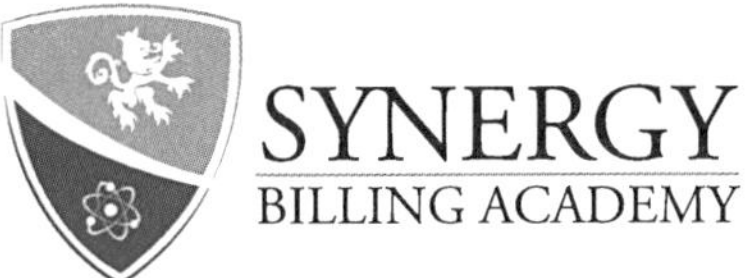

ICD-10-CM Chapter Categories[10]

Professionals will find the listing of family medicine, internal medicine, and pediatrics codes a little different in ICD-10-CM than what is currently found in ICD-9-CM. The following tables will show you all of the different sections related to family medicine, internal medicine, and pediatrics and the code representations for them.

Chapter 1 - ICD-10-CM Chapter Categories Table

Code	Description
A00-A09	Intestinal infectious diseases
A15-A19	Tuberculosis
A20-A28	Certain zoonotic bacterial diseases
A30-A49	Other bacterial diseases
A50-A64	Infections with a predominantly sexual mode of transmission
A65-A69	Other spirochetal diseases
A70-A74	Other diseases caused by chlamydia
A75-A79	Rickettsioses
A80-A89	Viral and prion infections of the central nervous system
A90-A99	Arthropod-borne viral fevers and viral hemorrhagic fevers
B00-B09	Viral infections characterized by skin and mucous membrane lesions
B10	Other human herpes viruses
B15-B19	Viral hepatitis
B20	Human immunodeficiency virus (HIV) disease
B25-B34	Other viral diseases
B35-B49	Mycoses
B50-B64	Protozoal diseases
B65-B83	Helminthiases
B85-B89	Pediculosis, acariasis, and other infestations
BB90-B94	Sequelae or infectious and parasitic diseases
B95-B97	Bacterial and viral infectious agents
B99	Other infectious diseases

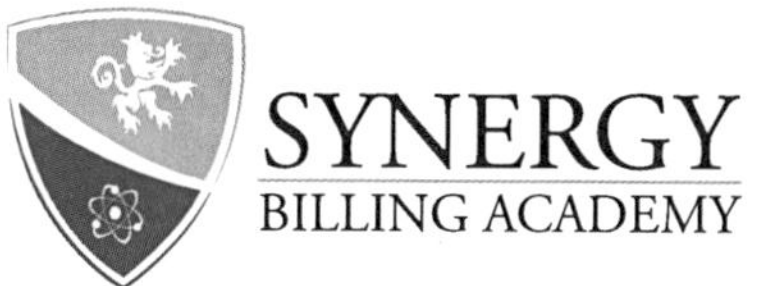

Chapter 4 - ICD-10-CM Chapter Categories Table

Code	Description
E00-E07	Disorders of thyroid gland
E08-E13	Diabetes mellitus
E15-E16	Other disorders of glucose regulation and pancreatic internal secretion
E20-E35	Disorders of other endocrine system
E36	Intraoperative complications of endocrine system
E40-E46	Malnutrition
E50-E64	Other nutritional deficiencies
E65-E68	Overweight, obesity, and other hyperalimentation
E70-E88	Metabolic disorders
E89	Postprocedural endocrine and metabolic complications and disorders, not elsewhere classified

Chapter 5 - ICD-10-CM Chapter Categories Table

Codes	Description
F01-F09	Mental disorders due to known physiological conditions
F10-F19	Mental and behavioral disorders due to psychoactive substance use
F20-F29	Schizophrenia, schizotypal, delusional, and other non-mood psychotic disorders
F30-F39	Mood [affective] disorders
F40-F48	Anxiety, dissociative, stress-related, somatoform, and other nonpsychotic mental disorders
F50-F59	Behavioral syndromes associated with physiological disturbances and physical factors
F60-F69	Disorders of adult personality and behavior
F70-F79	Intellectual disabilities
F80-F89	Pervasive and specific developmental disorders
F90-F98	Behavioral and emotional disorders with onset usually occurring in childhood and adolescence
F99	Unspecified mental disorder

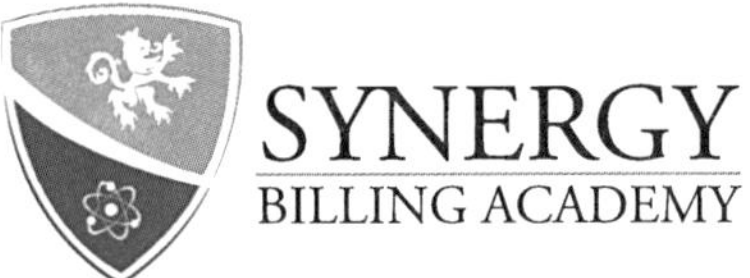

Chapter 7 - ICD-10-CM Chapter Categories Table

Code	Description
H00-H05	Disorders of eyelid, lacrimal system, and orbit
H10-H11	Disorders of conjunctiva
H15-H22	Disorders of sclera, cornea, iris, and ciliary body
H25-H28	Disorders of lens
H30-H36	Disorders of choroid and retina
H40-H42	Glaucoma
H43-H44	Disorders of vitreous body and globe
H46-H47	Disorders of optic nerve and visual pathways
H49-H52	Disorders of ocular muscles, binocular movement, accommodation, and refraction
H53-H54	Visual disturbances and blindness
H55-H57	Other disorders of eye and adnexa
H59	Intraoperative and postprocedural complications and disorders of eye and adnexa, not elsewhere classified

Chapter 8 - ICD-10-CM Chapter Categories Table

Code	Description
H60-H62	Diseases of external ear
H65-H75	Diseases of the middle ear and mastoid
H80-H83	Diseases of inner ear
H90-H94	Other disorders of ear
H95	Intraoperative and postprocedural complications and disorders of ear and mastoid process, not elsewhere classified

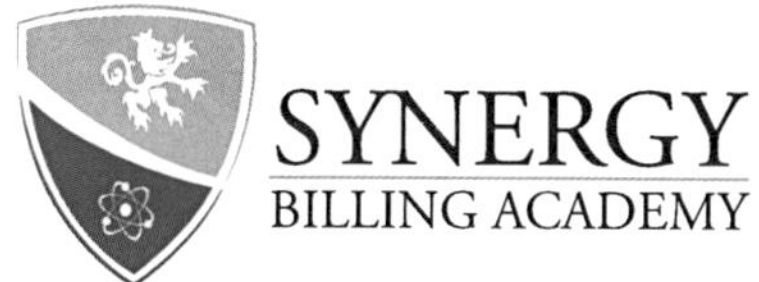

Chapter 9 - ICD-10-CM Chapter Categories Table

Code	Description
I00-I02	Acute rheumatic fever
I05-I09	Chronic rheumatic heart diseases
I10-I15	Hypertensive diseases
I20-I25	Ischemic heart diseases
I26-I28	Pulmonary heart disease and diseases of pulmonary circulation
I30-I52	Other forms of heart disease
I60-I69	Cerebrovascular diseases
I70-I79	Diseases of arteries, arterioles, and capillaries
I80-I89	Diseases of veins, lymphatic vessels, and lymph nodes, not elsewhere classified
I95-I99	Other and unspecified disorders of the circulatory system

Chapter 10 - ICD-10-CM Chapter Categories Table

Code	Descriptions
J00-J06	Acute upper respiratory infections
J09-J18	Influenza and pneumonia
J20-J22	Other acute lower respiratory infections
J30-J39	Other diseases of upper respiratory tract
J40-J47	Chronic lower respiratory diseases
J60-J70	Lung diseases due to external agents
J80-J84	Other respiratory diseases principally affecting the interstitium
J85-J86	Suppurative and necrotic conditions of the lower respiratory tract
J90-J94	Other diseases of the pleura
J95	Intraoperative and postprocedural complications and disorders of respiratory system, not elsewhere classified
J96-J99	Other diseases of the respiratory system

Chapter 11 - ICD-10-CM Chapter Categories Table

Code	Description
K00-K14	Diseases of oral cavity and salivary glands
K20-K31	Diseases of esophagus, stomach, and duodenum
K35-K38	Diseases of appendix
K40-K46	Hernia
K50-K52	Noninfective enteritis and colitis
K55-K64	Other diseases of intestines
K65-K68	Diseases of peritoneum and retroperitoneum
K70-K77	Diseases of liver
K80-K87	Disorders of gallbladder, biliary tract, and pancreas
K90-K95	Other diseases of digestive system

Chapter 13 - ICD-10-CM Chapter Categories Table

Code	Description
M00-M02	Infectious arthropathis
M05-M14	Inflammatory polyarthropathies
M15-M19	Osteoarthritis
M20-M25	Other joint disorders
M26-M27	Dentofacial anomalies [including malocclusion] and other disorders of jaw
M30-M36	Systemic connective tissue disorders
M40-M43	Deforming dorsopathies
M45-M49	Spondylopathies
M50-M54	Other dorsopathies
M60-M63	Disorders of muscles
M65-M67	Disorders of synovium and tendon
M70-M79	Other soft tissue disorders
M80-M85	Disorders of bone density and structure

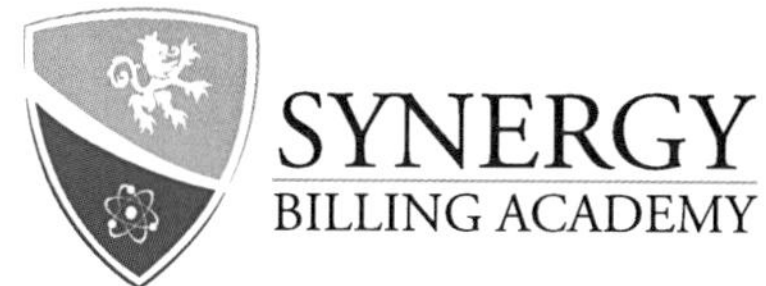

M86-M90	Other osteopathies
M91-M94	Chondropathies
M95	Other disorders of the musculoskeletal system and connective tissue
M96	Intraoperative and postprocedural complications and disorders of musculoskeletal system, not elsewhere classified
M99	Biomechanical lesions, not elsewhere classified

Chapter 14 - ICD-10-CM Chapter Categories Table

Code	Description
N00-N08	Glomerular diseases
N10-N16	Renal tubulo-interstitial diseases
N17-N19	Acute kidney failure and chronic kidney diseases
N20-N23	Urolithiasis
N25-N29	Other disorders of kidney and ureter
N30-N39	Other diseases of the urinary system
N40-N53	Diseases of male genital organs
N60-N65	Disorders of breast
N70-N77	Inflammatory diseases of female pelvic organs
N80-N98	Noninflammatory disorders of female genital tract
N99	Intraoperative and postprocedural complications and disorders of genitourinary system, not elsewhere classified

Chapter 15 - ICD-10-CM Chapter Categories Table

Code	Description
O00-O08	Pregnancy with abortive outcome
O09	Supervision of high risk pregnancy
O10-O16	Edema, proteinuria, and hypertensive disorders in pregnancy, childbirth, and the puerperium
O20-O29	Other maternal disorders predominantly related to pregnancy

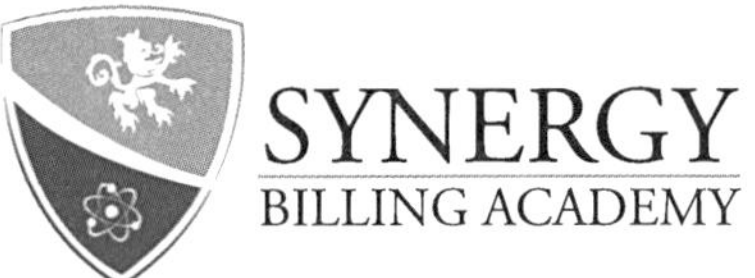

O30-O48	Maternal care related to the fetus and amniotic cavity and possible delivery problems
O60-O77	Complications of labor and delivery
O80, O82	Encounter for delivery
O85-O92	Complications predominantly related to the puerperium
O94-O9A	Other obstetric conditions, not elsewhere classified

Chapter 16 - ICD-10-CM Chapter Categories Table

Code	Description
P00-P04	Newborn affected by maternal factors and by complications of pregnancy, labor, and delivery
P05-P08	Disorders related to length of gestation and fetal growth
P09	Abnormal findings on neonatal screening
P19-P29	Respiratory and cardiovascular disorders specific to the perinatal period
P35-P39	Infections specific to the perinatal period
P50-P61	Hemorrhagic and hematological disorders of newborn
P70-P74	Transitory endocrine and metabolic disorders specific to newborn
P76-P78	Digestive system disorders of newborn
P80-P83	Conditions involving the integument and temperature regulation of newborn
P84	Other problems with newborn
P90-P96	Other disorders originating in the perinatal period

Chapter 17 - ICD-10-CM Chapter Categories Table

Code	Description
Q00-Q07	Congenital malformations of the nervous system
Q10-Q18	Congenital malformations of eye, ear, face, and neck
Q20-Q28	Congenital malformations of the circulatory system
Q30-Q34	Congenital malformations of the respiratory system
Q35-Q37	Cleft lip and cleft palate
Q38-Q45	Other congenital malformations of the digestive system

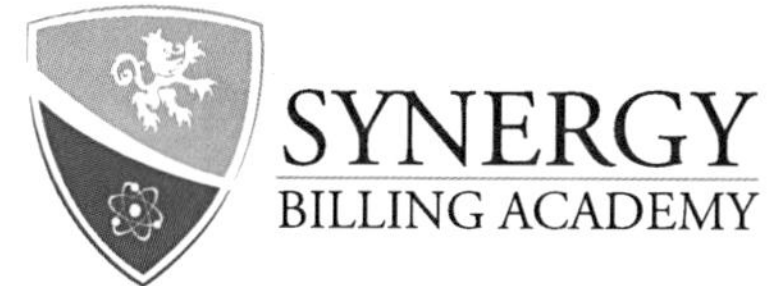

Q50-Q56	Congenital malformations of genital organs
Q60-Q64	Congenital malformations of the urinary system
Q65-Q79	Congenital malformations and deformations of the musculoskeletal system
Q80-Q89	Other congenital malformations
Q90-Q99	Chromosomal abnormalities, not elsewhere classified

Chapter 18 - ICD-10-CM Chapter Categories Table

Code	Description
R00-R09	Symptoms and signs involving the circulatory systems
R10-R19	Symptoms and signs involving the digestive system and abdomen
R20-R23	Symptoms and signs involving the skin and subcutaneous tissue
R25-R29	Symptoms and signs involving the nervous and musculoskeletal systems
R30-R39	Symptoms and signs involving the genitourinary system
R40-R46	Symptoms and signs involving cognition, perception, emotional state, and behavior
R47-R49	Symptoms and signs involving speech and voice
R50-R69	General symptoms and signs
R70-R79	Abnormal findings on examination of blood, without diagnosis
R80-R82	Abnormal findings on examination of urine, without diagnosis
R83-R89	Abnormal findings on examination of other body fluids, substances, and tissues without diagnosis
R90-R94	Abnormal findings on diagnostic imaging and in function studies, without diagnosis
R97	Abnormal tumor markers
R99	Ill-defined and unknown cause of mortality

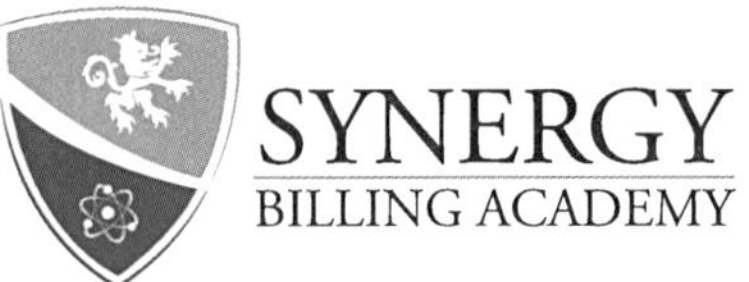

Chapter 19 - ICD-10-CM Chapter Categories Table

Code	Description
S00-S09	Injuries to the head
S10-S19	Injuries to the neck
S20-S29	Injuries to the thorax
S30-S39	Injuries to the abdomen, lower back, lumbar spine, pelvis, and external genitals
S40-S49	Injuries to the shoulder and upper arm
S50-S59	Injuries to the elbow and forearm
S60-S69	Injuries to the wrist, hand, and fingers
S70-S79	Injuries to the hip and thigh
S80-S89	Injuries to the knee and lower leg
S90-S99	Injuries to the ankle and foot
T07	Injuries involving multiple body regions
T14	Injury of unspecified body region
T15-T19	Effects of foreign body entering through natural orifice
T20-T32	Burns and corrosion • T20-T25 – Burns and corrosions of external body surface, specified by site • T26-T28 – Burns and corrosions confined to eye and internal organs • T30-T32 – Burns and corrosions of multiple and unspecified body regions
T33-T34	Frostbite
T36-T50	Poisoning by, adverse effect of an underdosing of drugs, medicaments, and biological substances
T51-T65	Toxic effects of substances chiefly nonmedicinal as to source
T66-T78	Other and unspecified effects of external causes
T79	Certain early complications of trauma
T80-T88	Complications of surgical and medical care, not elsewhere classified

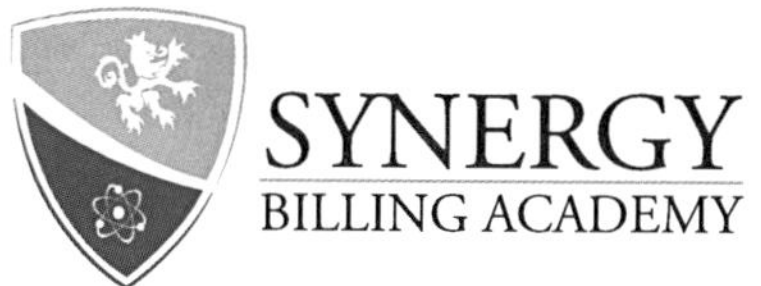

Chapter 20 - ICD-10-CM Chapter Categories Table

Code	Description
V00-X58	Accidents
V00-V99	Transport accidents
V00-V09	Pedestrian injured in transport accident
V10-V19	Pedal cycle rider injured in transport accident
V20-V29	Motorcycle rider injured in transport accident
V30-V39	Occupant of three-wheeled motor vehicle injured in transport accident
V40-V49	Car occupant injured in transport accident
V50-V59	Occupant of pickup truck or van injured in transport accident
V60-V69	Occupant of heavy transport vehicle injured in transport accident
V70-V79	Bus occupant injured in transport accident
V80-V89	Other land transport accidents
V90-V94	Water transport accidents
V95-V97	Air and space transport accidents
V98-V99	Other and unspecified transport accidents
W00-X58	Other external causes of accidental injury
W00 - W19	Slipping, tripping, stumbling, and falls
W20-W49	Exposure to inanimate mechanical forces
W50-W64	Exposure to animate mechanical forces
W65-W74	Accidental non-transport drowning and submersion
W85-W99	Exposure to electric current, radiation, and extreme ambient air temperature and pressure
X00-X08	Exposure to smoke, fire, and flames
X10-X19	Contact with heat and hot substances
X30-X39	Exposure to forces of nature
X52-X58	Accidental exposure to other specified factors
X71-X83	Intentional self-harm
X92-Y02	Assault
Y21-Y33	Event of undetermined intent
Y35-Y38	Legal intervention, operations of war, military operations, and terrorism

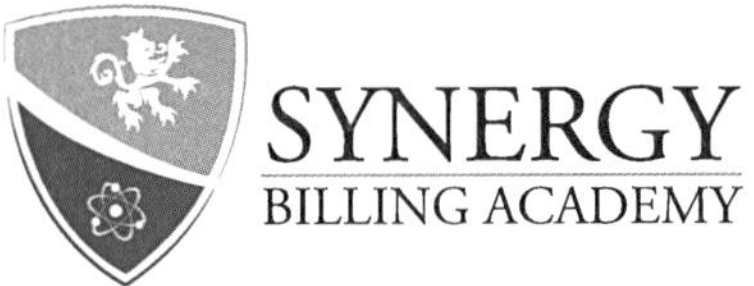

Y62-Y84	Complications of medical and surgical care
Y62-Y69	Misadventures to patients during surgical and medical care
Y70-Y82	Medical devices associated with adverse incidents in diagnostic and therapeutic use
Y83-Y84	Surgical and other medical procedures as the cause of abnormal reaction of the patient, or of later complication, without mention of misadventure at the time of the procedure
Y90-Y99	Supplementary factors related to causes of morbidity classified elsewhere

Chapter 21 - ICD-10-CM Chapter Categories Table

Code	Description
Z00-Z13	Persons encountering health services for examinations
Z14-Z15	Genetic carrier and genetic susceptibility to disease
Z16	Resistance to antimicrobial drugs
Z17	Estrogen receptor status
Z18	Retained foreign body fragment
Z20-Z28	Persons with potential health hazards related to communicable diseases
Z30-Z39	Persons encountering health services in circumstances related to reproduction
Z40-Z53	Encounters for other specific health care
Z55-Z65	Persons with potential health hazards related to socioeconomic and psychosocial circumstances
Z66	Do not resuscitate status
Z67	Blood type
Z68	Body mass index (BMI)
Z69-Z76	Persons encountering health services in other circumstances
Z77-Z99	Persons with potential health hazards related to family and personal history and certain conditions influencing health status

ICD-10-CM Guidelines [9]

As mentioned before, the National Center of Health Statistics (NCHS), along with the American Hospital Association (AHA), the American Health Information Management Association (AHIMA),

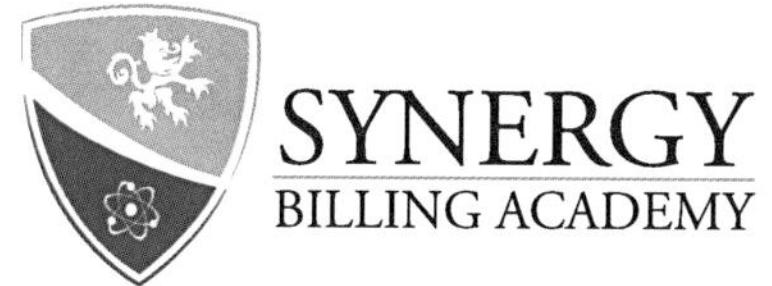

and the Centers for Medicare and Medicaid Services (CMS) developed and approved coding and reporting guidelines for ICD-10-CM; these organizations also maintain the manual.

In addition to general coding guidelines, there are guidelines for specific diagnoses and/or conditions in the classification. Unless otherwise indicated, these guidelines apply to all health care settings. Below are the official guidelines published by the NCHS in 2014 as they relate to the family medicine, internal medicine, and pediatrics chapters:

Chapter 1 - Guidelines

The NCHS has published the following guidelines:

A. Human Immunodeficiency Virus (HIV) Infections
B. Infectious Agents as the Cause Of Diseases Classified to Other Chapters
C. Infections Resistant to Antibiotics
D. Sepsis, Severe Sepsis, Septic Shock
E. Methicillin Resistant Staphylococcus Aureus (MRSA) Conditions

Chapter 1: Certain Infectious and Parasitic Diseases (A00-B99)

A. Human Immunodeficiency Virus (HIV) Infections

1. Code only confirmed cases

Code only confirmed cases of HIV infection/illness. This is an exception to the hospital inpatient guideline Section II, H.

In this context, "confirmation" does not require documentation of positive serology or culture for HIV; the provider's diagnostic statement that the patient is HIV positive or has an HIV-related illness is sufficient.

2. Selection and sequencing of HIV codes

a. Patient admitted for HIV-related condition

If a patient is admitted for an HIV-related condition, the principal diagnosis should be B20, Human immunodeficiency virus [HIV] disease, followed by additional diagnosis codes for all reported HIV-related conditions.

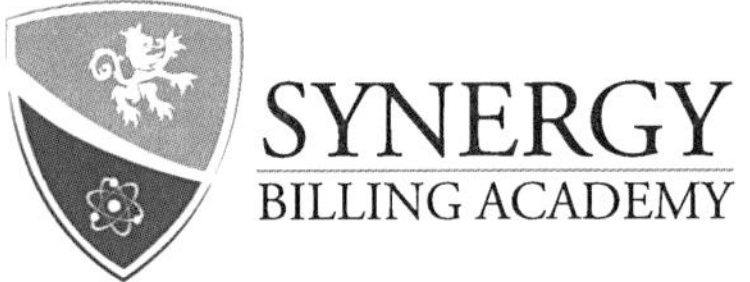

b. **Patient with HIV disease admitted for unrelated condition**

If a patient with HIV disease is admitted for an unrelated condition (such as a traumatic injury), the code for the unrelated condition (e.g., the nature of injury code) should be the principal diagnosis. Other diagnoses would be B20, followed by additional diagnosis codes for all reported HIV-related conditions.

c. **Whether the patient is newly diagnosed**

Whether the patient is newly diagnosed or has had previous admissions/ encounters for HIV conditions is irrelevant to the sequencing decision.

d. **Asymptomatic human immunodeficiency virus**

Z21, Asymptomatic human immunodeficiency virus [HIV] infection status, is to be applied when a patient without any documentation of symptoms is listed as being "HIV positive," "known HIV," "HIV test positive," or similar terminology. Do not use this code if the term "AIDS" is used or if the patient is treated for any HIV-related illness or is described as having any condition(s) resulting from his/ her HIV positive status; use B20 in these cases.

e. **Patients with inconclusive HIV serology**

Patients with inconclusive HIV serology, but no definitive diagnosis or manifestations of the illness, may be assigned code R75, Inconclusive laboratory evidence of human immunodeficiency virus [HIV].

f. **Previously diagnosed HIV-related illness**

Patients with any known prior diagnosis of an HIV-related illness should be coded to B20. Once a patient has developed an HIV-related illness, the patient should always be assigned code B20 on every subsequent admission/ encounter. Patients previously diagnosed with any HIV illness (B20) should never be assigned to R75 or Z21, Asymptomatic human immunodeficiency virus [HIV] infection status.

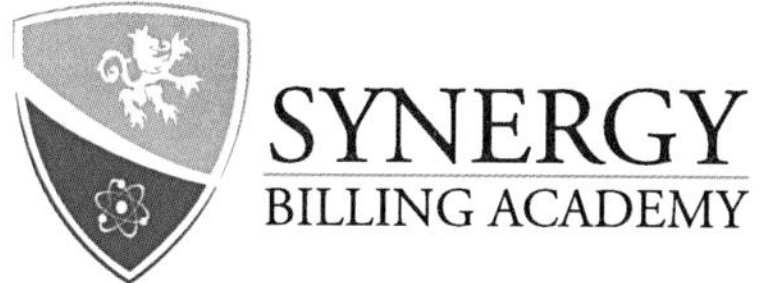

g. HIV infection in pregnancy, childbirth, and the puerperium

During pregnancy, childbirth, or the puerperium, a patient admitted (or presenting for a health care encounter) because of an HIV-related illness should receive a principal diagnosis code of O98.7-, Human immunodeficiency [HIV] disease complicating pregnancy, childbirth, and the puerperium, followed by B20 and the code(s) for the HIV-related illness(es).

Codes from Chapter 15 always take sequencing priority.

Patients with asymptomatic HIV infection status admitted (or presenting for a health care encounter) during pregnancy, childbirth, or the puerperium should receive codes of O98.7- and Z21.

h. Encounters for testing for HIV

If a patient is being seen to determine his/her HIV status, use code Z11.4, Encounter for screening for human immunodeficiency virus [HIV]. Use additional codes for any associated high-risk behavior.

If a patient with signs or symptoms is being seen for HIV testing, code the signs and symptoms. An additional counseling code, Z71.7, Human immunodeficiency virus [HIV] counseling, may be used if counseling is provided during the encounter for the test.

When a patient returns to be informed of his/her HIV test results and the test result is negative, use code Z71.7, Human immunodeficiency virus [HIV] counseling.

If the results are positive, see previous guidelines and assign codes as appropriate.

B. Infectious Agents as the Cause of Diseases Classified to Other Chapters

Certain infections are classified in chapters other than Chapter 1 and no organism is identified as part of the infection code. In these instances, it is necessary to use an additional code from Chapter 1 to identify the organism. A code from category B95, Streptococcus, Staphylococcus, and Enterococcus as the cause of diseases classified to other chapters; B96, Other bacterial

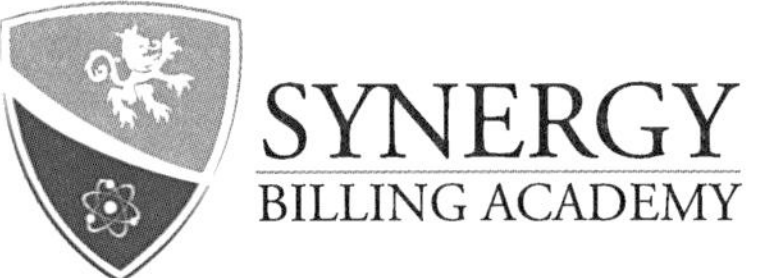

agents as the cause of diseases classified to other chapters; or B97, Viral agents as the cause of diseases classified to other chapters, is to be used as an additional code to identify the organism. An instructional note will be found at the infection code advising that an additional organism code is required.

C. Infections Resistant to Antibiotics

Many bacterial infections are resistant to current antibiotics. It is necessary to identify all infections documented as antibiotic resistant. Assign a code from category Z16, Resistance to antimicrobial drugs, following the infection code only if the infection code does not identify drug resistance.

D. Sepsis, Severe Sepsis, and Septic Shock

1. Coding of sepsis and severe sepsis

a. Sepsis

For a diagnosis of sepsis, assign the appropriate code for the underlying systemic infection. If the type of infection or causal organism is not further specified, assign code A41.9, Sepsis, unspecified organism.

A code from subcategory R65.2, Severe sepsis, should not be assigned unless severe sepsis or an associated acute organ dysfunction is documented.

i. Negative or inconclusive blood cultures and sepsis-negative or inconclusive blood cultures do not preclude a diagnosis of sepsis in patients with clinical evidence of the condition; however, the provider should be queried.

ii. The term urosepsis is a nonspecific term. It is not to be considered synonymous with sepsis. It has no default code in the Alphabetic Index. Should a provider use this term, he/she must be queried for clarification.

iii. Sepsis with organ dysfunction: If a patient has sepsis and associated acute organ dysfunction or multiple organ dysfunction (MOD), follow the instructions for coding severe sepsis.

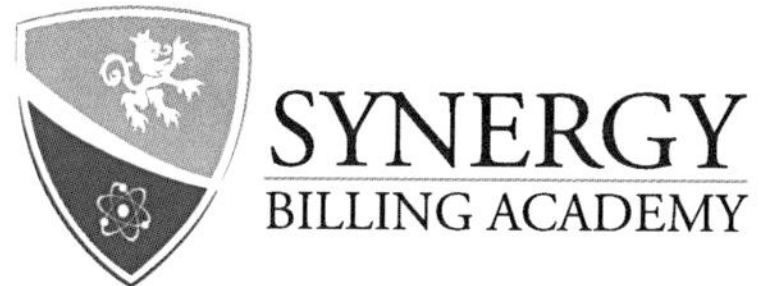

iv. Acute organ dysfunction that is not clearly associated with the sepsis: If a patient has sepsis and an acute organ dysfunction, but the medical record documentation indicates that the acute organ dysfunction is related to a medical condition other than the sepsis, do not assign a code from subcategory R65.2, Severe sepsis. An acute organ dysfunction must be associated with the sepsis in order to assign the severe sepsis code. If the documentation is not clear as to whether an acute organ dysfunction is related to the sepsis or another medical condition, query the provider.

b. Severe sepsis

The coding of severe sepsis requires a minimum of two codes: first a code for the underlying systemic infection, followed by a code from subcategory R65.2, Severe sepsis. If the causal organism is not documented, assign code A41.9, Sepsis, unspecified organism, for the infection. Additional code(s) for the associated acute organ dysfunction are also required.

Due to the complex nature of severe sepsis, some cases may require querying the provider prior to assigning the codes.

2. Septic shock

a. Septic shock generally refers to circulatory failure associated with severe sepsis, and therefore, it represents a type of acute organ dysfunction.

For cases of septic shock, the code for the systemic infection should be sequenced first, followed by code R65.21, Severe sepsis with septic shock, or code T81.12, Postprocedural septic shock. Any additional codes for the other acute organ dysfunctions should also be assigned. As noted in the sequencing instructions in the Tabular List, the code for septic shock cannot be assigned as a principal diagnosis.

3. Sequencing of severe sepsis

If severe sepsis is present on admission and meets the definition of principal diagnosis, the underlying systemic infection should be assigned as the principal diagnosis followed by the appropriate code from subcategory R65.2 as required by the sequencing rules in the Tabular List. A code from subcategory R65.2 can never be assigned as a principal diagnosis.

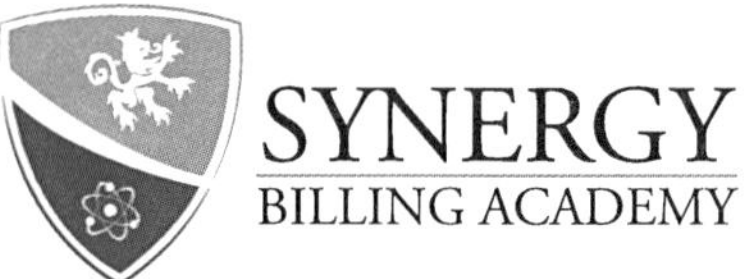

When severe sepsis develops during an encounter (when it was not present on admission), the underlying systemic infection and the appropriate code from subcategory R65.2 should be assigned as secondary diagnoses.

Severe sepsis may be present on admission but the diagnosis may not be confirmed until sometime after admission. If the documentation is not clear whether severe sepsis was present on admission, the provider should be queried.

4. **Sepsis and severe sepsis with a localized infection**

If the reason for admission is both sepsis or severe sepsis and a localized infection such as pneumonia or cellulitis, a code(s) for the underlying systemic infection should be assigned first and the code for the localized infection should be assigned as a secondary diagnosis. If the patient has severe sepsis, a code from subcategory R65.2 should also be assigned as a secondary diagnosis. If the patient is admitted with a localized infection such as pneumonia and sepsis/severe sepsis doesn't develop until after admission, the localized infection should be assigned first, followed by the appropriate sepsis/severe sepsis codes.

5. **Sepsis due to a postprocedural infection**

   a. **Documentation of causal relationship**

   As with all postprocedural complications, code assignment is based on the provider's documentation of the relationship between the infection and the procedure.

   b. **Sepsis due to a postprocedural infection**

   For such cases, the postprocedural infection code, such as T80.2, Infections following infusion, transfusion, and therapeutic injection; T81.4, Infection following a procedure; T88.0, Infection following immunization; or O86.0, Infection of obstetric surgical wound, should be coded first, followed by the code for the specific infection. If the patient has severe sepsis, the appropriate code from subcategory R65.2 should also be assigned with the additional code(s) for any acute organ dysfunction.

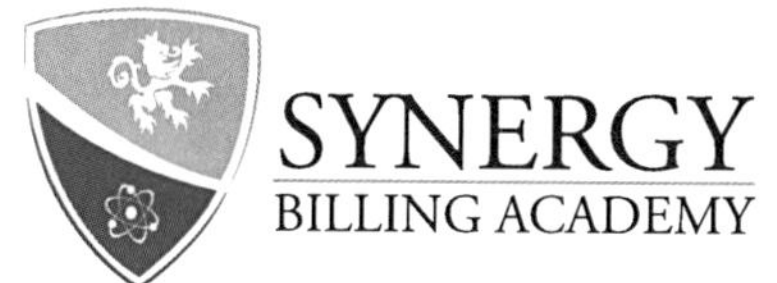

c. **Postprocedural infection and postprocedural septic shock**

In cases where a postprocedural infection has occurred and has resulted in severe sepsis and postprocedural septic shock, the code for the precipitating complication, such as code T81.4, Infection following a procedure, or O86.0, Infection of obstetrical surgical wound, should be coded first, followed by code R65.21, Severe sepsis with septic shock, and a code for the systemic infection.

6. **Sepsis and severe sepsis associated with a noninfectious process (condition)**

In some cases, a noninfectious process (condition) such as trauma may lead to an infection that can result in sepsis or severe sepsis. If sepsis or severe sepsis is documented as associated with a noninfectious condition, such as a burn or serious injury, and this condition meets the definition for principal diagnosis, the code for the noninfectious condition should be sequenced first, followed by the code for the resulting infection. If severe sepsis is present, a code from subcategory R65.2 should also be assigned with any associated organ dysfunction(s) codes. It is not necessary to assign a code from subcategory R65.1, Systemic inflammatory response syndrome (SIRS) of non-infectious origin, for these cases.

If the infection meets the definition of principal diagnosis, it should be sequenced before the non-infectious condition. When both the associated non-infectious condition and the infection meet the definition of principal diagnosis, either may be assigned as principal diagnosis.

Only one code from category R65, Symptoms and signs specifically associated with systemic inflammation and infection, should be assigned. Therefore, when a non-infectious condition leads to an infection resulting in severe sepsis, assign the appropriate code from subcategory R65.2, Severe sepsis. Do not additionally assign a code from subcategory R65.1, Systemic inflammatory response syndrome (SIRS) of non-infectious origin.

See Section I.C.18. SIRS due to non-infectious process

7. **Sepsis and septic shock complicating abortion, pregnancy, childbirth, and the puerperium**

See Section I.C.15. Sepsis and septic shock complicating abortion, pregnancy, childbirth, and the puerperium

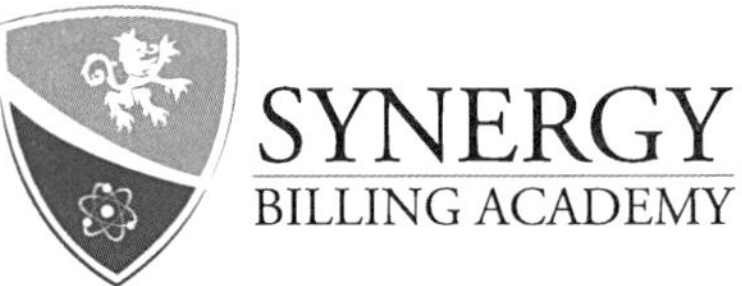

8. **Newborn sepsis**

   **See Section I.C.16. f. Bacterial sepsis of newborn*

E. **Methicillin Resistant Staphylococcus aureus (MRSA) Conditions**

1. **Selection and sequencing of MRSA codes**

   a. **Combination codes for MRSA infection**

   When a patient is diagnosed with an infection due to methicillin resistant Staphylococcus aureus (MRSA), and that infection has a combination code that includes the causal organism (e.g., sepsis, pneumonia) assign the appropriate combination code for the condition (e.g., code A41.02, Sepsis due to Methicillin resistant Staphylococcus aureus, or code J15.212, Pneumonia due to Methicillin resistant Staphylococcus aureus). Do not assign code B95.62, Methicillin resistant Staphylococcus aureus infection as the cause of diseases classified elsewhere, as an additional code because the combination code includes the type of infection and the MRSA organism. Do not assign a code from subcategory Z16.11, Resistance to penicillins, as an additional diagnosis.

   **See Section C.1. for instructions on coding and sequencing of sepsis and severe sepsis.*

   b. **Other codes for MRSA infection**

   When there is documentation of a current infection (e.g., wound infection, stitch abscess, urinary tract infection) due to MRSA, and that infection does not have a combination code that includes the causal organism, assign the appropriate code to identify the condition along with code B95.62, Methicillin resistant Staphylococcus aureus infection as the cause of diseases classified elsewhere for the MRSA infection. Do not assign a code from subcategory Z16.11, Resistance to penicillins.

   c. **Methicillin susceptible Staphylococcus aureus (MSSA) and MRSA colonization**

   The condition or state of being colonized or carrying MSSA or MRSA is called colonization or carriage, while an individual person is described as being

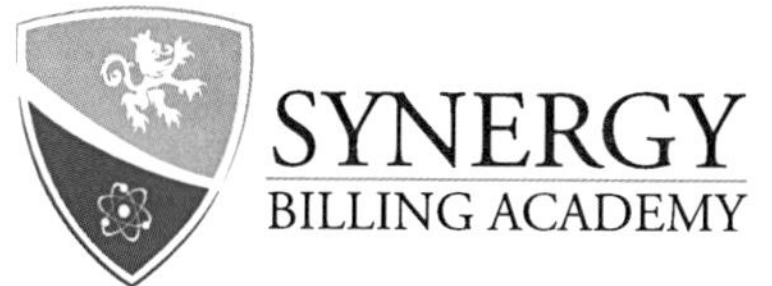

colonized or being a carrier. Colonization means that MSSA or MRSA is present on or in the body without necessarily causing illness. A positive MRSA colonization test might be documented by the provider as "MRSA screen positive" or "MRSA nasal swab positive."

Assign code Z22.322, Carrier or suspected carrier of Methicillin resistant Staphylococcus aureus, for patients documented as having MRSA colonization. Assign code Z22.321, Carrier or suspected carrier of Methicillin susceptible Staphylococcus aureus, for patients documented as having MSSA colonization. Colonization is not necessarily indicative of a disease process or as the cause of a specific condition the patient may have unless documented as such by the provider.

d. MRSA colonization and infection

If a patient is documented as having both MRSA colonization and infection during a hospital admission, code Z22.322, Carrier or suspected carrier of Methicillin resistant Staphylococcus aureus, and a code for the MRSA infection may both be assigned.

Chapter 4 - Guidelines

New guidelines that clarify code usage are found under specific codes.

- Under E34.0, Carcinoid syndrome, the note states, "May be used as an additional code to identify functional activity associated with a carcinoid tumor." No such note appears under the ICD-9-CM code 259.2 for this same condition.

The NCHS has published the following guidelines:

A. Diabetes mellitus
    1. Type of diabetes
    2. Type of diabetes mellitus not documented
    3. Diabetes mellitus and the use of insulin
    4. Diabetes mellitus in pregnancy and gestational diabetes
    5. Complications due to insulin pump malfunction
        a. Underdose of insulin due to insulin pump failure
        b. Overdose of insulin due to insulin pump failure

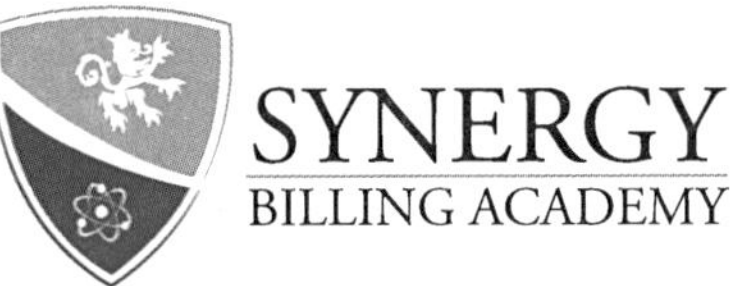

6. Secondary diabetes mellitus
    a. Secondary diabetes mellitus and the use of insulin
    b. Assigning and sequencing secondary diabetes codes and their causes
        i. Secondary diabetes mellitus due to pancreatectomy
        ii. Secondary diabetes due to drugs

Chapter 4: Endocrine, Nutritional, and Metabolic Diseases (E00-E89)

a. Diabetes mellitus

The diabetes mellitus codes are combination codes that include the type of diabetes mellitus, the body system affected, and the complications affecting that body system. Use as many codes within a particular category as are necessary to describe all of the complications of the disease. They should be sequenced based on the reason for a particular encounter. Assign as many codes from categories E08–E13 as needed to identify all of a patient's associated conditions.

1. Type of diabetes

The age of a patient is not the sole determining factor, though most type 1 diabetics develop the condition before reaching puberty. For this reason, type 1 diabetes mellitus is also referred to as juvenile diabetes.

2. Type of diabetes mellitus not documented

If the type of diabetes mellitus is not documented in the medical record, the default is E11.-, Type 2 diabetes mellitus.

3. Diabetes mellitus and the use of insulin

If the documentation in a medical record does not indicate the type of diabetes but does indicate that the patient uses insulin, code E11, Type 2 diabetes mellitus, should be assigned. Code Z79.4, Long-term (current) use of insulin, should also be assigned to indicate that the patient uses insulin. Code Z79.4 should not be assigned if insulin is given temporarily to bring a type 2 patient's blood sugar under control during an encounter.

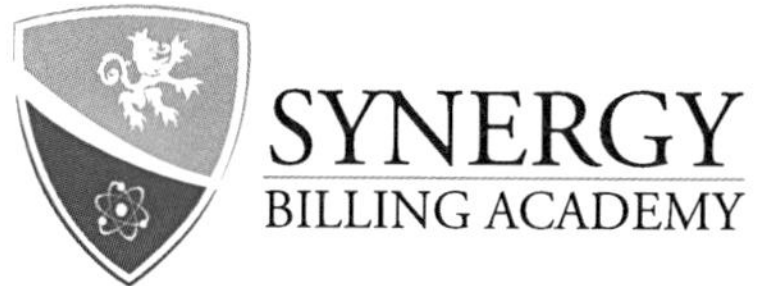

4. **Diabetes mellitus in pregnancy and gestational diabetes**

   **See Section I.C.15. Diabetes mellitus in pregnancy.*
   **See Section I.C.15. Gestational (pregnancy-induced) diabetes*

5. **Complications due to insulin pump malfunction**

   a. **Underdose of insulin due to insulin pump failure**

   An underdose of insulin due to an insulin pump failure should be assigned to a code from subcategory T85.6, Mechanical complication of other specified internal and external prosthetic devices, implants, and grafts, that specifies the type of pump malfunction as the principal or first-listed code, followed by code T38.3x6-, Underdosing of insulin and oral hypoglycemic [antidiabetic] drugs. Additional codes for the type of diabetes mellitus and any associated complications due to the underdosing should also be assigned.

   b. **Overdose of insulin due to insulin pump failure**

   The principal or first-listed code for an encounter due to an insulin pump malfunction resulting in an overdose of insulin should also be T85.6-, Mechanical complication of other specified internal and external prosthetic devices, implants, and grafts, followed by code T38.3x1-, Poisoning by insulin and oral hypoglycemic [antidiabetic] drugs, accidental (unintentional).

6. **Secondary diabetes mellitus**

   Codes under categories E08, Diabetes mellitus due to underlying condition; E09, Drug, or chemical-induced diabetes mellitus; and E13, Other specified diabetes mellitus, identify complications/manifestations associated with secondary diabetes mellitus. Secondary diabetes is always caused by another condition or event (e.g., cystic fibrosis, malignant neoplasm of pancreas, pancreatectomy, adverse effect of drug, or poisoning).

   a. **Secondary diabetes mellitus and the use of insulin**

   For patients who routinely use insulin, code Z79.4, Long-term (current) use of insulin, should also be assigned. Code Z79.4 should not be assigned if insulin

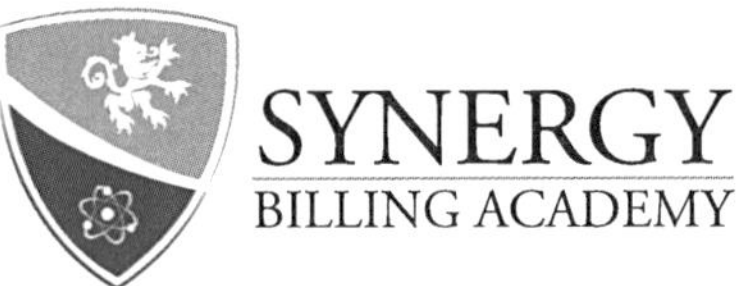

is given temporarily to bring a patient's blood sugar under control during an encounter.

b. Assigning and sequencing secondary diabetes codes and their causes

The sequencing of the secondary diabetes codes in relationship to codes for the cause of the diabetes is based on the Tabular List instructions for categories E08, E09, and E13.

i. Secondary diabetes mellitus due to pancreatectomy

For postpancreatectomy diabetes mellitus (lack of insulin due to the surgical removal of all or part of the pancreas), assign code E89.1, Postprocedural hypoinsulinemia. Assign a code from category E13 and a code from subcategory Z90.41-, Acquired absence of pancreas, as additional codes.

ii. Secondary diabetes due to drugs

Secondary diabetes may be caused by an adverse effect of correctly administered medications, poisoning, or sequela of poisoning. See section I.C.19.e for coding of adverse effects and poisoning, and section I.C.20 for external cause code reporting.

Chapter 5 - Guidelines

Many changes were made to Chapter 5, including organization and terminology, which resulted in some guideline adjustments as well. In ICD-10-CM, beneath code F54, Psychological and behavioral factors associated with disorders or diseases classified elsewhere, there is a note that states to "code first the associated physical disorder." The equivalent ICD-9-CM code, 316, has a note to "use additional code to identify the associated physical condition."

The NCHS has published the following guidelines:

A. Pain Disorders Related to Psychological Factors
B. Mental and Behavioral Disorders Due to Psychoactive Substance Use
    1. In remission
    2. Psychoactive substance use, abuse, and dependence
    3. Psychoactive substance use

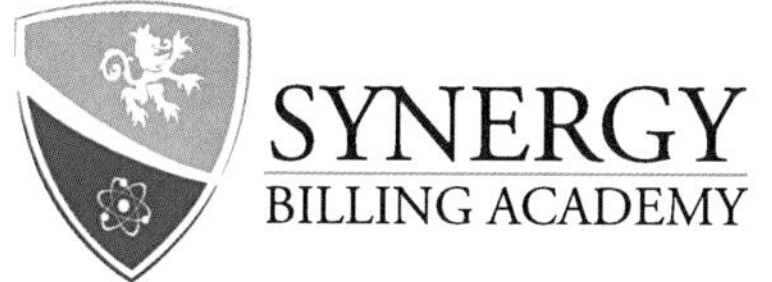

5. Chapter 5: Mental, Behavioral, and Neurodevelopmental Disorders (F01–F99)

A. Pain Disorders Related to Psychological Factors

Assign code F45.41 for pain that is exclusively related to psychological disorders. As indicated by the Excludes1 note under category G89, a code from category G89 should not be assigned with code F45.41.

Code F45.42, Pain disorders with related psychological factors, should be used with a code from category G89, Pain, not elsewhere classified, if there is documentation of a psychological component for a patient with acute or chronic pain.

*See Section I.C.6. Pain

b. Mental and Behavioral Disorders Due to Psychoactive Substance Use

1. In remission

Selection of codes for “in remission” for categories F10-F19, Mental and behavioral disorders due to psychoactive substance use (categories F10-F19 with -.21), requires the provider’s clinical judgment. The appropriate codes for “in remission” are assigned only on the basis of provider documentation (as defined in the Official Guidelines for Coding and Reporting).

2. Psychoactive substance use, abuse and dependence

When the provider documentation refers to use, abuse, and dependence of the same substance (e.g. alcohol, opioids, cannabis, etc.), only one code should be assigned to identify the pattern of use based on the following hierarchy:

- If both use and abuse are documented, assign only the code for abuse.
- If both abuse and dependence are documented, assign only the code for dependence.
- If use, abuse, and dependence are all documented, assign only the code for dependence.
- If both use and dependence are documented, assign only the code for dependence..

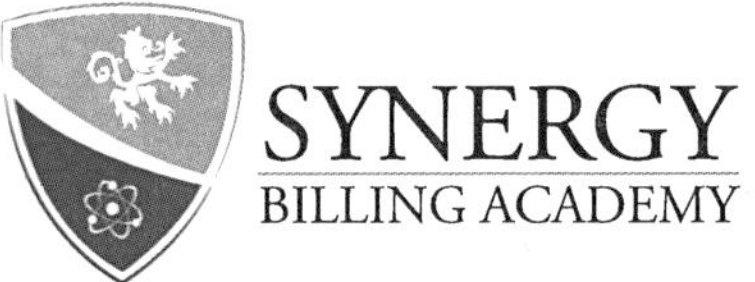

3. **Psychoactive Substance Use**

   As with all other diagnoses, the codes for psychoactive substance use (F10.9-, F11.9-, F12.9-, F13.9-, F14.9-, F15.9-, and F16.9-) should only be assigned based on provider documentation; they should only be used when they meet the definition of a reportable diagnosis (see Section III, Reporting Additional Diagnoses). The codes are to be used only when the psychoactive substance use is associated with a mental or behavioral disorder, and such a relationship is documented by the provider.

Chapter 7 – Guidelines

The NCHS has published chapter-specific guidelines for Chapter 7:

A. Glaucoma
   1. Assigning Glaucoma Codes
   2. Bilateral Glaucoma with Same Type and Stage
   3. Bilateral Glaucoma Stage with Different Types or Stages
   4. Patient Admitted with Glaucoma and Stage Evolves During the Admission
   5. Indeterminate Stage Glaucoma

7. Chapter 7: Diseases of the Eye and Adnexa (H00-H59)

A. Glaucoma

1. **Assigning Glaucoma Codes**

   Assign as many codes from category H40, Glaucoma, as needed to identify the type of glaucoma, the affected eye, and the glaucoma stage.

2. **Bilateral glaucoma with same type and stage**

   When a patient has bilateral glaucoma and both eyes are documented as having the same type and stage and there is a code for bilateral glaucoma, report only the code for the type of glaucoma, bilateral, with the 7th character for the stage.

   When a patient has bilateral glaucoma and both eyes are documented as having the same type and stage and the classification does not provide a code for bilateral

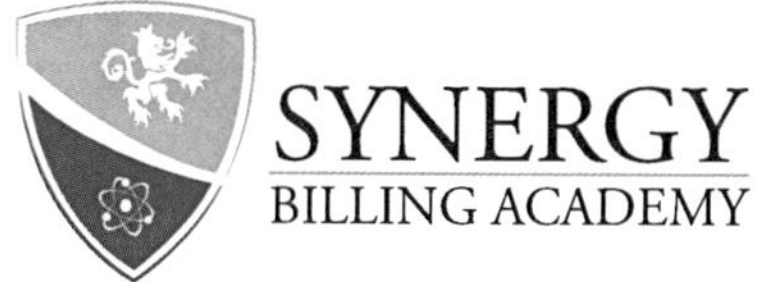

glaucoma (e.g., subcategories H40.10, H40.11, and H40.20), report only one code for the type of glaucoma with the appropriate 7th character for the stage.

3. **Bilateral glaucoma stage with different types or stages**

   When a patient has bilateral glaucoma and each eye is documented as having a different type or stage and the classification distinguishes laterality, assign the appropriate code for each eye rather than the code for bilateral glaucoma.

   When a patient has bilateral glaucoma and each eye is documented as having a different type and the classification does not distinguish laterality (e.g., subcategories H40.10, H40.11, and H40.20), assign one code for each type of glaucoma with the appropriate 7th character for the stage.

   When a patient has bilateral glaucoma and each eye is documented as having the same type, but different stage, and the classification does not distinguish laterality (e.g., subcategories H40.10, H40.11, and H40.20), assign a code for the type of glaucoma for each eye with the 7th character for the specific glaucoma stage documented for each eye.

4. **Patient admitted with glaucoma and stage evolves during the admission**

   If a patient is admitted with glaucoma and the stage progresses during the admission, assign the code for highest stage documented.

5. **Indeterminate stage glaucoma**

   Assignment of the 7th character "4" for "indeterminate stage" should be based on the clinical documentation. The 7th character "4" is used for glaucomas whose stage cannot be clinically determined. This 7th character should not be confused with the 7th character "0," unspecified, which should be assigned only when there is no documentation regarding the stage of the glaucoma.

Chapter 8 – Guidelines

8. Chapter 8: Diseases of the Ear and Mastoid Process (H60-H95)

At this time, there are no chapter-specific guidelines related to related to Chapter 8, Diseases of the Ears and Mastoid Process, but the space is reserved for future expansion.

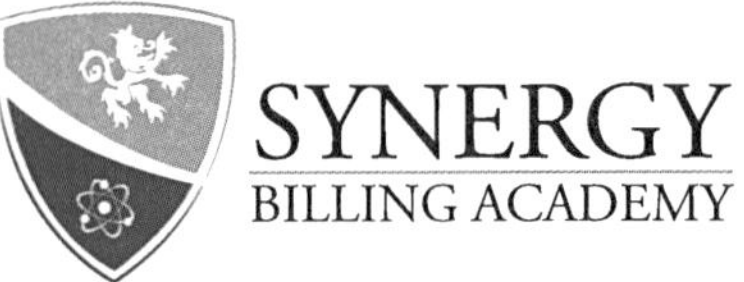

Chapter 9 – Guidelines

The NCHS has published chapter-specific guidelines for Chapter 9 of ICD-10-CM:

A. Hypertension
B. Atherosclerotic Coronary Artery Disease and Angina
C. Intraoperative and Postprocedural Cerebrovascular Accident
D. Sequelae of Cerebrovascular Disease
E. Acute Myocardial Infarction (AMI)

9. Chapter 9: Diseases of the Circulatory System (I00-I99)

A. Hypertension

1. Hypertension with heart disease

Heart conditions classified to I50.- or I51.4–I51.9, are assigned to a code from category I11, Hypertensive heart disease, when a causal relationship is stated (due to hypertension) or implied (hypertensive). Use an additional code from category I50, Heart failure, to identify the type of heart failure in those patients with heart failure. The same heart conditions (I50.- and I51.4–I51.9) with hypertension, but without a stated causal relationship, are coded separately. Sequence according to the circumstances of the admission/encounter.

2. Hypertensive chronic kidney disease

Assign codes from category I12, Hypertensive chronic kidney disease, when both hypertension and a condition classifiable to category N18, Chronic kidney disease (CKD), are present. Unlike hypertension with heart disease, ICD-10-CM presumes a cause-and-effect relationship and classifies chronic kidney disease with hypertension as hypertensive chronic kidney disease.

The appropriate code from category N18 should be used as a secondary code with a code from category I12 to identify the stage of chronic kidney disease.

See Section I.C.14. Chronic kidney disease.

If a patient has hypertensive chronic kidney disease and acute renal failure, an additional code for the acute renal failure is required.

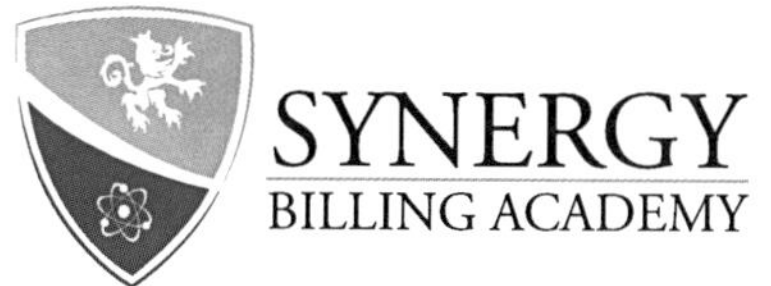

3. **Hypertensive heart and chronic kidney disease**

   Assign codes from combination category I13, Hypertensive heart and chronic kidney disease, when both hypertensive kidney disease and hypertensive heart disease are stated in the diagnosis. Assume a relationship between the hypertension and the chronic kidney disease whether or not the condition is so designated. If heart failure is present, assign an additional code from category I50 to identify the type of heart failure.

   The appropriate code from category N18, Chronic kidney disease, should be used as a secondary code with a code from category I13 to identify the stage of chronic kidney disease.

   See Section I.C.14. Chronic kidney disease.

   The codes in category I13, Hypertensive heart and chronic kidney disease, are combination codes that include hypertension, heart disease, and chronic kidney disease. The Includes note at I13 specifies that the conditions included at I11 and I12 are included together in I13. If a patient has hypertension, heart disease, and chronic kidney disease, then a code from I13 should be used, not individual codes for hypertension, heart disease, and chronic kidney disease or codes from I11 or I12.

   For patients with both acute renal failure and chronic kidney disease, an additional code for acute renal failure is required.

4. **Hypertensive cerebrovascular disease**

   For hypertensive cerebrovascular disease, first assign the appropriate code from categories I60–I69, followed by the appropriate hypertension code.

5. **Hypertensive retinopathy**

   Subcategory H35.0, Background retinopathy and retinal vascular changes, should be used with a code from category I10–I15, Hypertensive disease, to include the systemic hypertension. The sequencing is based on the reason for the encounter.

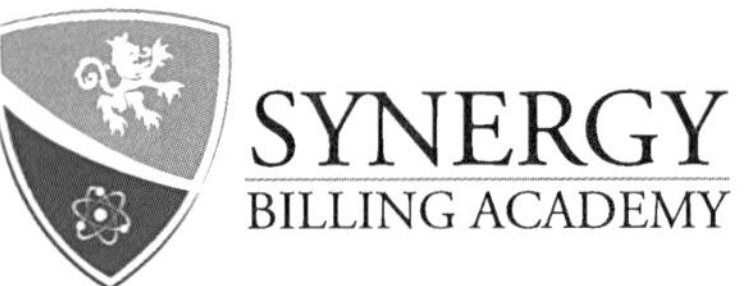

6. **Hypertension, secondary**

   Secondary hypertension is due to an underlying condition. Two codes are required: one to identify the underlying etiology and one from category I15 to identify the hypertension. Sequencing of codes is determined by the reason for admission/encounter.

7. **Hypertension, transient**

   Assign code R03.0, Elevated blood pressure reading without diagnosis of hypertension, unless patient has an established diagnosis of hypertension. Assign code O13.-, Gestational [pregnancy-induced] hypertension without significant proteinuria, or O14.-, Pre-eclampsia, for transient hypertension of pregnancy.

8. **Hypertension, controlled**

   This diagnostic statement usually refers to an existing state of hypertension under control by therapy. Assign the appropriate code from categories I10–I15, Hypertensive diseases.

9. **Hypertension, uncontrolled**

   Uncontrolled hypertension may refer to untreated hypertension or hypertension not responding to current therapeutic regimen. In either case, assign the appropriate code from categories I10–I15, Hypertensive diseases.

B. Atherosclerotic Coronary Artery Disease and Angina

ICD-10-CM has combination codes for atherosclerotic heart disease with angina pectoris. The subcategories for these codes are I25.11, Atherosclerotic heart disease of native coronary artery with angina pectoris, and I25.7, Atherosclerosis of coronary artery bypass graft(s) and coronary artery of transplanted heart with angina pectoris.

When using one of these combination codes, it is not necessary to use an additional code for angina pectoris. A causal relationship can be assumed in a patient with both atherosclerosis and angina pectoris, unless the documentation indicates the angina is due to something other than the atherosclerosis.

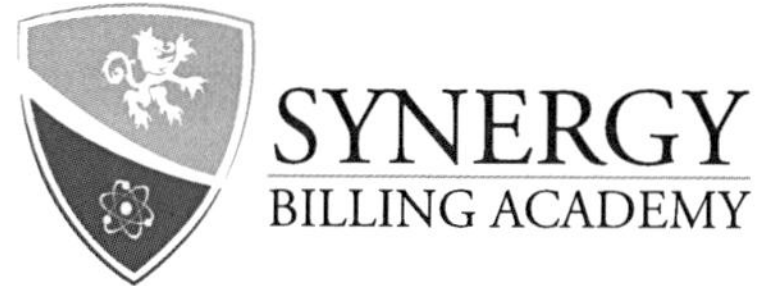

If a patient with coronary artery disease is admitted due to an acute myocardial infarction (AMI), the AMI should be sequenced before the coronary artery disease.

See Section I.C.9. Acute myocardial infarction (AMI).

D. Intraoperative and Postprocedural Cerebrovascular Accident

Medical record documentation should clearly specify the cause-and-effect relationship between the medical intervention and the cerebrovascular accident in order to assign a code for intraoperative or postprocedural cerebrovascular accident.

Proper code assignment depends on whether the accident was an infarction or hemorrhage and whether it occurred intraoperatively or postoperatively. If it was a cerebral hemorrhage, code assignment depends on the type of procedure performed.

D. Sequelae of Cerebrovascular Disease

1. Category I69, Sequelae of cerebrovascular disease

   Category I69 is used to indicate conditions classifiable to categories I60–I67 as the causes of sequela (neurologic deficits) themselves classified elsewhere. These late effects include neurologic deficits that persist after initial onset of conditions classifiable to categories I60–I67. The neurologic deficits caused by cerebrovascular disease may be present from the onset or may arise at any time after the onset of the condition classifiable to categories I60–I67.

   Codes from category I69, Sequelae of cerebrovascular disease, that specify hemiplegia, hemiparesis, and monoplegia identify whether the dominant or nondominant side is affected. Should the affected side be documented, but not specified as dominant or nondominant, and the classification system does not indicate a default, code selection is as follows:

   - For ambidextrous patients, the default should be dominant.
   - If the left side is affected, the default is non-dominant.
   - If the right side is affected, the default is dominant.

2. **Codes from category I69 with codes from I60–I67**

   Codes from category I69 may be assigned on a health care record with codes from

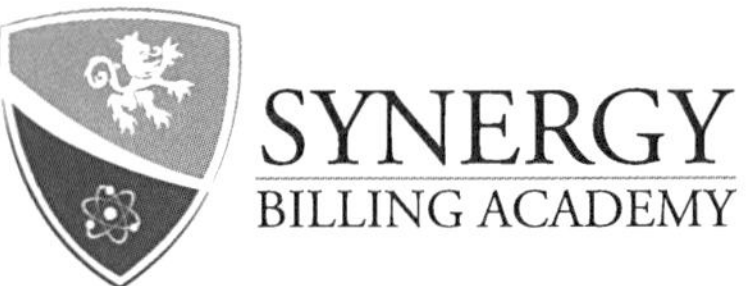

I60–I67 if the patient has a current cerebrovascular disease and deficits from an old cerebrovascular disease.

3. **Codes from category I69 and personal history of transient ischemic attack (TIA) and cerebral infarction (Z86.73)**

   Codes from category I69 should not be assigned if the patient does not have neurologic deficits.

   See Section I.C.21.4. History (of) for use of personal history codes.

E. Acute Myocardial Infarction (AMI)

1. **ST elevation myocardial infarction (STEMI) and non-ST elevation myocardial infarction (NSTEMI)**

   The ICD-10-CM codes for acute myocardial infarction (AMI) identify the site, such as anterolateral wall or true posterior wall. Subcategories I21.0–I21.2 and code I21.3 are used for ST elevation myocardial infarction (STEMI). Code I21.4, Non-ST elevation (NSTEMI) myocardial infarction, is used for non-ST elevation myocardial infarction (NSTEMI) and nontransmural MIs.

   If NSTEMI evolves to STEMI, assign the STEMI code. If STEMI converts to NSTEMI due to thrombolytic therapy, it is still coded as STEMI.

   For encounters occurring while the myocardial infarction is equal to, or less than, four weeks old, including transfers to another acute setting or a postacute setting, and the patient requires continued care for the myocardial infarction, codes from category I21 may continue to be reported. For encounters after the four-week time frame, if the patient is still receiving care related to the myocardial infarction, the appropriate aftercare code should be assigned, rather than a code from category I21. For old or healed myocardial infarctions not requiring further care, code I25.2, Old myocardial infarction, may be assigned.

2. **Acute myocardial infarction, unspecified**

   Code I21.3, ST elevation (STEMI) myocardial infarction of unspecified site, is the default for unspecified acute myocardial infarction. If only STEMI or transmural MI without the site is documented, assign code I21.3.

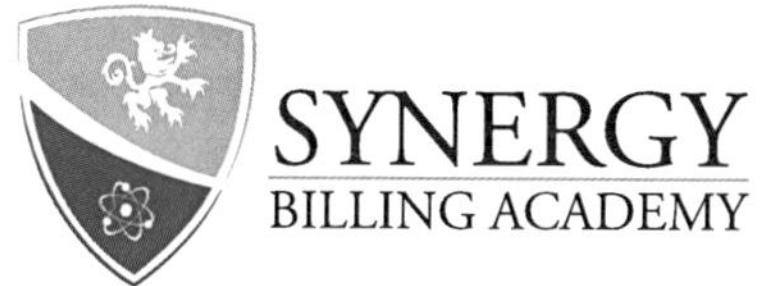

3. **AMI documented as nontransmural or subendocardial but site provided**

   If an AMI is documented as nontransmural or subendocardial, but the site is provided, it is still coded as a subendocardial AMI.

   See Section I.C.21.3 for information on coding status post administration of tPA in a different facility within the last 24 hours.

4. **Subsequent acute myocardial infarction**

   A code from category I22, Subsequent ST elevation (STEMI) and non-ST elevation (NSTEMI) myocardial infarction, is to be used when a patient who has suffered an AMI has a new AMI within the four-week time frame of the initial AMI. A code from category I22 must be used in conjunction with a code from category I21. The sequencing of the I22 and I21 codes depends on the circumstances of the encounter.

Chapter 10 – Guidelines

Guidelines for code usage may also be category-specific. Under ICD-10-CM category J10, Influenza, is a note to use an additional code to identify the virus. No such note appears under the ICD-9-CM category (487) for this same condition.

The NCHS has published chapter-specific guidelines for Chapter 10 of ICD-10-CM:

A. Chronic Obstructive Pulmonary Disease [COPD] and Asthma
B. Acute Respiratory Failure
C. Influenza Due to Certain Identified Influenza Viruses
D. Ventilator-Associated Pneumonia

10. Chapter 10: Diseases of the Respiratory System (J00-J99)

A. Chronic Obstructive Pulmonary Disease [COPD] and Asthma

1. **Acute exacerbation of chronic obstructive bronchitis and asthma**

   The codes in categories J44 and J45 distinguish between uncomplicated cases and those in acute exacerbation. An acute exacerbation is a worsening or decompensation of a chronic condition. An acute exacerbation is not equivalent to an infection superimposed on a chronic condition, though an exacerbation may be triggered by an infection.

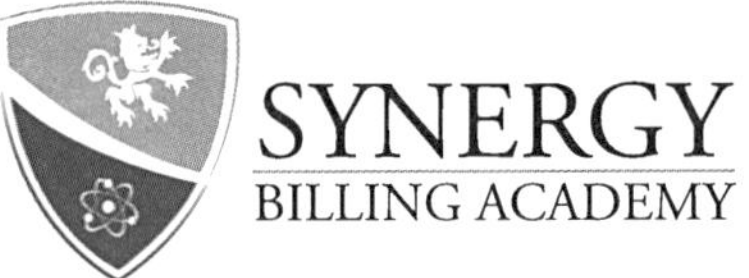

B. Acute Respiratory Failure

1. Acute respiratory failure as principal diagnosis

A code from subcategory J96.0, Acute respiratory failure, or subcategory J96.2, Acute and chronic respiratory failure, may be assigned as a principal diagnosis when it is the condition established after study to be chiefly responsible for occasioning the admission to the hospital, and the selection is supported by the Alphabetic Index and Tabular List. However, chapter-specific coding guidelines (such as obstetrics, poisoning, HIV, newborn) that provide sequencing direction take precedence.

2. Acute respiratory failure as secondary diagnosis

Respiratory failure may be listed as a secondary diagnosis if it occurs after admission, or if it is present on admission but does not meet the definition of principal diagnosis.

3. Sequencing of acute respiratory failure and another acute condition

When a patient is admitted with respiratory failure and another acute condition, (e.g., myocardial infarction, cerebrovascular accident, aspiration pneumonia), the principal diagnosis will not be the same in every situation. This applies whether the other acute condition is a respiratory or nonrespiratory condition. Selection of the principal diagnosis will be dependent on the circumstances of admission. If both the respiratory failure and the other acute condition are equally responsible for occasioning the admission to the hospital and there are no chapter-specific sequencing rules, the guideline regarding two or more diagnoses that equally meet the definition for principal diagnosis (Section II, C.) may be applied.

If the documentation is not clear as to whether acute respiratory failure and another condition are equally responsible for occasioning the admission, query the provider for clarification.

C. Influenza Due to Certain Identified Influenza Viruses

Code only confirmed cases of influenza due to certain identified influenza viruses (category J09), and due to other identified influenza virus (category J10). This is an exception to the hospital inpatient guideline Section II, H. (Uncertain Diagnosis).

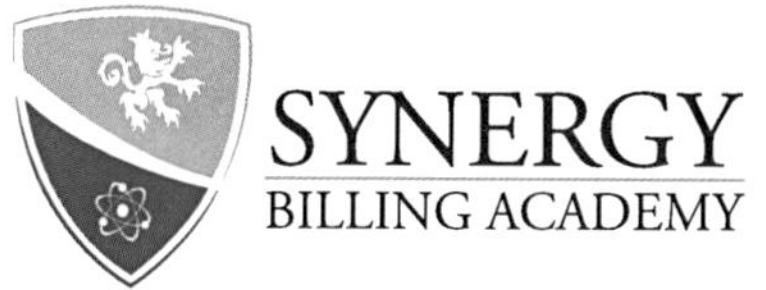

In this context, "confirmation" does not require documentation of positive laboratory testing specific for avian or other novel influenza A or other identified influenza virus. However, coding should be based on the provider's diagnostic statement that the patient has avian influenza or other novel influenza A, for category J09, or has another particular identified strain of influenza, such as H1N1 or H3N2, but not identified as novel or variant, for category J10.

If the provider records "suspected," "possible," or "probable" avian influenza, or novel influenza or other identified influenza, then the appropriate influenza code from category J11, Influenza due to unidentified influenza virus, should be assigned. A code from category J09, Influenza due to certain identified influenza viruses, should not be assigned, nor should a code from category J10, Influenza due to other identified influenza virus.

D. Ventilator-Associated Pneumonia

1. Documentation of ventilator-associated pneumonia

As with all procedural or postprocedural complications, code assignment is based on the provider's documentation of the relationship between the condition and the procedure.

Code J95.851, Ventilator-associated pneumonia, should be assigned only when the provider has documented ventilator-associated pneumonia (VAP). An additional code to identify the organism (e.g., *Pseudomonas aeruginosa*, code B96.5) should also be assigned. Do not assign an additional code from categories J12–J18 to identify the type of pneumonia.

Code J95.851 should not be assigned for cases where the patient has pneumonia and is on a mechanical ventilator and the provider has not specifically stated that the pneumonia is ventilator-associated pneumonia. If the documentation is unclear as to whether the patient has a pneumonia that is a complication attributable to the mechanical ventilator, query the provider.

2. Ventilator-associated pneumonia develops after admission

A patient may be admitted with one type of pneumonia (e.g., code J13, Pneumonia due to Streptococcus pneumonia) and subsequently develop VAP. In this instance, the principal diagnosis would be the appropriate code from categories J12–J18 for the

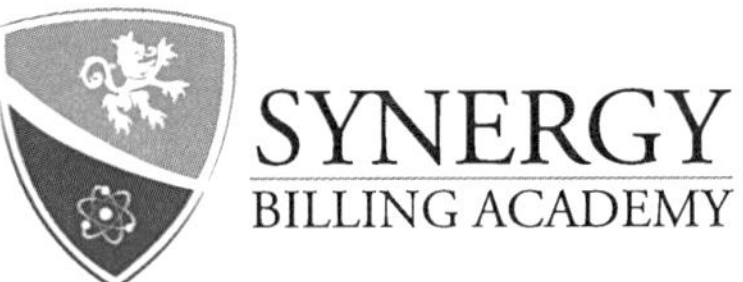

pneumonia diagnosed at the time of admission. Code J95.851, Ventilator-associated pneumonia, would be assigned as an additional diagnosis when the provider has also documented the presence of ventilator-associated pneumonia.

Chapter 11 – Guidelines

Guideline modifications were made to specific codes in this chapter.

No instructional notes are found at the start of the subchapter for hernias in ICD-9-CM. However, this is not the case in ICD-10-CM. The note "Hernia with both gangrene and obstruction is classified to hernia with gangrene" applies to all conditions coded to categories K40-K46.

11. Chapter 11: Diseases of the Digestive System (K00-K95)

Reserved for future guideline expansion.

Chapter 13 – Guidelines

The NCHS has published chapter-specific guidelines for Chapter 13 of ICD-10-CM:

A. Site and Laterality
B. Acute Traumatic Versus Chronic or Recurrent Musculoskeletal Conditions
C. Coding of Pathologic Fractures
D. Osteoporosis

Chapter 13: Diseases of the Musculoskeletal System and Connective Tissue (M00-M99)

A. Site and Laterality

Most of the codes within Chapter 13 have site and laterality designations. The site represents the bone, joint, or the muscle involved. For some conditions where more than one bone, joint, or muscle is usually involved, such as osteoarthritis, there is a "multiple sites" code available. For categories where no multiple site code is provided and more than one bone, joint, or muscle is involved, multiple codes should be used to indicate the different sites involved.

1. Bone versus joint

For certain conditions, the bone may be affected at the upper or lower end, (e.g., M87,

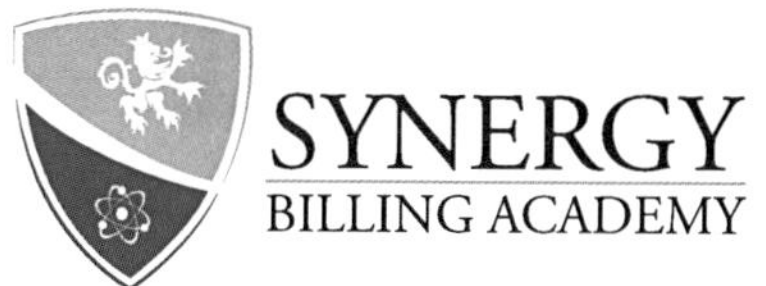

Avascular necrosis of bone, or M80 or M81, Osteoporosis). Though the portion of the bone affected may be at the joint, the site designation will be the bone, not the joint.

B. Acute traumatic versus chronic or recurrent musculoskeletal conditions

Many musculoskeletal conditions are a result of previous injury or trauma to a site, or are recurrent conditions. Bone, joint, or muscle conditions that are the result of a healed injury are usually found in Chapter 13. Recurrent bone, joint, or muscle conditions are also usually found in Chapter 13. Any current, acute injury should be coded with the appropriate injury code from Chapter 19. Chronic or recurrent conditions should generally be coded with a code from Chapter 13. If it is difficult to determine from the documentation in the record which code is best to describe a condition, query the provider.

C. Coding of Pathologic Fractures

The 7th character "A" is for use as long as the patient is receiving active treatment for the fracture. Examples of active treatment are: surgical treatment, emergency department encounter, or evaluation and treatment by a new physician. The 7th character "D" is to be used for encounters after the patient has completed active treatment. The other 7th characters, listed under each subcategory in the Tabular List, are to be used for subsequent encounters for the treatment of problems associated with healing, such as malunions, nonunions, and sequelae.

Care for complications of surgical treatment for fracture repairs during the healing or recovery phase should be coded with the appropriate complication codes.

See Section I.C.19. Coding of traumatic fractures.

D. Osteoporosis

Osteoporosis is a systemic condition, meaning that all bones of the musculoskeletal system are affected. Therefore, site is not a component of the codes under category M81, Osteoporosis without current pathological fracture. The site codes under category M80, Osteoporosis with current pathological fracture, identify the site of the fracture, not the osteoporosis.

1. Osteoporosis without pathological fracture

Category M81, Osteoporosis without current pathological fracture, is for use for patients with osteoporosis who do not currently have a pathological fracture due to

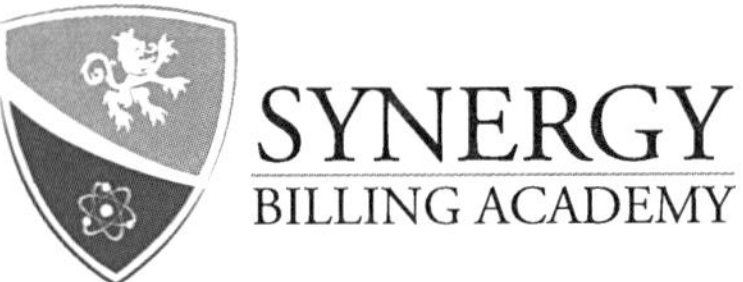

the osteoporosis, even if they have had a fracture in the past. For patients with a history of osteoporosis fractures, status code Z87.310, Personal history of (healed) osteoporosis fracture, should follow the code from M81.

2) **Osteoporosis with current pathological fracture**

Category M80, Osteoporosis with current pathological fracture, is for patients who have a current pathological fracture at the time of an encounter. The codes under M80 identify the site of the fracture. A code from category M80, not a traumatic fracture code, should be used for any patient with known osteoporosis who suffers a fracture, even if the patient had a minor fall or trauma, if that fall or trauma would not usually break a normal, healthy bone.

Chapter 14 - Guidelines

Several notes have been made available to indicate that additional codes are needed and should be used in Chapter 14.

- N17, Acute kidney failure: Code also associated underlying condition
- N18, Chronic kidney disease (CKD): Code first any associated:
  - Diabetic chronic kidney disease (E08.22, E09.22, E10.22, E11.22, E13.22)
  - Hypertensive chronic kidney disease (I12.-, I13.-)
  - Use additional code to identify kidney transplant status, if applicable (Z94.0)
- N30, Cystitis: Use additional code to identify infectious agents (B95-B97)
- N31, Neuromuscular dysfunction of bladder, NEC: Use additional code to identify any associated urinary incontinence (N39.3–N39.4-)
- N33, Bladder disorders in diseases classified elsewhere: Code first underlying disease, such as schistosomiasis (B65.0–B6.9)
- N40.1, Enlarged prostate with lower urinary tract symptoms (LUTS): Use additional code for associated symptoms, when specified:
  - Incomplete bladder emptying (R39.14)
  - Nocturia (R35.1)
  - Straining on urination (R39.16)
  - Urinary frequency (R35.0)
  - Urinary hesitancy (R39.11)
  - Urinary incontinence (N39.1-)
  - Urinary obstruction (N13.8)
  - Urinary retention (R33.8)

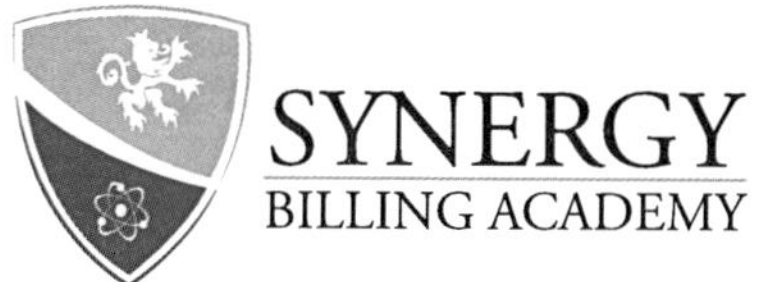

- Urinary urgency (R39.15)
- Weak urinary stream (R39.12)

The NCHS has published chapter-specific guidelines for Chapter 14 of ICD-10-CM:

A. Chronic Kidney Disease
    1. Stages of chronic kidney disease (CKD)
    2. Chronic kidney disease and kidney transplant status
    3. Chronic kidney disease with other conditions

Chapter 14: Diseases of Genitourinary System (N00-N99)

A. Chronic kidney disease

1. Stages of chronic Kidney Disease (CKD)

The ICD-10-CM classifies CKD based on severity. The severity of CKD is designated by stages 1–5. Stage 2, code N18.2, equates to mild CKD; stage 3, code N18.3, equates to moderate CKD; and stage 4, code N18.4, equates to severe CKD. Code N18.6, End-stage renal disease (ESRD), is assigned when the provider has documented end-stage renal disease (ESRD).

If both a stage of CKD and ESRD are documented, assign code N18.6 only.

2. Chronic kidney disease and kidney transplant status

Patients who have undergone a kidney transplant may still have some form of chronic kidney disease (CKD) because the kidney transplant may not fully restore kidney function. Therefore, the presence of CKD alone does not constitute a transplant complication. Assign the appropriate N18 code for the patient's stage of CKD and code Z94.0, Kidney transplant status. If a transplant complication such as failure or rejection or other transplant complication is documented, see section I.C.19.g for information on coding complications of a kidney transplant. If the documentation is unclear as to whether the patient has a complication of the transplant, query the provider.

3. Chronic kidney disease with other conditions

Patients with CKD may also suffer from other serious conditions, most commonly diabetes mellitus and hypertension. The sequencing of the CKD code in relationship

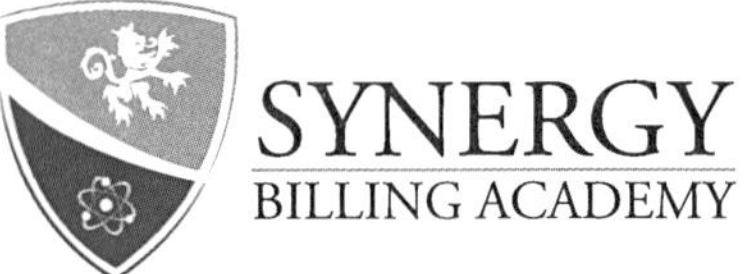

to codes for other contributing conditions is based on the conventions in the Tabular List.

See I.C.9. Hypertensive chronic kidney disease.

See I.C.19. Chronic kidney disease and kidney transplant complications.

Chapter 15 - Guidelines

The NCHS has published chapter-specific guidelines for this chapter:

A. General Rules for Obstetric Cases
B. Selection of OB Principal or First-Listed Diagnosis
C. Pre-Existing Conditions Versus Conditions Due to the Pregnancy
D. Pre-Existing Hypertension in Pregnancy
E. Fetal Conditions Affecting the Management of the Mother
F. HIV Infection in Pregnancy, Childbirth, and the Puerperium
G. Diabetes Mellitus in Pregnancy
H. Long-Term Use of Insulin
I. Gestational (Pregnancy Induced) Diabetes
J. Sepsis and Septic Shock Complicating Abortion, Pregnancy, Childbirth, and the Puerperium
K. Puerperal Sepsis
L. Alcohol and Tobacco Use During Pregnancy, Childbirth, and the Puerperium
M. Poisoning, Toxic Effects, Adverse Effects, and Underdosing in a Pregnant Patient
N. Code O80, Normal Delivery
O. The Peripartum and Postpartum Periods
P. Code O94, Sequelae of Complication of Pregnancy, Childbirth, and the Puerperium
Q. Termination of Pregnancy and Spontaneous Abortions
R. Abuse in a Pregnant Patient

A. General Rules for Obstetric Cases

1. Codes from Chapter 15 and sequencing priority

Obstetric cases require codes from Chapter 15, codes in the range O00-O9A, Pregnancy, Childbirth, and the Puerperium. Chapter 15 codes have sequencing priority over codes from other chapters. Additional codes from other chapters may be

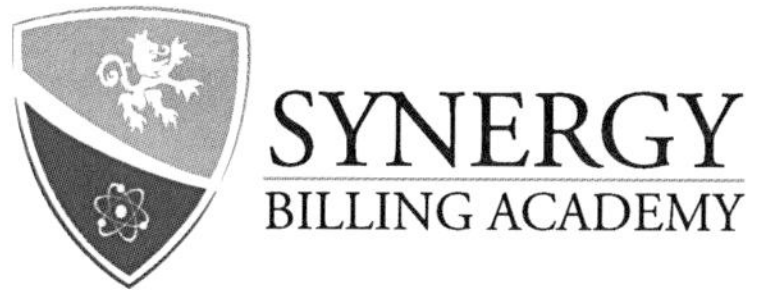

used in conjunction with Chapter 15 codes to further specify conditions. Should the provider document that the pregnancy is incidental to the encounter, then code Z33.1, Pregnant state, incidental, should be used in place of any Chapter 15 codes. It is the provider's responsibility to state that the condition being treated is not affecting the pregnancy.

2. **Chapter 15 codes used only on the maternal record**

   Chapter 15 codes are to be used only on the maternal record, never on the record of the newborn.

3. **Final character for trimester**

   The majority of codes in Chapter 15 have a final character indicating the trimester of pregnancy. The time frames for the trimesters are indicated at the beginning of the chapter. If trimester is not a component of a code, it is because the condition always occurs in a specific trimester, or the concept of trimester of pregnancy is not applicable. Certain codes have characters for only certain trimesters, because the condition does not occur in all trimesters, but it may occur in more than just one.

   Assignment of the final character for trimester should be based on the provider's documentation of the trimester (or number of weeks) for the current admission/ encounter. This applies to the assignment of trimester for pre-existing conditions as well as those that develop during or are due to the pregnancy. The provider's documentation of the number of weeks may be used to assign the appropriate code identifying the trimester.

   Whenever delivery occurs during the current admission and there is an "in childbirth" option for the obstetric complication being coded, the "in childbirth" code should be assigned.

4. **Selection of trimester for inpatient admissions that encompass more than one trimester**

   In instances when a patient is admitted to a hospital for complications of pregnancy during one trimester and remains in the hospital into a subsequent trimester, the trimester character for the antepartum complication code should be assigned based on the trimester when the complication developed, not the trimester of the discharge.

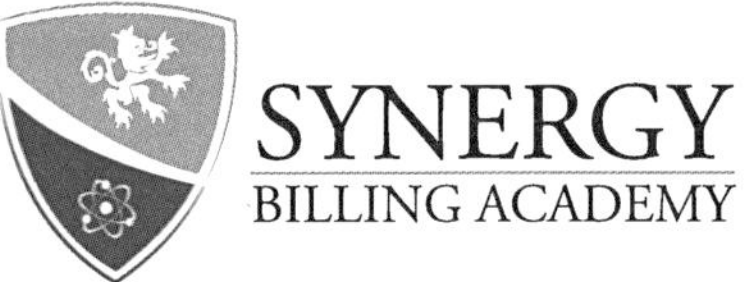

If the condition developed prior to the current admission/encounter or represents a pre-existing condition, the trimester character for the trimester at the time of the admission/encounter should be assigned.

5. **Unspecified trimester**

   Each category that includes codes for trimester has a code for "unspecified trimester." The "unspecified trimester" code should rarely be used, such as when the documentation in the record is insufficient to determine the trimester and it is not possible to obtain clarification.

6. **7th character for fetus identification**

   Where applicable, a 7th character is to be assigned for certain categories (i.e., O31, O32, O33.3 - O33.6, O35, O36, O40, O41, O60.1, O60.2, O64, and O69) to identify the fetus for which the complication code applies.

   Assign 7th character "0":

   - For single gestations
   - When the documentation in the record is insufficient to determine the fetus affected and it is not possible to obtain clarification.
   - When it is not possible to clinically determine which fetus is affected.

B. Selection of OB Principal or First-Listed Diagnosis

1. **Routine outpatient prenatal visits**

   For routine outpatient prenatal visits when no complications are present, a code from category Z34, Encounter for supervision of normal pregnancy, should be used as the first-listed diagnosis. These codes should not be used in conjunction with Chapter 15 codes.

2. **Prenatal outpatient visits for high-risk patients**

   For routine prenatal outpatient visits for patients with high-risk pregnancies, a code from category O09, Supervision of high-risk pregnancy, should be used as the first-listed diagnosis. Secondary Chapter 15 codes may be used in conjunction with these codes if appropriate.

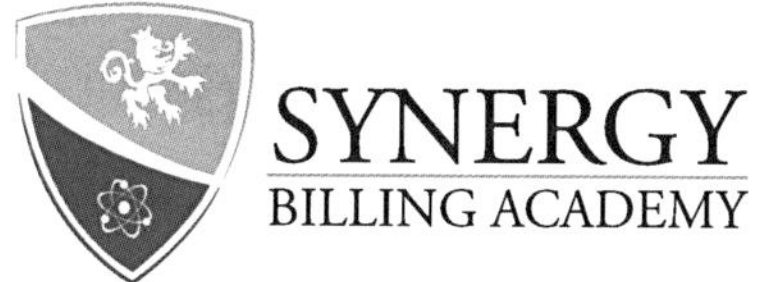

3. **Episodes when no delivery occurs**

   In episodes when no delivery occurs, the principal diagnosis should correspond to the principal complication of the pregnancy which necessitated the encounter. Should more than one complication exist, all of which are treated or monitored, any of the complication codes may be sequenced first.

4. **When a delivery occurs**

   When a delivery occurs, the principal diagnosis should correspond to the main circumstances or complication of the delivery. In cases of cesarean delivery, the principal diagnosis should be the condition established after study that was responsible for the patient's admission. If the patient was admitted with a condition that resulted in performing a cesarean procedure, that condition should be selected as the principal diagnosis. If the reason for the admission/encounter was unrelated to the condition resulting in the cesarean delivery, the condition related to the reason for the admission/ encounter should be selected as the principal diagnosis.

5. **Outcome of delivery**

   A code from category Z37, Outcome of delivery, should be included on every maternal record when a delivery has occurred. These codes are not to be used on subsequent records or on the newborn's record.

c. **Pre-Existing Conditions Versus Conditions Due to the Pregnancy**

Certain categories in Chapter 15 distinguish between conditions of the mother that existed prior to pregnancy (pre-existing) and those that are a direct result of pregnancy. When assigning codes from Chapter 15, it is important to assess if a condition was pre-existing prior to pregnancy or developed during or due to the pregnancy in order to assign the correct code.

Categories that do not distinguish between pre-existing and pregnancy-related conditions may be used for either. It is acceptable to use codes specifically for the puerperium with codes complicating pregnancy and childbirth if a condition arises postpartum during the delivery encounter.

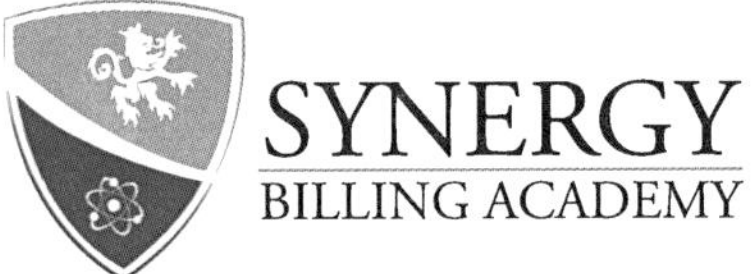

D. **Pre-Existing Hypertension in Pregnancy**

Category O10, Pre-existing hypertension complicating pregnancy, childbirth, and the puerperium, includes codes for hypertensive heart and hypertensive chronic kidney disease. When assigning one of the O10 codes that includes hypertensive heart disease or hypertensive chronic kidney disease, it is necessary to add a secondary code from the appropriate hypertension category to specify the type of heart failure or chronic kidney disease.

See Section I.C.9. Hypertension.

E. **Fetal Conditions Affecting the Management of the Mother**

1. **Codes from categories O35 and O36**

Codes from categories O35, Maternal care for known or suspected fetal abnormality and damage, and O36, Maternal care for other fetal problems, are assigned only when the fetal condition is actually responsible for modifying the management of the mother, such as by requiring diagnostic studies, additional observation, special care, or termination of pregnancy. The fact that the fetal condition exists does not justify assigning a code from this series to the mother's record.

2. **In utero surgery**

In cases when surgery is performed on the fetus, a diagnosis code from category O35, Maternal care for known or suspected fetal abnormality and damage, should be assigned identifying the fetal condition. Assign the appropriate procedure code for the procedure performed.

No code from Chapter 16, the perinatal codes, should be used on the mother's record to identify fetal conditions. Surgery performed in utero on a fetus is still to be coded as an obstetric encounter.

F. **HIV Infection in Pregnancy, Childbirth, and the Puerperium**

During pregnancy, childbirth, or the puerperium, a patient admitted because of an HIV-related illness should receive a principal diagnosis from subcategory O98.7-, Human immunodeficiency [HIV] disease complicating pregnancy, childbirth, and the puerperium, followed by the code(s) for the HIV-related illness(es).

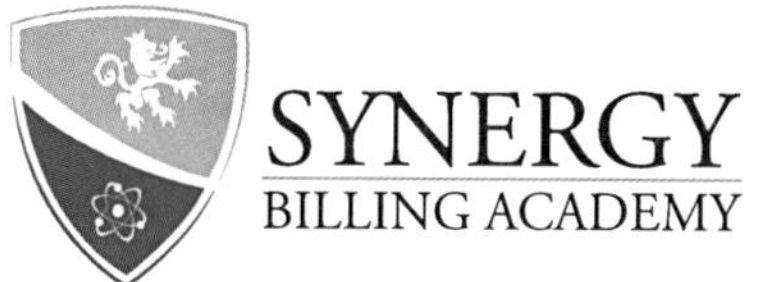

Patients with asymptomatic HIV infection status admitted during pregnancy, childbirth, or the puerperium should receive codes of O98.7- and Z21, Asymptomatic human immunodeficiency virus [HIV] infection status.

G. Diabetes Mellitus in Pregnancy

Diabetes mellitus is a significant complicating factor in pregnancy. Pregnant women who are diabetic should be assigned a code from category O24, Diabetes mellitus in pregnancy, childbirth, and the puerperium, first, followed by the appropriate diabetes code(s) (E08-E13) from Chapter 4.

H. Long-Term Use of Insulin

Code Z79.4, Long-term (current) use of insulin, should also be assigned if the diabetes mellitus is being treated with insulin.

I. Gestational (Pregnancy-Induced) Diabetes

Gestational (pregnancy induced) diabetes can occur during the second and third trimesters of pregnancy in women who were not diabetic prior to pregnancy. Gestational diabetes can cause complications in the pregnancy similar to those of pre-existing diabetes mellitus. It also puts the woman at greater risk of developing diabetes after the pregnancy. Codes for gestational diabetes are in subcategory O24.4, Gestational diabetes mellitus. No other code from category O24, Diabetes mellitus in pregnancy, childbirth, and the puerperium, should be used with a code from O24.4.

The codes under subcategory O24.4 include diet-controlled and insulin-controlled. If a patient with gestational diabetes is treated with both diet and insulin, only the code for insulin-controlled is required.

Code Z79.4, Long-term (current) use of insulin, should not be assigned with codes from subcategory O24.4.

An abnormal glucose tolerance in pregnancy is assigned a code from subcategory O99.81, Abnormal glucose complicating pregnancy, childbirth, and the puerperium.

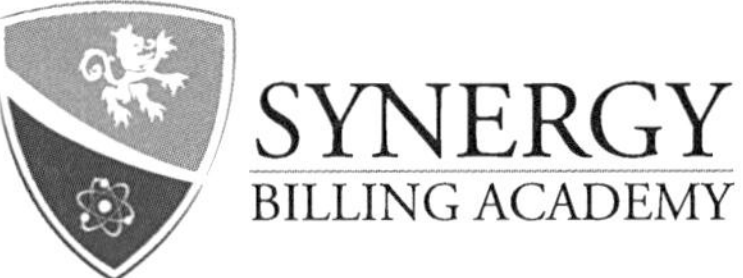

J. **Sepsis and Septic Shock Complicating Abortion, Pregnancy, Childbirth, and the Puerperium**

When assigning a Chapter 15 code for sepsis complicating abortion, pregnancy, childbirth, and the puerperium, a code for the specific type of infection should be assigned as an additional diagnosis. If severe sepsis is present, a code from subcategory R65.2, Severe sepsis, and code(s) for associated organ dysfunction(s) should also be assigned as additional diagnoses.

K. **Puerperal Sepsis**

Code O85, Puerperal sepsis, should be assigned with a secondary code to identify the causal organism (e.g., for a bacterial infection, assign a code from category B95-B96, Bacterial infections in conditions classified elsewhere). A code from category A40, Streptococcal sepsis, or A41, Other sepsis, should not be used for puerperal sepsis. If applicable, use additional codes to identify severe sepsis (R65.2-) and any associated acute organ dysfunction.

L. **Alcohol and Tobacco Use During Pregnancy, Childbirth, and the Puerperium**

1. **Alcohol use during pregnancy, childbirth, and the puerperium**

   Codes under subcategory O99.31, Alcohol use complicating pregnancy, childbirth, and the puerperium, should be assigned for any pregnancy case when a mother uses alcohol during the pregnancy or postpartum. A secondary code from category F10, Alcohol-related disorders, should also be assigned to identify manifestations of the alcohol use.

2. **Tobacco use during pregnancy, childbirth and the puerperium**

   Codes under subcategory O99.33, Smoking (tobacco) complicating pregnancy, childbirth, and the puerperium, should be assigned for any pregnancy case when a mother uses any type of tobacco product during the pregnancy or postpartum. A secondary code from category F17, Nicotine dependence, should also be assigned to identify the type of nicotine dependence.

M. **Poisoning, Toxic Effects, Adverse Effects, and Underdosing in a Pregnant Patient**

A code from subcategory O9A.2, Injury, poisoning, and certain other consequences of external causes complicating pregnancy, childbirth, and the puerperium, should be sequenced first,

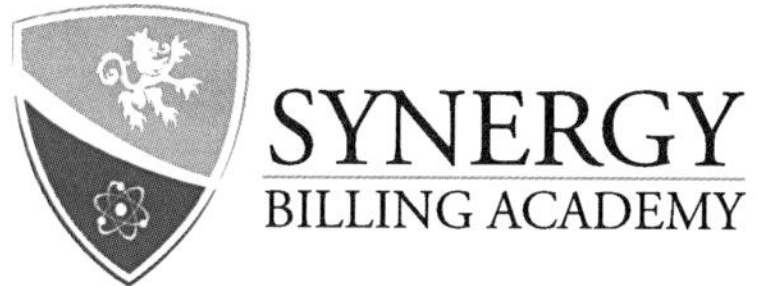

followed by the appropriate injury, poisoning, toxic effect, adverse effect, or underdosing code, and then the additional code(s) that specifies the condition caused by the poisoning, toxic effect, adverse effect, or underdosing.

See Section I.C.19. Adverse effects, poisoning, underdosing, and toxic effects.

N. Code O80, Normal Delivery

1. Encounter for full-term uncomplicated delivery

Code O80 should be assigned when a woman is admitted for a full-term normal delivery and delivers a single, healthy infant without any complications antepartum, during the delivery, or postpartum during the delivery episode. Code O80 is always a principal diagnosis. It is not to be used if any other code from Chapter 15 is needed to describe a current complication of the antenatal, delivery, or perinatal period. Additional codes from other chapters may be used with code O80 if they are not related to or are in any way complicating the pregnancy.

2. Uncomplicated delivery with resolved antepartum complication

Code O80 may be used if the patient had a complication at some point during the pregnancy, but the complication is not present at the time of the admission for delivery.

3. Outcome of delivery for O80

Z37.0, Single live birth, is the only outcome of delivery code appropriate for use with O80.

O. The Peripartum and Postpartum Periods

1. Peripartum and postpartum periods

The postpartum period begins immediately after delivery and continues for six weeks. The peripartum period is defined as the last month of pregnancy to five months postpartum.

2. Peripartum and postpartum complication

A postpartum complication is any complication occurring within the six-week period after the birth.

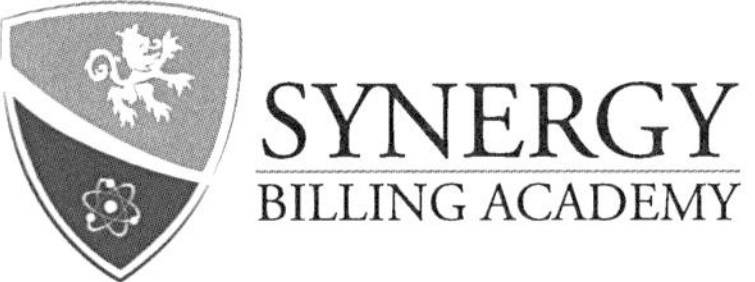

3. **Pregnancy-related complications after six-week period**

   Chapter 15 codes may also be used to describe pregnancy-related complications after the peripartum or postpartum period if the provider documents that a condition is pregnancy related.

4. **Admission for routine postpartum care following delivery outside hospital**

   When the mother delivers outside the hospital prior to admission and is admitted for routine postpartum care and no complications are noted, code Z39.0, Encounter for care and examination of mother immediately after delivery, should be assigned as the principal diagnosis.

5. **Pregnancy-associated cardiomyopathy**

   Pregnancy-associated cardiomyopathy, code O90.3, is unique in that it may be diagnosed in the third trimester of pregnancy but may continue to progress months after delivery. For this reason, it is referred to as peripartum cardiomyopathy. Code O90.3 is only for use when the cardiomyopathy develops as a result of pregnancy in a woman who did not have pre-existing heart disease.

P. Code O94, Sequelae of Complications of Pregnancy, Childbirth, and the Puerperium

1. **Code O94**

   Code O94, Sequelae of complication of pregnancy, childbirth, and the puerperium, is for use in those cases when an initial complication of a pregnancy develops sequelae requiring care or treatment at a future date.

2. **After the initial postpartum period**

   This code may be used at any time after the initial postpartum period.

3. **Sequencing of code O94**

   This code, like all sequela codes, is to be sequenced following the code describing the sequelae of the complication.

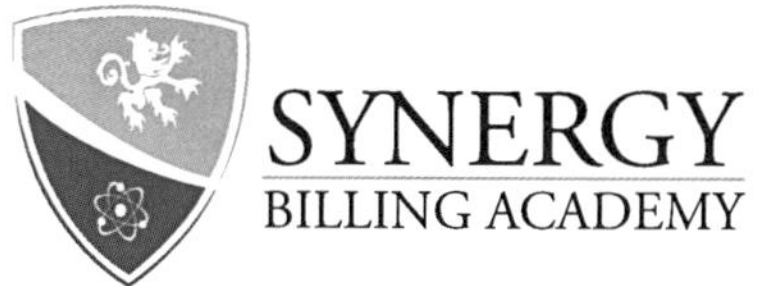

Q. Termination of Pregnancy and Spontaneous Abortions

1. Abortion with liveborn fetus

When an attempted termination of pregnancy results in a liveborn fetus, assign code Z33.2, Encounter for elective termination of pregnancy, and a code from category Z37, Outcome of Delivery.

2. Retained products of conception following an abortion

Subsequent encounters for retained products of conception following a spontaneous abortion or elective termination of pregnancy are assigned the appropriate code from category O03, Spontaneous abortion, or codes O07.4, Failed attempted termination of pregnancy without complication, and Z33.2, Encounter for elective termination of pregnancy. This coding is appropriate even when the patient was discharged previously with a discharge diagnosis of complete abortion.

3. Complications leading to abortion

Codes from Chapter 15 may be used as additional codes to identify any documented complications of the pregnancy in conjunction with codes in categories O07 and O08.

R. Abuse of a Pregnant Patient

For suspected or confirmed cases of abuse of a pregnant patient, a code from subcategories O9A.3, Physical abuse complicating pregnancy, childbirth, and the puerperium; O9A.4, Sexual abuse complicating pregnancy, childbirth, and the puerperium; or O9A.5, Psychological abuse complicating pregnancy, childbirth, and the puerperium, should be sequenced first, followed by the appropriate codes (if applicable) to identify any associated current injury due to physical abuse, sexual abuse, as well the perpetrator of abuse.

See Section I.C.19. Adult and child abuse, neglect, and other maltreatment.

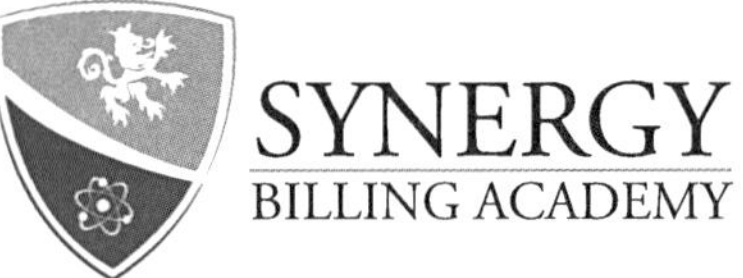

Chapter 16 - Guidelines

The NCHS has published chapter-specific guidelines for this chapter:

A. General Perinatal Rules
B. Observation and Evaluation of Newborns for Suspected Conditions Not Found
C. Coding Additional Perinatal Diagnoses
D. Prematurity and Fetal Growth Retardation
E. Low Birth Weight and Immaturity Status
F. Bacterial Sepsis of Newborn
G. Stillbirth

Chapter 16: Certain Conditions Originating in the Perinatal Period (P00-P96)

For coding and reporting purposes, the perinatal period is defined as before birth through the 28th day following birth. The following guidelines are provided for reporting purposes.

A. General Perinatal Rules

1. Use of Chapter 16 codes

Codes in this chapter are never for use on the maternal record. Codes from Chapter 15, the obstetric chapter, are never permitted on the newborn record. Chapter 16 codes may be used throughout the life of the patient if the condition is still present.

2. Principal diagnosis for birth record

When coding the birth episode in a newborn's record, assign a code from category Z38, Liveborn infants according to place of birth and type of delivery, as the principal diagnosis. A code from category Z38 is assigned only once, to a newborn at the time of birth. If a newborn is transferred to another institution, a code from category Z38 should not be used at the receiving hospital.

A code from category Z38 is used only on the newborn record, not on the mother's record.

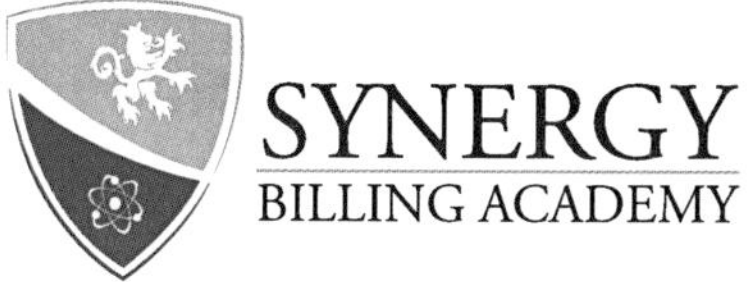

3. **Use of codes from other chapters with codes from Chapter 16**

   Codes from other chapters may be used with codes from Chapter 16 if the codes from the other chapters provide more specific detail. Codes for signs and symptoms may be assigned when a definitive diagnosis has not been established. If the reason for the encounter is a perinatal condition, the code from Chapter 16 should be sequenced first.

4. **Use of Chapter 16 codes after the perinatal period**

   Should a condition originate in the perinatal period and continue throughout the life of the patient, the perinatal code should continue to be used regardless of the patient's age.

5. **Birth process or community-acquired conditions**

   If a newborn has a condition that may be either due to the birth process or community-acquired and the documentation does not indicate which, the default is due to the birth process and the code from Chapter 16 should be used. If the condition is community-acquired, a code from Chapter 16 should not be assigned.

6. **Code all clinically significant conditions**

   All clinically significant conditions noted on routine newborn examination should be coded. A condition is clinically significant if it requires:

   - clinical evaluation; or
   - therapeutic treatment; or
   - diagnostic procedures; or
   - extended length of hospital stay; or
   - increased nursing care and/or monitoring; or
   - has implications for future health care needs.

   Note: The perinatal guidelines listed above are the same as the general coding guidelines for "additional diagnoses," except for the final point regarding implications for future health care needs. Codes should be assigned for conditions that have been specified by the provider as having implications for future health care needs.

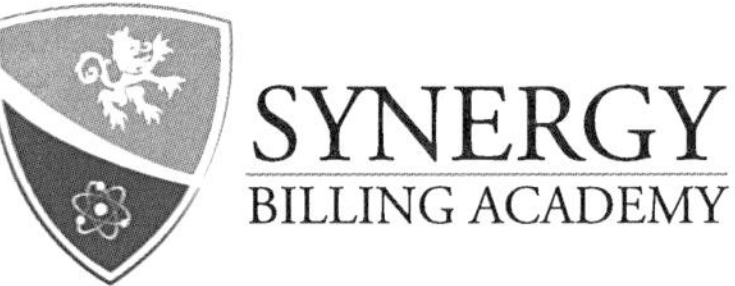

B. **Observation and Evaluation of Newborns for Suspected Conditions Not Found**

Reserved for future expansion.

C. **Coding Additional Perinatal Diagnoses**

1. **Assigning codes for conditions that require treatment**

   Assign codes for conditions that require treatment or further investigation, prolong the length of stay, or require resource utilization.

2. **Codes for conditions specified as having implications for future health care needs**

   Assign codes for conditions that have been specified by the provider as having implications for future health care needs.

   Note: This guideline should not be used for adult patients.

D. **Prematurity and Fetal Growth Retardation**

Providers utilize different criteria in determining prematurity. A code for prematurity should not be assigned unless it is documented. Assignment of codes in categories P05, Disorders of newborn related to slow fetal growth and fetal malnutrition, and P07, Disorders of newborn related to short gestation and low birth weight, not elsewhere classified, should be based on the recorded birth weight and estimated gestational age. Codes from category P05 should not be assigned with codes from category P07.

When both birth weight and gestational age are available, two codes from category P07 should be assigned, with the code for birth weight sequenced before the code for gestational age.

E. **Low Birth Weight and Immaturity Status**

Codes from category P07, Disorders of newborn related to short gestation and low birth weight, not elsewhere classified, are for use for a child or adult who was premature or had a low birth weight as a newborn when this is affecting the patient's current health status.

See Section I.C.21. Factors influencing health status and contact with health services, status.

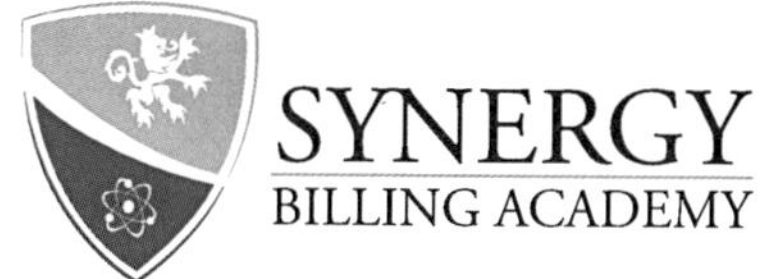

F. **Bacterial Sepsis of Newborn**

Category P36, Bacterial sepsis of newborn, includes congenital sepsis. If a perinate is documented as having sepsis without documentation of congenital or community-acquired status, the default is congenital and a code from category P36 should be assigned. If the P36 code includes the causal organism, an additional code from category B95, Streptococcus, Staphylococcus, and Enterococcus as the cause of diseases classified elsewhere; or B96, Other bacterial agents as the cause of diseases classified elsewhere, should not be assigned. If the P36 code does not include the causal organism, assign an additional code from category B96. If applicable, use additional codes to identify severe sepsis (R65.2-) and any associated acute organ dysfunction.

G. **Stillbirth**

Code P95, Stillbirth, is only for use in institutions that maintain separate records for stillbirths. No other code should be used with P95. Code P95 should not be used on the mother's record.

Chapter 17 – Guidelines

The NCHS has published chapter-specific guidelines for this chapter.

When a malformation/deformation or chromosomal abnormality does not have a unique code assignment, assign additional code(s) for any manifestations that may be present.

When the code assignment specifically identifies the malformation/deformation or chromosomal abnormality, manifestations that are inherent components of the anomaly should not be coded separately. Additional codes should be assigned for manifestations that are not inherent components.

Codes from Chapter 17 may be used throughout the life of the patient. If a congenital malformation or deformity has been corrected, a personal history code should be used to identify the history of the malformation or deformity. Although present at birth, malformation/deformation or chromosomal abnormality may not be identified until later in life. Whenever the condition is diagnosed by the physician, it is appropriate to assign a code from codes Q00-Q99.For the birth admission, the appropriate code from category Z38, Liveborn infants, according to place of birth and type of delivery, should be sequenced as the principal diagnosis, followed by any congenital anomaly codes, Q00–Q99.

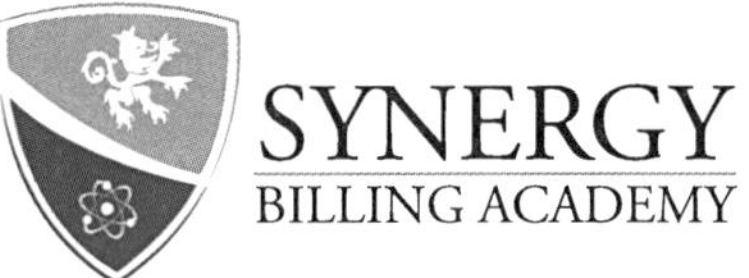

Chapter 17: Congenital Malformations, Deformations, and Chromosomal Abnormalities (Q00-Q99)

Assign an appropriate code(s) from categories Q00-Q99, Congenital malformations, deformations, and chromosomal abnormalities, when a malformation/deformation or chromosomal abnormality is documented. A malformation/deformation or chromosomal abnormality may be the principal/ first-listed diagnosis on a record or a secondary diagnosis.

Chapter 18 – Guidelines

A lengthy guideline appears at the beginning of the chapter. This guideline outlines the conditions classified to this particular chapter. Additionally, guidelines for code usage appear at the subchapter level.

Many of the new blocks and categories in Chapter 18 have extensive Excludes1 notes such as the one found under R09, Other symptoms involving the circulatory and respiratory system. New guidelines that clarify code usage are also found under specific codes. Code R52, Pain unspecified, includes inclusive terms and Excludes1 notes.

The NCHS has published chapter-specific guidelines for Chapter 18 of ICD-10-CM:

A. Use of Symptom Codes
B. Use of a Symptom Code with a Definitive Diagnosis Code
C. Combination Codes That Include Symptoms
D. Repeated Falls
E. Coma Scale
F. Functional Quadriplegia
G. SIRS Due to Noninfectious Process
H. Death NOS

18. Chapter 18: Symptoms, Signs, and Abnormal Clinical and Laboratory Findings, Not Elsewhere Classified (R00-R99)

Chapter 18 includes symptoms, signs, abnormal results of clinical or other investigative procedures, and ill-defined conditions regarding which no diagnosis classifiable elsewhere is recorded. Signs and symptoms that point to a specific diagnosis have been assigned to a category in other chapters of the classification.

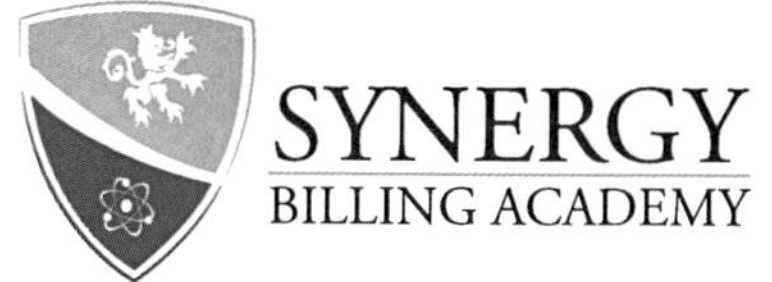

A. Use of Symptom Codes

Codes that describe symptoms and signs are acceptable for reporting purposes when a related definitive diagnosis has not been established (confirmed) by the provider.

B. Use of a Symptom Code with a Definitive Diagnosis Code

Codes for signs and symptoms may be reported in addition to a related definitive diagnosis when the sign or symptom is not routinely associated with that diagnosis, such as the various signs and symptoms associated with complex syndromes. The definitive diagnosis code should be sequenced before the symptom code.

Signs or symptoms that are associated routinely with a disease process should not be assigned as additional codes, unless otherwise instructed by the classification.

C. Combination Codes That Include Symptoms

ICD-10-CM contains a number of combination codes that identify both the definitive diagnosis and common symptoms of that diagnosis. When using one of these combination codes, an additional code should not be assigned for the symptom.

D. Repeated Falls

Code R29.6, Repeated falls, is for use for encounters when a patient has recently fallen and the reason for the fall is being investigated.

Code Z91.81, History of falling, is for use when a patient has fallen in the past and is at risk for future falls. When appropriate, both codes R29.6 and Z91.81 may be assigned together.

E. Coma Scale

The coma scale codes (R40.2-) can be used in conjunction with traumatic brain injury codes, acute cerebrovascular disease, or sequelae of cerebrovascular disease codes. These codes are primarily for use by trauma registries, but they may be used in any setting where this information is collected. The coma scale codes should be sequenced after the diagnosis code(s).

These codes, one from each subcategory, are needed to complete the scale. The 7th character indicates when the scale was recorded. The 7th character should match for all three codes.

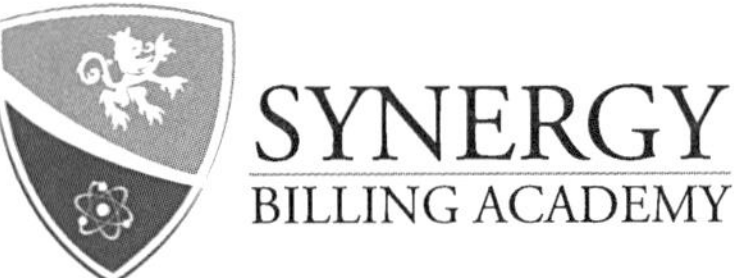

At a minimum, report the initial score documented on presentation at your facility. This may be a score from the emergency medicine technician (EMT) or one assigned in the emergency department. If desired, a facility may choose to capture multiple coma scale scores.

Assign code R40.24, Glasgow coma scale, total score, when only the total score is documented in the medical record and not the individual score(s).

F. Functional Quadriplegia

Functional quadriplegia (code R53.2) is the lack of ability to use one's limbs or to ambulate due to extreme debility. It is not associated with neurologic deficit or injury, and code R53.2 should not be used for cases of neurologic quadriplegia. It should only be assigned if functional quadriplegia is specifically documented in the medical record.

G. SIRS due to Noninfectious Process

The systemic inflammatory response syndrome (SIRS) can develop as a result of certain non-infectious disease processes, such as trauma, malignant neoplasm, or pancreatitis. When SIRS is documented with a noninfectious condition and no subsequent infection is documented, the code for the underlying condition, such as an injury, should be assigned, followed by code R65.10, Systemic inflammatory response syndrome (SIRS) of non-infectious origin without acute organ dysfunction; or code R65.11, Systemic inflammatory response syndrome (SIRS) of non-infectious origin with acute organ dysfunction. If an associated acute organ dysfunction is documented, the appropriate code(s) for the specific type of organ dysfunction(s) should be assigned in addition to code R65.11. If acute organ dysfunction is documented, but it cannot be determined if the acute organ dysfunction is associated with SIRS or due to another condition (e.g., directly due to the trauma), the provider should be queried.

H. Death NOS

Code R99, Ill-defined and unknown cause of mortality, is only for use in the very limited circumstance when a patient who has already died is brought into an emergency department or other health care facility and is pronounced dead upon arrival. It does not represent the discharge disposition of death.

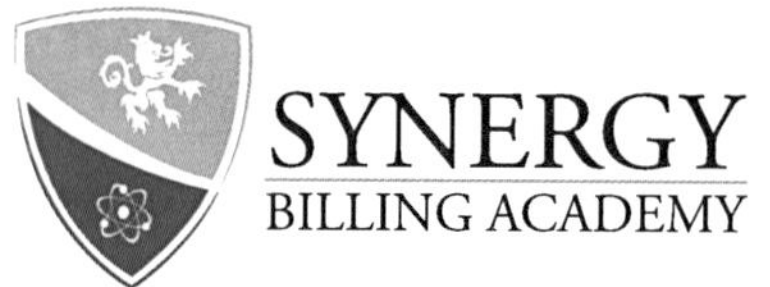

Chapter 19 – Guidelines

The following guideline appears at the beginning of Chapter 19: "Use secondary code(s) from Chapter 20, External causes of morbidity, to indicate cause of injury. Codes within the T section that include the external cause do not require an additional external cause code."

The note in ICD-9-CM defines "complicated" as used in the fourth-digit subdivisions to mean those open wounds with infection. ICD-10-CM contains a note under the different categories for open wounds and directs professionals to also code any associated wound infection.

A similar change has occurred to the instruction for complications of surgical and medical care, not elsewhere classified (T80-T88). In ICD-9-CM, there is no guideline under this subchapter. However, ICD-10-CM includes a note stating to use an additional code (Y62-Y82) to identify devices involved and details of circumstances.

The NCHS has published chapter-specific guidelines for Chapter 19:

A. Application of 7th Characters in Chapter 19
B. Coding of Injuries
C. Coding of Traumatic Fractures
D. Coding of Burns and Corrosions
E. Adverse Effects, Poisoning, Underdosing, and Toxic Effects
F. Adult and Child Abuse, Neglect, and Other Maltreatment
G. Complications of Care

19. Chapter 19: Injury, Poisoning, and Certain Other Consequences of External Causes (S00-T88)

A. Application of 7th Characters in Chapter 19

Most categories in Chapter 19 have a 7th character requirement for each applicable code. Most categories in this chapter have three 7th character values (with the exception of fractures): A, initial encounter; D, subsequent encounter; and S, sequela. Categories for traumatic fractures have additional 7th character values.

7th character "A," Initial encounter, is used while the patient is receiving active treatment for the condition. Examples of active treatment are: surgical treatment, emergency department encounter, or evaluation and treatment by a new physician.

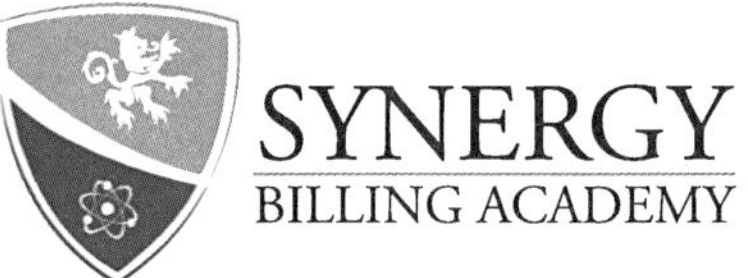

7th character "D," Subsequent encounter, is used for encounters after the patient has received active treatment of the condition and is now receiving routine care for the condition during the healing or recovery phase. Examples of subsequent care are: cast change or removal, removal of external or internal fixation device, medication adjustment, or other aftercare and follow-up visits following treatment of the injury or condition.

The aftercare Z Codes should not be used for aftercare for conditions such as injuries or poisonings, where 7th characters are provided to identify subsequent care. For example, for aftercare of an injury, assign the acute injury code with the 7th character "D" (subsequent encounter).

7th character "S," Sequela, is for use for complications or conditions that arise as a direct result of a condition, such as scar formation after a burn. The scars are sequelae of the burn. When using 7th character "S," it is necessary to use both the injury code that precipitated the sequela and the code for the sequela itself. The "S" is added only to the injury code, not the sequela code. The 7th character "S" identifies the injury responsible for the sequela. The specific type of sequela (e.g., scar) is sequenced first, followed by the injury code.

B. Coding of Injuries

When coding injuries, assign separate codes for each injury unless a combination code is provided, in which case the combination code is assigned. Code T07, Unspecified multiple injuries, should not be assigned in the inpatient setting unless information for a more specific code is not available. Traumatic injury codes (S00–T14.9) are not to be used for normal, healing surgical wounds or to identify complications of surgical wounds.

The code for the most serious injury, as determined by the provider and the focus of treatment, is sequenced first.

1. **Superficial injuries**

   Superficial injuries such as abrasions or contusions are not coded when associated with more severe injuries of the same site.

2. **Primary injury with damage to nerves/blood vessels**

   When a primary injury results in minor damage to peripheral nerves or blood vessels, the primary injury is sequenced first with additional code(s) for injuries to nerves and

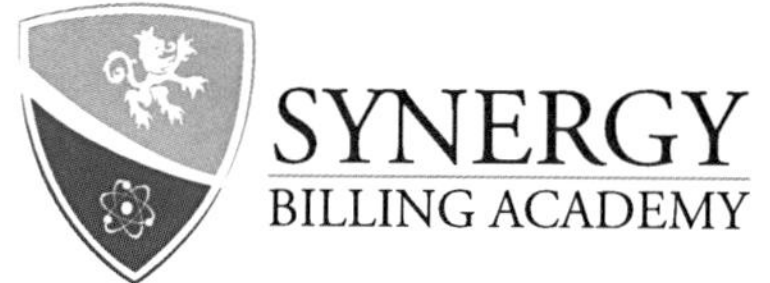

spinal cord (such as category S04), and/or injury to blood vessels (such as category S15). When the primary injury is to the blood vessels or nerves, that injury should be sequenced first.

C. Coding of Traumatic Fractures

The principles of multiple coding of injuries should be followed when coding fractures. Fractures of specified sites are coded individually by site in accordance with both the provisions within categories S02, S12, S22, S32, S42, S49, S52, S59, S62, S72, S79, S82, S89, and S92 and the level of detail furnished by medical record content.

A fracture not indicated as open or closed should be coded to closed. A fracture not indicated whether displaced or not displaced should be coded to displaced.

More specific guidelines are as follows:

1. Initial vs. Subsequent Encounter for Fractures

Traumatic fractures are coded using the appropriate 7th character for initial encounter (A, B, C) while the patient is receiving active treatment for the fracture. Examples of active treatment are: surgical treatment, emergency department encounter, or evaluation and treatment by a new physician. The appropriate 7th character for initial encounter should also be assigned for a patient who delayed seeking treatment for the fracture or nonunion.

Fractures are coded using the appropriate 7th character for subsequent care for encounters after the patient has completed active treatment of the fracture and is now receiving routine care for the fracture during the healing or recovery phase. Examples of fracture aftercare are: cast change or removal, removal of external or internal fixation device, medication adjustment, or follow-up visits following fracture treatment.

Care for complications of surgical treatment for fracture repairs during the healing or recovery phase should be coded with the appropriate complication codes.

Care of complications of fractures, such as malunion and nonunion, should be reported with the appropriate 7th character for subsequent care with nonunion (K, M, N,) or subsequent care with malunion (P, Q, R).

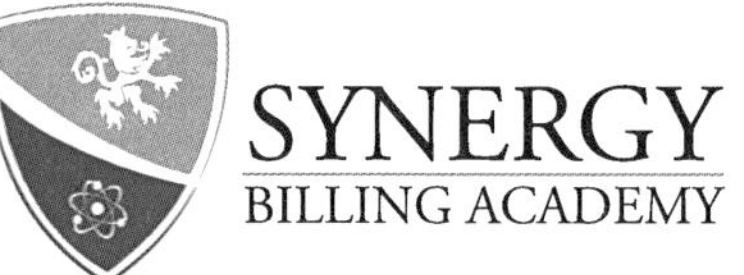

A code from category M80, not a traumatic fracture code, should be used for any patient with known osteoporosis who suffers a fracture, even if the patient had a minor fall or trauma, if that fall or trauma would not usually break a normal, healthy bone.

See Section I.C.13. Osteoporosis.

The aftercare Z Codes should not be used for aftercare for traumatic fractures. For aftercare of a traumatic fracture, assign the acute fracture code with the appropriate 7th character.

2. **Multiple fractures sequencing**

Multiple fractures are sequenced in accordance with the severity of the fracture.

D. Coding of Burns and Corrosions

The ICD-10-CM makes a distinction between burns and corrosions. The burn codes are for thermal burns, except sunburns, that come from a heat source, such as a fire or hot appliance. The burn codes are also for burns resulting from electricity and radiation. Corrosions are burns due to chemicals. The guidelines are the same for burns and corrosions.

Current burns (T20-T25) are classified by depth, extent, and agent (X Code). Burns are classified by depth as first degree (erythema), second degree (blistering), and third degree (full-thickness involvement). Burns of the eye and internal organs (T26-T28) are classified by site, but not by degree.

1. **Sequencing of burn and related condition codes**

Sequence first the code that reflects the highest degree of burn when more than one burn is present.

a. When the reason for the admission or encounter is for treatment of external multiple burns, sequence first the code that reflects the burn of the highest degree.
b. When a patient has both internal and external burns, the circumstances of admission govern the selection of the principal or first-listed diagnosis.
c. When a patient is admitted for burn injuries and other related conditions such as smoke inhalation and/or respiratory failure, the circumstances of admission govern the selection of the principal or first-listed diagnosis.

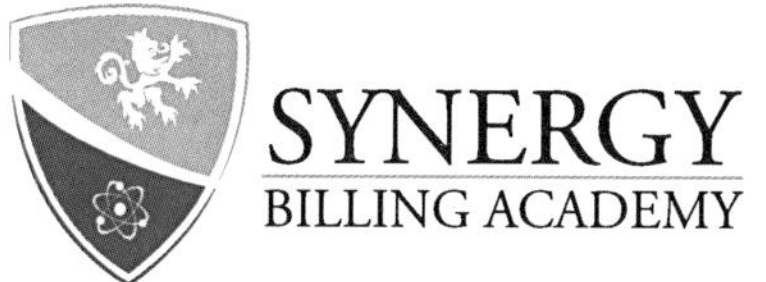

2. **Burns of the same local site**

   Classify burns of the same local site (three-character category level, T20-T28) but of different degrees to the subcategory identifying the highest degree recorded in the diagnosis.

3. **Non-healing burns**

   Non-healing burns are coded as acute burns.

   Necrosis of burned skin should be coded as a non-healed burn.

4. **Infected Burn**

   For any documented infected burn site, use an additional code for the infection.

5. **Assign separate codes for each burn site**

   When coding burns, assign separate codes for each burn site. Category T30, Burn and corrosion, body region unspecified, is extremely vague and should rarely be used.

6. **Burns and corrosions classified according to extent of body surface involved**

   Assign codes from category T31, Burns classified according to extent of body surface involved, or T32, Corrosions classified according to extent of body surface involved, when the site of the burn is not specified or when there is a need for additional data. It is advisable to use category T31 as additional coding when needed to provide data for evaluating burn mortality, such as that needed by burn units. It is also advisable to use category T31 as an additional code for reporting purposes when there is mention of a third-degree burn involving 20 percent or more of the body surface.

   Categories T31 and T32 are based on the classic "rule of nines" in estimating body surface involved: head and neck are assigned 9 percent, each arm 9 percent, each leg 18 percent, the anterior trunk 18 percent, posterior trunk 18 percent, and genitalia 1 percent. Providers may change these percentage assignments where necessary to accommodate infants and children who have proportionately larger heads than adults, and patients who have large buttocks, thighs, or abdomen that have been burned.

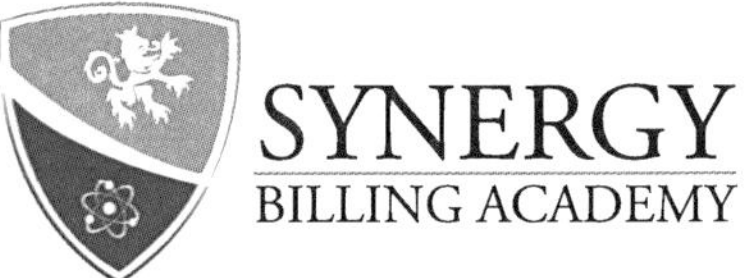

7. **Encounters for treatment of sequela of burns**

   Encounters for the treatment of the late effects of burns or corrosions (e.g., scars or joint contractures) should be coded with a burn or corrosion code with the 7th character "S" for sequela.

8. **Sequelae with a late effect code and current burn**

   When appropriate, both a code for a current burn or corrosion with 7th character "A" or "D" and a burn or corrosion code with 7th character "S" may be assigned on the same record (when both a current burn and sequelae of an old burn exist). Burns and corrosions do not heal at the same rate and a current healing wound may still exist with sequela of a healed burn or corrosion.

9. **Use of an external cause code with burns and corrosions**

   An external cause code should be used with burns and corrosions to identify the source and intent of the burn, as well as the place where it occurred.

E. Adverse Effects, Poisoning, Underdosing, and Toxic Effects

Codes in categories T36-T65 are combination codes that include the substance that was taken as well as the intent. No additional external cause code is required for poisonings, toxic effects, adverse effects, and underdosing codes.

1. **Do not code directly from the Table of Drugs**

   Do not code directly from the Table of Drugs and Chemicals. Always refer back to the Tabular List.

2. **Use as many codes as necessary**

   Use as many codes as necessary to describe completely all drugs, medicinal, or biological substances involved.

3. **Describing the same causative agent**

   If the same code would describe the causative agent for more than one adverse reaction, poisoning, toxic effect, or underdosing, assign the code only once.

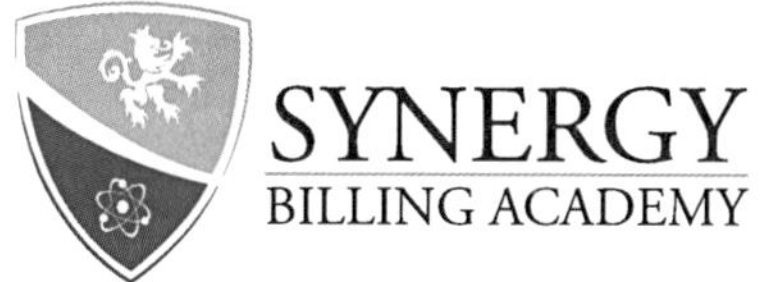

4. **Two or more drugs, medicinal, or biological substances**

   If two or more drugs, medicinal, or biological substances are reported, code each individually unless a combination code is listed in the Table of Drugs and Chemicals.

5. **The occurrence of drug toxicity is classified in ICD-10-CM as follows:**

   a. **Adverse Effect**

      When coding an adverse effect of a drug that has been correctly prescribed and properly administered, assign the appropriate code for the nature of the adverse effect followed by the appropriate code for the adverse effect of the drug (T36-T50). The code for the drug should have a 5th or 6th character "5" (for example, T36.0X5-) Examples of the nature of an adverse effect are tachycardia, delirium, gastrointestinal hemorrhaging, vomiting, hypokalemia, hepatitis, renal failure, or respiratory failure.

   b. **Poisoning**

      When coding a poisoning or reaction to the improper use of a medication (e.g., overdose, wrong substance given or taken in error, wrong route of administration), first assign the appropriate code from categories T36-T50. The poisoning codes have an associated intent as their 5th or 6th character (accidental, intentional self-harm, assault, and undetermined). Use additional code(s) for all manifestations of poisonings.

      If there is also a diagnosis of abuse or dependence of the substance, the abuse or dependence is assigned as an additional code.

      Examples of poisoning include:

      i. **Error was made in drug prescription**

         Errors made in drug prescription or in the administration of the drug by provider, nurse, patient, or other person.

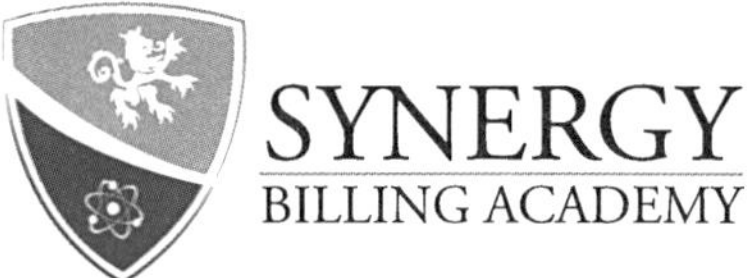

ii. Overdose of a drug intentionally taken

If an overdose of a drug was intentionally taken or administered and resulted in drug toxicity, it would be coded as a poisoning.

iii. Nonprescribed drug taken with correctly prescribed and properly administered drug

If a nonprescribed drug or medicinal agent was taken in combination with a correctly prescribed and properly administered drug, any drug toxicity or other reaction resulting from the interaction of the two drugs would be classified as a poisoning.

iv. Interaction of drug(s) and alcohol

When a reaction results from the interaction of a drug(s) and alcohol, this would be classified as poisoning.

See Section I.C.4. if poisoning is the result of insulin pump malfunctions.

c. Underdosing

Underdosing refers to taking less of a medication than is prescribed by a provider or a manufacturer's instruction. For underdosing, assign the code from categories T36-T50 (5th or 6th character "6").

Codes for underdosing should never be assigned as principal or first-listed codes. If a patient has a relapse or exacerbation of the medical condition for which the drug is prescribed because of the reduction in dose, then the medical condition itself should be coded.

Noncompliance (Z91.12-, Z91.13-) or complication of care (Y63.6-Y63.9) codes are to be used with an underdosing code to indicate intent, if known.

d. Toxic Effects

When a harmful substance is ingested or comes in contact with a person, this is classified as a toxic effect. The toxic effect codes are in categories T51-T65.

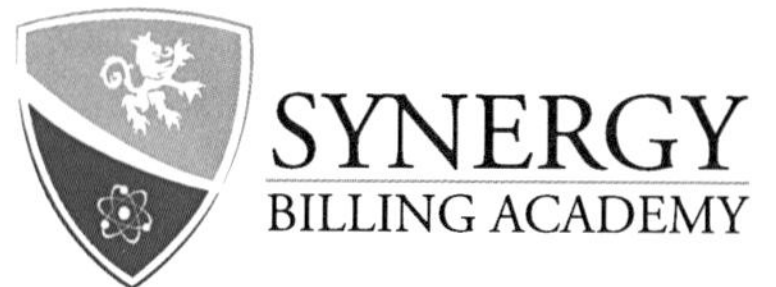

Toxic effect codes have an associated intent: accidental, intentional self-harm, assault, and undetermined.

F. Adult and Child Abuse, Neglect, and Other Maltreatment

Sequence first the appropriate code from categories T74.- (Adult and child abuse, neglect, and other maltreatment, confirmed) or T76.- (Adult and child abuse, neglect, and other maltreatment, suspected) for abuse, neglect, and other maltreatment, followed by any accompanying mental health or injury code(s).

If the documentation in the medical record states abuse or neglect, it is coded as confirmed (T74.-). It is coded as suspected if it is documented as suspected (T76.-).

For cases of confirmed abuse or neglect, an external cause code from the assault section (X92-Y08) should be added to identify the cause of any physical injuries. A perpetrator code (Y07) should be added when the perpetrator of the abuse is known. For suspected cases of abuse or neglect, do not report external cause or perpetrator code.

If a suspected case of abuse, neglect, or mistreatment is ruled out during an encounter, code Z04.71, Encounter for examination and observation following alleged physical adult abuse, ruled out, or code Z04.72, Encounter for examination and observation following alleged child physical abuse, ruled out, should be used, rather than a code from T76.

If a suspected case of alleged rape or sexual abuse is ruled out during an encounter, code Z04.41, Encounter for examination and observation following alleged physical adult abuse, ruled out, or code Z04.42, Encounter for examination and observation following alleged rape or sexual abuse, ruled out, should be used, rather than code from T76.

See Section I.C.15. Abuse in a pregnant patient.

G. Complications of Care

1. General guidelines for complications of care

a. Documentation of complications of care

See Section I.B.16. for information on documentation of complications of care.

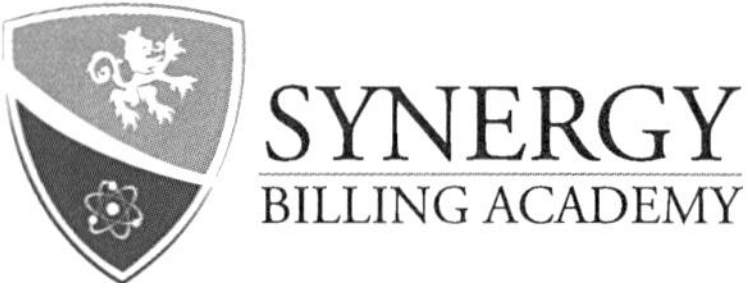

2. **Pain due to medical devices**

   Pain associated with devices, implants, or grafts left in a surgical site (for example, a painful hip prosthesis) is assigned to the appropriate code(s) found in Chapter 19, Injury, Poisoning, and Certain Other Consequences of External Causes. Specific codes for pain due to medical devices are found in the T Code section of the ICD-10-CM. Use additional code(s) from category G89 to identify acute or chronic pain due to presence of the device, implant, or graft (G89.18 or G89.28).

3. **Transplant complications**

   a. **Transplant complications other than kidney**

      Codes under category T86, Complications of transplanted organs and tissues, are for use for both complications and rejection of transplanted organs. A transplant complication code is only assigned if the complication affects the function of the transplanted organ. Two codes are required to fully describe a transplant complication: the appropriate code from category T86 and a secondary code that identifies the complication.

      Pre-existing conditions or conditions that develop after the transplant are not coded as complications unless they affect the function of the transplanted organs.

      See I.C.21. for transplant organ removal status.

      See I.C.2. for malignant neoplasm associated with transplanted organ.

   b. **Kidney transplant complications**

      Patients who have undergone kidney transplant may still have some form of chronic kidney disease (CKD) because the kidney transplant may not fully restore kidney function. Code T86.1- should be assigned for documented complications of a kidney transplant, such as transplant failure or rejection or other transplant complication. Code T86.1- should not be assigned for post-kidney transplant patients who have CKD unless a transplant complication such as transplant failure or rejection is documented. If the documentation is unclear as to whether the patient has a complication of the transplant, query the provider.

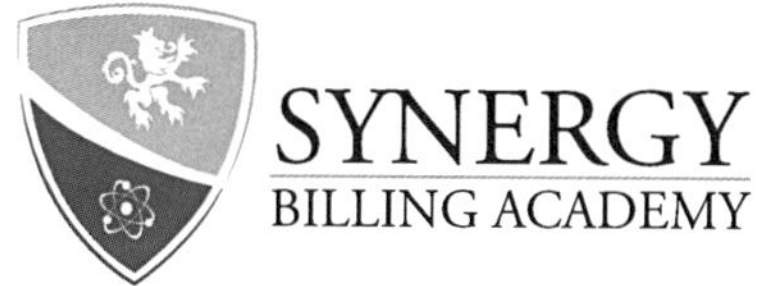

Conditions other than CKD that affect the function of the transplanted kidney should be assigned a code from subcategory T86.1, Complications of transplanted organ, kidney, and a secondary code that identifies the complication.

For patients with CKD following a kidney transplant, but who do not have a complication such as failure or rejection, see section I.C.14, Chronic kidney disease and kidney transplant status.

4. **Complication codes that include the external cause**

   As with certain other T Codes, some of the complications of care codes have the external cause included in the code. The code includes the nature of the complication as well as the type of procedure that caused the complication. No external cause code indicating the type of procedure is necessary for these codes.

5. **Complications of care codes within the body system chapters**

   Intraoperative and postprocedural complication codes are found within the body system chapters with codes specific to the organs and structures of that body system. These codes should be sequenced first, followed by a code(s) for the specific complication, if applicable.

Chapter 20 – Guidelines

New notes have been added to this chapter to indicate which categories require the 7th character to indicate whether the episode of care being identified was the initial, subsequent, or a secondary consequence or result (sequelae).

While there is an instructional note found at the start of category E849, place of occurrence, in ICD-9-CM, it has been expanded in ICD-10-CM. The new guidelines state to use Y92 in conjunction with the activity code; the place of occurrence should be recorded only at the initial encounter for treatment.

The NCHS has published chapter-specific guidelines for Chapter 20:

A. General External Cause Coding Guidelines
B. Place of Occurrence Guideline

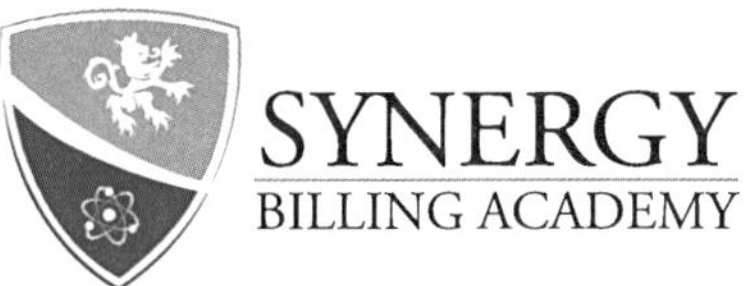

C. Activity Code
D. Place of Occurrence, Activity, and Status Codes Used with Other External Cause Code
E. Limitation of External Cause Codes by Reporting Format
F. Multiple External Cause Coding Guidelines
G. Child and Adult Abuse Guideline
H. Unknown or Undetermined Intent Guideline
I. Sequelae (Late Effects) of External Cause Guidelines
J. Terrorism Guidelines
K. External Cause Status

20. Chapter 20: External Causes of Morbidity (V00-Y99)

The external causes of morbidity codes should never be sequenced as the first-listed or principal diagnosis.

External cause codes are intended to provide data for injury research and evaluation of injury prevention strategies. These codes capture how the injury or health condition happened (cause), the intent (unintentional or accidental; or intentional, such as suicide or assault), the place where the event occurred, the activity of the patient at the time of the event, and the person's status (e.g., civilian, military).

There is no national requirement for mandatory ICD-10-CM external cause code reporting. Unless a provider is subject to a state-based external cause code reporting mandate or these codes are required by a particular payer, reporting of ICD-10-CM codes in Chapter 20, External Causes of Morbidity, is not required. In the absence of a mandatory reporting requirement, providers are encouraged to voluntarily report external cause codes, as they provide valuable data for injury research and evaluation of injury prevention strategies.

A. General External Cause Coding Guidelines

1. Used with any code in the ranges of A00.0-T88.9 and Z00-Z99

An external cause code may be used with any code in the ranges of A00.0-T88.9 and Z00-Z99, Classification that is a health condition due to an external cause. Though external cause codes are most applicable to injuries, they are also valid for use with such things as infections or diseases due to an external source, and other health conditions, such as a heart attack that occurs during strenuous physical activity.

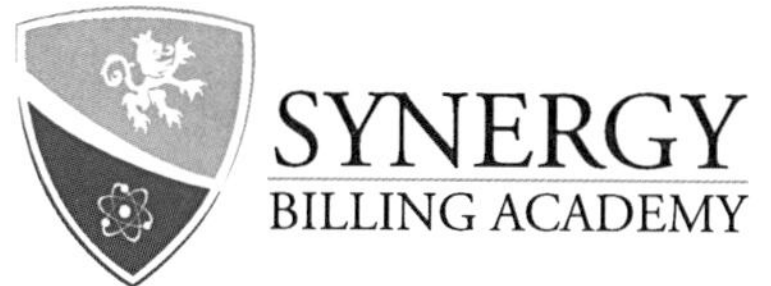

2. **External cause code used for length of treatment**

   Assign the external cause code, with the appropriate 7th character (initial encounter, subsequent encounter, or sequela) for each encounter for which the injury or condition is being treated.

3. **Use the full range of external cause codes**

   Use the full range of external cause codes to completely describe the cause, the intent, the place of occurrence, the patient's status, and, if applicable, the activity of the patient at the time of the event for all injuries and other health conditions due to an external cause.

4. **Assign as many external cause codes as necessary**

   Assign as many external cause codes as necessary to fully explain each cause. If only one external code can be recorded, assign the code most related to the principal diagnosis.

5. **The selection of the appropriate external cause code**

   The selection of the appropriate external cause code is guided by the Alphabetic Index of External Causes and by Includes and Excludes notes in the Tabular List.

6. **External cause code can never be a principal diagnosis**

   An external cause code can never be a principal (first-listed) diagnosis.

7. **Combination external cause codes**

   Certain of the external cause codes are combination codes that identify sequential events that result in an injury, such as a fall which results in striking against an object. The injury may be due to either event or both. The combination external cause code used should correspond to the sequence of events regardless of which caused the most serious injury.

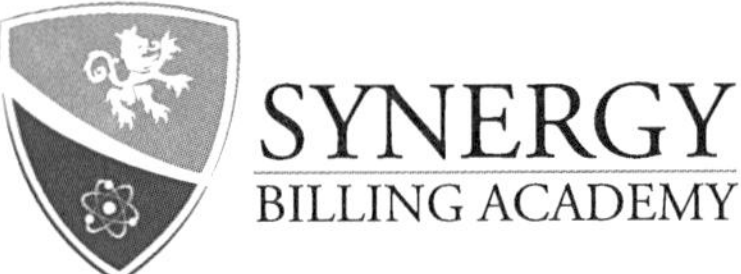

8. **No external cause code needed in certain circumstances**

   No external cause code from Chapter 20 is needed if the external cause and intent are included in a code from another chapter (e.g., T36.0X1, Poisoning by penicillins, accidental (unintentional)).

B. **Place of Occurrence Guideline**

Codes from category Y92, Place of occurrence of the external cause, are secondary codes for use after other external cause codes to identify the location of the patient at the time of injury or other condition.

A place of occurrence code is used only once, at the initial encounter for treatment. No 7th characters are used for Y92. Only one code from Y92 should be recorded on a medical record.

Do not use place of occurrence code Y92.9 if the place is not stated or is not applicable.

C. **Activity Code**

Assign a code from category Y93, Activity code, to describe the activity of the patient at the time the injury or other health condition occurred.

An activity code is used only once, at the initial encounter for treatment. Only one code from Y93 should be recorded on a medical record.

The activity codes are not applicable to poisonings, adverse effects, misadventures, or sequela.

Do not assign Y93.9, Unspecified activity, if the activity is not stated.

A code from category Y93 is appropriate for use with external cause and intent codes if identifying the activity provides additional information about the event.

D. **Place of Occurrence, Activity, and Status Codes Used with Other External Cause Codes**

When applicable, place of occurrence, activity, and external cause status codes are sequenced after the main external cause code(s). Regardless of the number of external cause codes assigned, there should be only one place of occurrence code, one activity code, and one external cause status code assigned to an encounter.

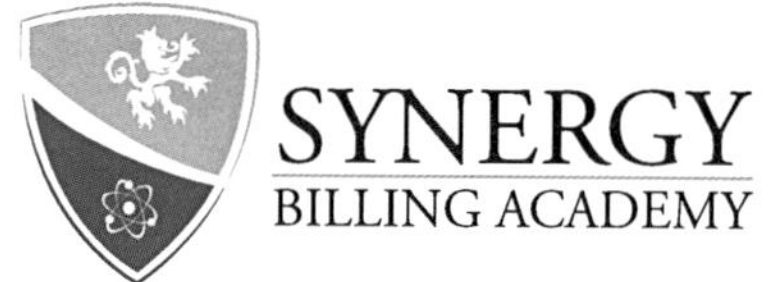

E. Limitation of External Cause Codes by Reporting Format

If the reporting format limits the number of external cause codes that can be used in reporting clinical data, report the code for the cause/intent most related to the principal diagnosis. If the format permits capture of additional external cause codes, the cause/intent, including medical misadventures, of the additional events should be reported rather than the codes for place, activity, or external status.

F. Multiple External Cause Coding Guidelines

More than one external cause code is required to fully describe the external cause of an illness or injury. The assignment of external cause codes should be sequenced in the following priority: if two or more events cause separate injuries, an external cause code should be assigned for each cause.

The first-listed external cause code will be selected in the following order:

External codes for child and adult abuse take priority over all other external cause codes.

See Section I.C.19., Adult and Child abuse guidelines.

External cause codes for terrorism events take priority over all other external cause codes except child and adult abuse.

External cause codes for cataclysmic events take priority over all other external cause codes except child and adult abuse and terrorism.

External cause codes for transport accidents take priority over all other external cause codes except cataclysmic events, child and adult abuse, and terrorism.

Activity and external cause status codes are assigned following all causal (intent) external cause codes.

The first-listed external cause code should correspond to the cause of the most serious diagnosis due to an assault, accident, or self-harm, following the order of hierarchy listed above.

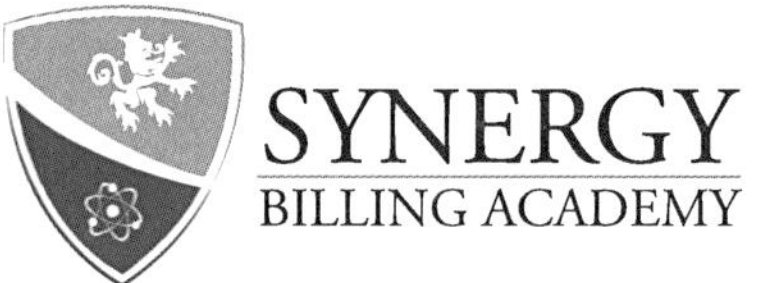

G. Child and Adult Abuse Guideline

Adult and child abuse, neglect, and maltreatment are classified as assault. Any of the assault codes may be used to indicate the external cause of any injury resulting from the confirmed abuse.

For confirmed cases of abuse, neglect, and maltreatment, when the perpetrator is known, a code from Y07, Perpetrator of maltreatment and neglect, should accompany any other assault codes.

See Section I.C.19. Adult and child abuse, neglect, and other maltreatment.

H. Unknown or Undetermined Intent Guideline

If the intent (e.g., accident, self-harm, assault) of the cause of an injury or other condition is unknown or unspecified, code the intent as accidental intent. All transport accident categories assume accidental intent.

1. Use of undetermined intent

External cause codes for events of undetermined intent are only for use if the documentation in the record specifies that the intent cannot be determined.

i. Sequelae (late effects) of external cause guidelines

1. Sequelae external cause codes

Sequela are reported using the external cause code with the 7th character "S" for sequela. These codes should be used with any report of a late effect or sequela resulting from a previous injury.

2. Sequela external cause code with a related current injury

A sequela external cause code should never be used with a related current nature of injury code.

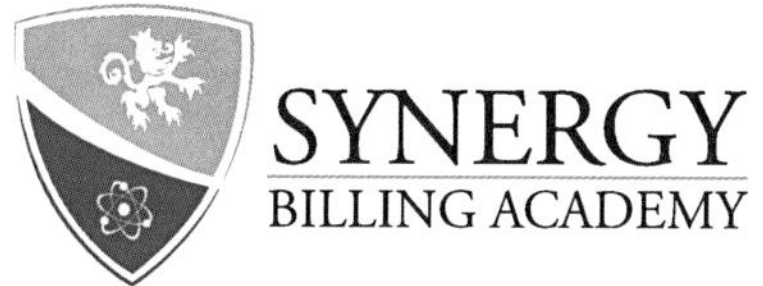

3. **Use of sequela external cause codes for subsequent visits**

   Use a late effect external cause code for subsequent visits when a late effect of the initial injury is being treated. Do not use a late effect external cause code for subsequent visits for follow-up care (e.g., to assess healing, to receive rehabilitative therapy) of the injury when no late effect of the injury has been documented.

J. Terrorism Guidelines

1. **Cause of injury identified by the Federal Bureau of Investigations (FBI) as terrorism**

   When the cause of an injury is identified by the Federal Bureau of Investigations (FBI) as terrorism, the first-listed external cause code should be a code from category Y38, Terrorism. The definition of terrorism employed by the FBI is found at the inclusion note at the beginning of category Y38. Use an additional code for place of occurrence (Y92.-). More than one Y38 code may be assigned if the injury is the result of more than one mechanism of terrorism.

2. **Cause of an injury is suspected to be the result of terrorism**

   When the cause of an injury is suspected to be the result of terrorism, a code from category Y38 should not be assigned. Suspected cases should be classified as assault.

3. **Code Y38.9, Terrorism, secondary effects**

   Assign code Y38.9, Terrorism, secondary effects, for conditions occurring subsequent to the terrorist event. This code should not be assigned for conditions that are due to the initial terrorist act.

   It is acceptable to assign code Y38.9 with another code from Y38 if there is an injury due to the initial terrorist event and an injury that is a subsequent result of the terrorist event.

K. External Cause Status

A code from category Y99, External cause status, should be assigned whenever any other

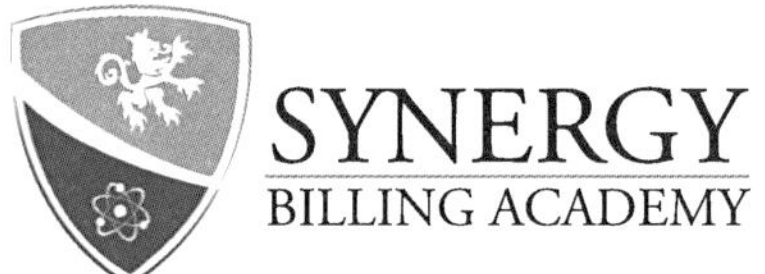

external cause code is assigned for an encounter, including an activity code, except for the events noted below. Assign a code from category Y99, External cause status, to indicate the work status of the person at the time the event occurred. The status code indicates whether the event occurred during military activity, while a non-military person was at work, or while an individual including a student or volunteer was involved in a non-work activity at the time of the causal event.

A code from Y99, External cause status, should be assigned, when applicable, with other external cause codes, such as transport accidents and falls. The external cause status codes are not applicable to poisonings, adverse effects, misadventures, or late effects.

Do not assign a code from category Y99 if no other external cause codes (e.g., cause, activity) are applicable for the encounter.

An external cause status code is used only once, at the initial encounter for treatment. Only one code from Y99 should be recorded on a medical record.

Do not assign code Y99.9, Unspecified external cause status, if the status is not stated.

Chapter 21 – Guidelines

The NCHS has published the following guidelines:

A. Use of Z Codes in any Health Care Setting
B. Z Codes Indicate a Reason for an Encounter
C. Categories of Z Codes
    1. Contact/Exposure
    2. Inoculations and Vaccinations
    3. Status
    4. History (Of)
    5. Screening
    6. Observation
    7. Aftercare
    8. Follow-Up
    9 Donor
    10. Counseling
    11. Encounters for Obstetrical and Reproductive Services
    12. Newborns and Infants

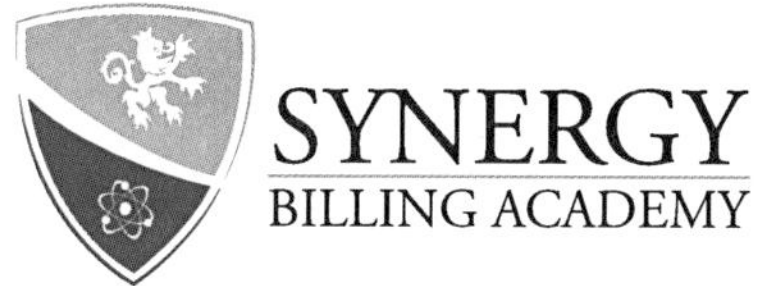

13. Routine and Administrative Examinations
14. Miscellaneous Z Codes
    I. Prophylactic Organ Removal
15. Nonspecific Z Codes
16. Z Codes That May Only Be Principal/First-Listed Diagnosis

21. Chapter 21: Factors Influencing Health Status and Contact with Health Services (Z00-Z99)

Note: The chapter-specific guidelines provide additional information about the use of Z Codes for specified encounters.

A. Use of Z Codes in any Health Care Setting

Z Codes are for use in any health care setting. Z Codes may be used as either a first-listed (principal diagnosis code in the inpatient setting) or secondary code, depending on the circumstances of the encounter. Certain Z Codes may only be used as first-listed or principal diagnosis.

B. Z Codes Indicate a Reason for an Encounter

Z codes are not procedure codes. A corresponding procedure code must accompany a Z Code to describe any procedure performed.

C. Categories of Z Codes

1. Contact/Exposure

Category Z20 indicates contact with, and suspected exposure to, communicable diseases. These codes are for patients who do not show any sign or symptom of a disease but are suspected to have been exposed to it by close personal contact with an infected individual or are in an area where a disease is epidemic.

Category Z77 indicates contact with and suspected exposures hazardous to health.

Contact/exposure codes may be used as a first-listed code to explain an encounter for testing, or, more commonly, as a secondary code to identify a

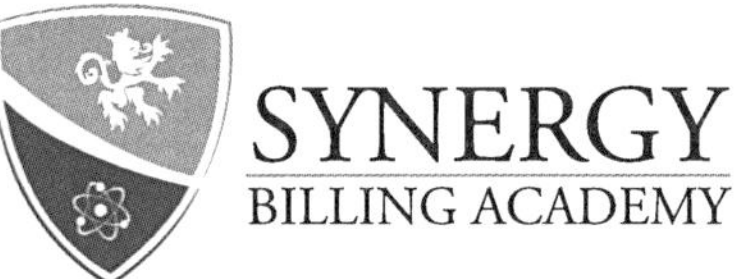

potential risk.

2. **Inoculations and vaccinations**

   Code Z23 is for encounters for inoculations and vaccinations. It indicates that a patient is being seen to receive a prophylactic inoculation against a disease. Procedure codes are required to identify the actual administration of the injection and the type(s) of immunizations given. Code Z23 may be used as a secondary code if the inoculation is given as a routine part of preventive health care, such as a well-baby visit.

3. **Status**

   Status codes indicate that a patient is either a carrier of a disease or has the sequelae or residual of a past disease or condition. This includes such things as the presence of prosthetic or mechanical devices resulting from past treatment. A status code is informative, because the status may affect the course of treatment and its outcome. A status code is distinct from a history code. The history code indicates that the patient no longer has the condition.

   A status code should not be used with a diagnosis code from one of the body system chapters if the diagnosis code includes the information provided by the status code. For example, code Z94.1, Heart transplant status, should not be used with a code from subcategory T86.2, Complications of heart transplant. The status code does not provide additional information. The complication code indicates that the patient is a heart transplant patient.

   For encounters for weaning from a mechanical ventilator, assign a code from subcategory J96.1, Chronic respiratory failure, followed by code Z99.11, Dependence on respirator [ventilator] status.

The status Z Codes/categories are:

- Z14, Genetic carrier
  - Genetic carrier status indicates that a person carries a gene, associated with a particular disease, which may be passed to offspring who may develop that disease. The person does not have the disease and is not at risk of developing the disease.
- Z15, Genetic susceptibility to disease

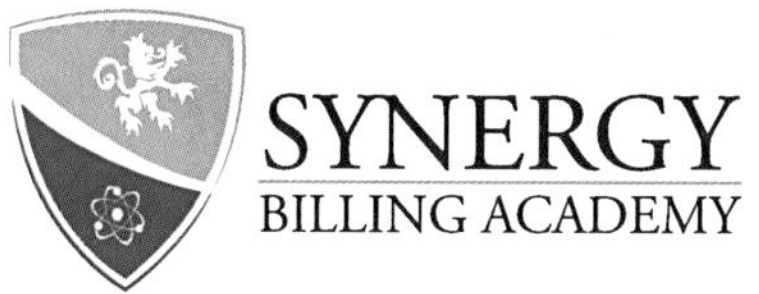

  - Genetic susceptibility indicates that a person has a gene that increases the risk of that person developing the disease.
  - Codes from category Z15 should not be used as principal or first-listed codes. If the patient has the condition to which he/she is susceptible, and that condition is the reason for the encounter, the code for the current condition should be sequenced first. If the patient is being seen for follow-up after completing treatment for this condition, and the condition no longer exists, a follow-up code should be sequenced first, followed by the appropriate personal history and genetic susceptibility codes. If the purpose of the encounter is genetic counseling associated with procreative management, code Z31.5, Encounter for genetic counseling, should be assigned as the first-listed code, followed by a code from category Z15. Additional codes should be assigned for any applicable family or personal history.
- Z16, Resistance to antimicrobial drugs
  - This code indicates that a patient has a condition that is resistant to antimicrobial drug treatment. Sequence the infection code first.
- Z17, Estrogen receptor status
- Z18, Retained foreign body fragments
- Z21, Asymptomatic HIV infection status
  - This code indicates that a patient has tested positive for HIV but has manifested no signs or symptoms of the disease.
- Z22, Carrier of infectious disease
  - Carrier status indicates that a person harbors the specific organisms of a disease without manifest symptoms and is capable of transmitting the infection.
- Z28.3, Underimmunization status
- Z33.1, Pregnant state, incidental
  - This code is a secondary code only for use when the pregnancy is in no way complicating the reason for visit. Otherwise, a code from the obstetric chapter is required.
- Z66, Do not resuscitate
  - This code may be used when it is documented by the provider that a patient is on do not resuscitate status at any time during the stay.
- Z67, Blood type
- Z68, Body mass index (BMI)

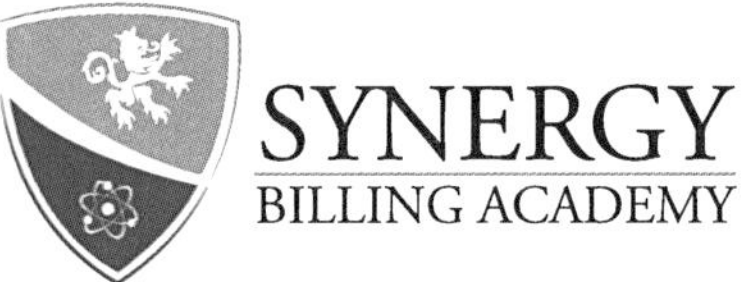

- Z74.01, Bed confinement status
- Z76.82, Awaiting organ transplant status
- Z78, Other specified health status
  - Code Z78.1, Physical restraint status, may be used when it is documented by the provider that a patient has been put in restraints during the current encounter. Please note that this code should not be reported when it is documented by the provider that a patient is temporarily restrained during a procedure.
- Z79, Long-term (current) drug therapy
  - Codes from this category indicate a patient's continuous use of a prescribed drug (including such things as aspirin therapy) for the long-term treatment of a condition or for prophylactic use. It is not for use for patients who have addictions to drugs. This subcategory is not for use of medications for detoxification or maintenance programs to prevent withdrawal symptoms in patients with drug dependence (e.g., methadone maintenance for opiate dependence). Assign the appropriate code for the drug dependence instead.
  - Assign a code from Z79 if the patient is receiving a medication for an extended period as a prophylactic measure (such as for the prevention of deep vein thrombosis) or as treatment of a chronic condition (such as arthritis) or a disease requiring a lengthy course of treatment (such as cancer). Do not assign a code from category Z79 for medication being administered for a brief period of time to treat an acute illness or injury (such as a course of antibiotics to treat acute bronchitis).
- Z88, Allergy status to drugs, medicaments, and biological substances
  - Except: Z88.9, Allergy status to unspecified drugs, medicaments, and biological substances status
- Z89, Acquired absence of limb
- Z90, Acquired absence of organs, not elsewhere classified
- Z91.0-, Allergy status, other than to drugs and biological substances
- Z92.82, Status post administration of tPA (rtPA) in a different facility within the last 24 hours prior to admission to a current facility
  - Assign code Z92.82, Status post administration of tPA (rtPA) in a different facility within the last 24 hours prior to admission to current facility, as a secondary diagnosis when a patient is received by transfer into a facility and documentation indicates

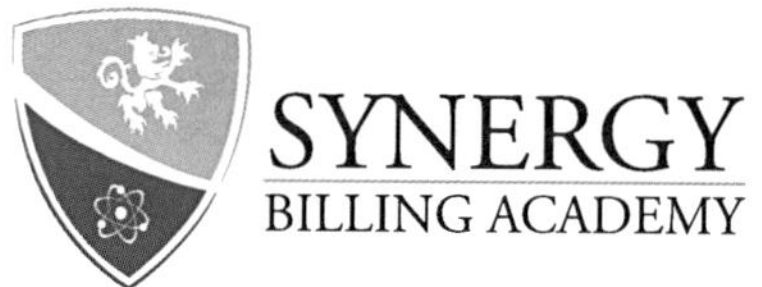

they were administered tissue plasminogen activator (tPA) within the last 24 hours prior to admission to the current facility.
  - This guideline applies even if the patient is still receiving the tPA at the time he or she is received into the current facility.
  - The appropriate code for the condition for which the tPA was administered (such as cerebrovascular disease or myocardial infarction) should be assigned first.
  - Code Z92.82 is only applicable to the receiving facility record and not to the transferring facility record.
- Z93, Artificial opening status
- Z94, Transplanted organ and tissue status
- Z95, Presence of cardiac and vascular implants and grafts
- Z96, Presence of other functional implants
- Z97, Presence of other devices
- Z98, Other postprocedural states
  - Assign code Z98.85, Transplanted organ removal status, to indicate that a transplanted organ has been previously removed. This code should not be assigned for the encounter in which the transplanted organ is removed. The complication necessitating removal of the transplant organ should be assigned for that encounter.
  - See section I.C19. for information on the coding of organ transplant complications.
- Z99, Dependence on enabling machines and devices, not elsewhere classified
  - Note: Categories Z89-Z90 and Z93-Z99 are for use only if there are no complications or malfunctions of the organ or tissue replaced, the amputation site, or the equipment on which the patient is dependent.

4. History (of)

There are two types of history Z Codes, personal and family. Personal history codes explain a patient's past medical condition that no longer exists and is not currently being treated, but that has the potential for recurrence and therefore may require continued monitoring.

Family history codes are for use when a patient has a family member(s) who

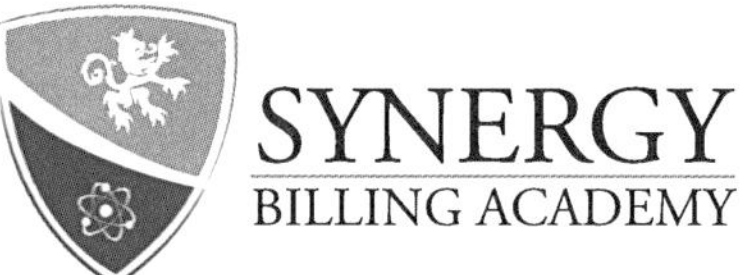

has had a particular disease that causes the patient to be at higher risk of also developing the disease.

Personal history codes may be used in conjunction with follow-up codes and family history codes may be used in conjunction with screening codes to explain the need for a test or procedure. History codes are also acceptable on any medical record regardless of the reason for visit. A history of an illness, even if no longer present, is important information that may alter the type of treatment ordered.

The history Z Code categories are:

- Z80, Family history of primary malignant neoplasm
- Z81, Family history of mental and behavioral disorders
- Z82, Family history of certain disabilities and chronic diseases (leading to disablement)
- Z83, Family history of other specific disorders
- Z84, Family history of other conditions
- Z85, Personal history of malignant neoplasm
- Z86, Personal history of certain other diseases
- Z87, Personal history of other diseases and conditions
- Z91.4-, Personal history of psychological trauma, not elsewhere classified
- Z91.5, Personal history of self-harm
- Z91.8-, Other specified personal risk factors, not elsewhere classified
    - Except: Z91.83, Wandering in diseases classified elsewhere
- Z92, Personal history of medical treatment
    - Except: Z92.0, Personal history of contraception
    - Except: Z92.82, Status post administration of tPA (rtPA) in a different facility within the last 24 hours prior to admission to a current facility

5. **Screening**

Screening is the testing for disease or disease precursors in seemingly well individuals so that early detection and treatment can be provided for those who test positive for the disease (e.g., screening mammogram).

The testing of a person to rule out or confirm a suspected diagnosis because the patient has some sign or symptom is a diagnostic examination, not a screening. In these cases, the sign or symptom is used to explain the reason for the test.

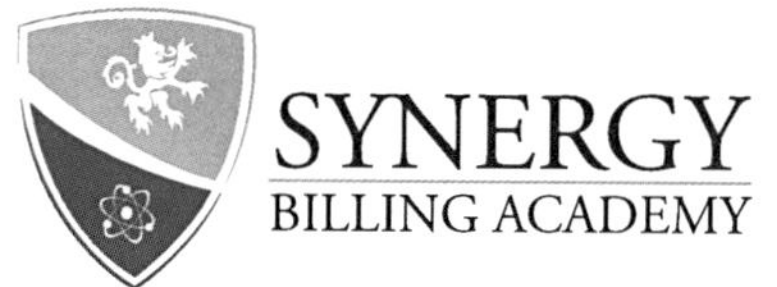

A screening code may be a first-listed code if the reason for the visit is specifically the screening exam. It may also be used as an additional code if the screening is done during an office visit for other health problems. A screening code is not necessary if the screening is inherent to a routine examination, such as a pap smear done during a routine pelvic examination.

Should a condition be discovered during the screening, then the code for the condition may be assigned as an additional diagnosis.
The Z Code indicates that a screening exam is planned. A procedure code is required to confirm that the screening was performed.
The screening Z Codes/categories are:

- Z11, Encounter for screening for infectious and parasitic diseases
- Z12, Encounter for screening for malignant neoplasms
- Z13, Encounter for screening for other diseases and disorders
  - Except: Z13.9, Encounter for screening, unspecified
- Z36, Encounter for antenatal screening for mother

6. Observation

There are two observation Z Code categories. They are for use in very limited circumstances when a person is being observed for a suspected condition that is ruled out. The observation codes are not for use if an injury or illness or any signs or symptoms related to the suspected condition are present. In such cases, the diagnosis/symptom code is used with the corresponding external cause code.

The observation codes are to be used as principal diagnosis only. Additional codes may be used in addition to the observation code but only if they are unrelated to the suspected condition being observed.

Codes from subcategory Z03.7, Encounter for suspected maternal and fetal conditions ruled out, may either be used as a first-listed or as an additional code assignment depending on the case. They are for use in very limited circumstances on a maternal record when an encounter is for a suspected maternal or fetal condition that is ruled out during that encounter (for example, a maternal or fetal condition may be suspected due to an abnormal test result). These codes should not be used when the condition is confirmed. In those cases, the confirmed condition should be coded. In addition, these codes are not for use if an illness or any signs or symptoms related to the suspected condition or problem are present. In such cases, the diagnosis/symptom code is used.

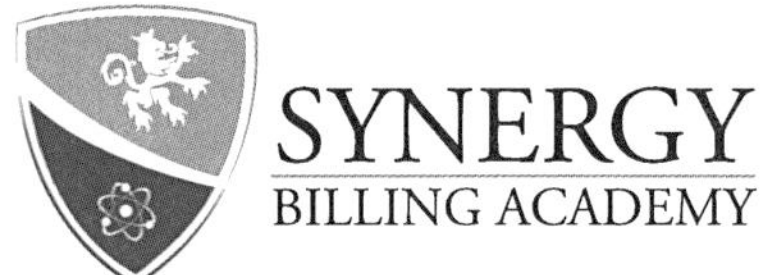

Additional codes may be used in addition to the code from subcategory Z03.7, but only if they are unrelated to the suspected condition being evaluated. Codes from subcategory Z03.7 may not be used for encounters for antenatal screening of mother. *See Section I.C.21. Screening.*

For encounters for suspected fetal condition that are inconclusive following testing and evaluation, assign the appropriate code from category O35, O36, O40, or O41. The observation Z Code categories are:

- Z03, Encounter for medical observation for suspected diseases and conditions ruled out
- Z04, Encounter for examination and observation for other reasons
  - Except: Z04.9, Encounter for examination and observation for unspecified reason

7. Aftercare

Aftercare visit codes cover situations when the initial treatment of a disease has been performed and the patient requires continued care during the healing or recovery phase, or for the long-term consequences of the disease. The diagnosis code is to be used in these cases. Exceptions to this rule are codes Z51.0, Encounter for antineoplastic radiation therapy, and codes from subcategory Z51.1, Encounter for antineoplastic chemotherapy and immunotherapy. These codes are to be first-listed, followed by the diagnosis code when a patient's encounter is solely to receive radiation therapy, chemotherapy, or immunotherapy for the treatment of a neoplasm. If the reason for the encounter is more than one type of antineoplastic therapy, code Z51.0 and a code from subcategory Z51.1 may be assigned together, in which case one of these codes would be reported as a secondary diagnosis.

The aftercare Z Codes should also not be used for aftercare for injuries. For aftercare of an injury, assign the acute injury code with the appropriate 7th character (for subsequent encounter).

The aftercare codes are generally first-listed to explain the specific reason for the encounter. An aftercare code may be used as an additional code when some type of aftercare is provided in addition to the reason for admission and no diagnosis code is applicable. An example of this would be the closure of a colostomy during an encounter for treatment of another condition.

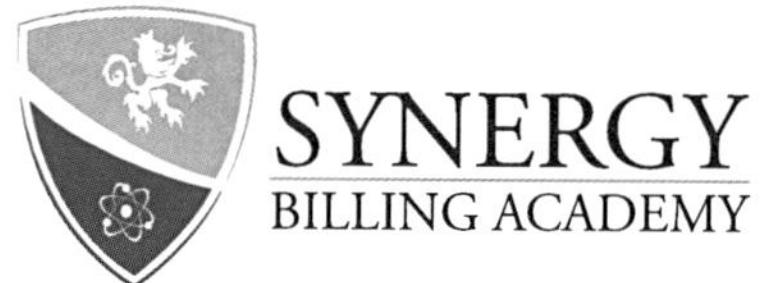

Aftercare codes should be used in conjunction with other aftercare codes or diagnosis codes to provide better detail on the specifics of an aftercare encounter visit, unless otherwise directed by the classification. Should a patient receive multiple types of antineoplastic therapy during the same encounter, code Z51.0, Encounter for antineoplastic radiation therapy, and codes from subcategory Z51.1, Encounter for antineoplastic chemotherapy and immunotherapy, may be used together on a record. The sequencing of multiple aftercare codes depends on the circumstances of the encounter.

Certain aftercare Z Code categories need a secondary diagnosis code to describe the resolving condition or sequela(e). For others, the condition is included in the code title.

Additional Z Code aftercare category terms include fitting and adjustment and attention to artificial openings.

Status Z Codes may be used with aftercare Z Codes to indicate the nature of the aftercare. For example, code Z95.1, Presence of aortocoronary bypass graft, may be used with code Z48.812, Encounter for surgical aftercare following surgery on the circulatory system, to indicate the surgery for which the aftercare is being performed. A status code should not be used when the aftercare code indicates the type of status, such as using Z43.0, Encounter for attention to tracheostomy, with Z93.0, Tracheostomy status.

The aftercare Z Codes are:

- Z42, Encounter for plastic and reconstructive surgery following medical procedure or healed injury
- Z43, Encounter for attention to artificial openings
- Z44, Encounter for fitting and adjustment of external prosthetic device
- Z45, Encounter for adjustment and management of implanted device
- Z46, Encounter for fitting and adjustment of other devices
- Z47, Orthopedic aftercare
- Z48 Encounter for other postprocedural aftercare
- Z49 Encounter for care involving renal dialysis
- Z51 Encounter for other aftercare

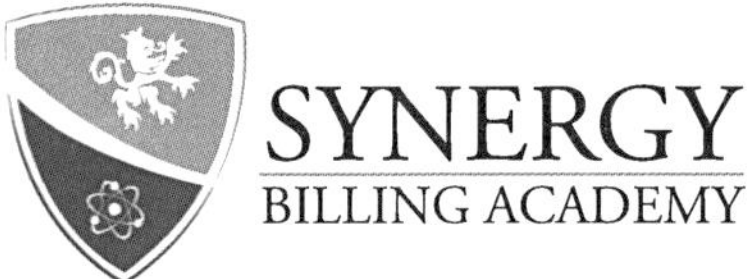

8. **Follow-up**

The follow-up codes are used to explain continuing surveillance following completed treatment of a disease, condition, or injury. They imply that the condition has been fully treated and no longer exists. They should not be confused with aftercare codes or injury codes with a 7th character for subsequent encounter, which explain ongoing care of a healing condition or its sequela(e).

Follow-up codes may be used in conjunction with history codes to provide the full picture of the healed condition and its treatment. The follow-up code is sequenced first, followed by the history code.

A follow-up code may be used to explain multiple visits. Should a condition be found to have recurred on the follow-up visit, then the diagnosis code for the condition should be assigned in place of the follow-up code.

The follow-up Z Code categories are:

- Z08, Encounter for follow-up examination after completed treatment for malignant neoplasm
- Z09, Encounter for follow-up examination after completed treatment for conditions other than malignant neoplasm
- Z39, Encounter for maternal postpartum care and examination

9. **Donor**

Codes in category Z52, Donors of organs and tissues, are used for living individuals who are donating blood or other body tissue. These codes are only for individuals donating for others, not for self-donations. They are not used to identify cadaveric donations.

10. **Counseling**

Counseling Z Codes are used when a patient or family member receives assistance in the aftermath of an illness or injury, or when support is required in coping with family or social problems. They are not used in conjunction with a diagnosis code when the counseling component of care is considered integral to standard treatment.

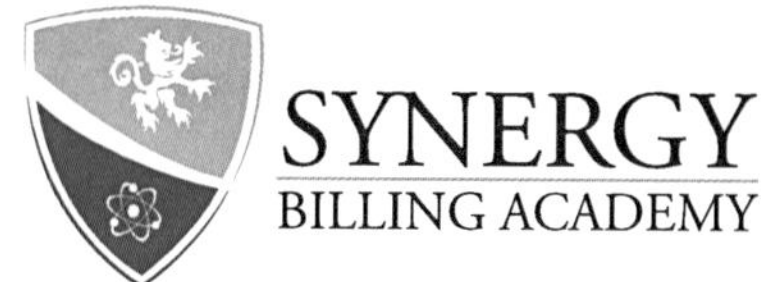

The counseling Z Codes/categories are:

- Z30.0-, Encounter for general counseling and advice on contraception
- Z31.5, Encounter for genetic counseling
- Z31.6-, Encounter for general counseling and advice on procreation
- Z32.2, Encounter for childbirth instruction
- Z32.3, Encounter for childcare instruction
- Z69, Encounter for mental health services for victim and perpetrator of abuse
- Z70, Counseling related to sexual attitude, behavior, and orientation
- Z71, Persons encountering health services for other counseling and medical advice, not elsewhere classified
- Z76.81, Expectant mother prebirth pediatrician visit

11. Encounters for obstetrical and reproductive services

See Section I.C.15. on Pregnancy, Childbirth, and the Puerperium for further instruction on the use of these codes.

Z Codes for pregnancy are for use in those circumstances when none of the problems or complications included in the codes from the Obstetrics chapter exist (a routine prenatal visit or postpartum care). Codes in category Z34, Encounter for supervision of normal pregnancy, are always first-listed and are not to be used with any other code from the OB chapter.

Codes in category Z3A, Weeks of gestation, may be assigned to provide additional information about the pregnancy. The date of the admission should be used to determine weeks of gestation for inpatient admissions that encompass more than one gestational week.

The outcome of delivery, category Z37, should be included on all maternal delivery records. It is always a secondary code. Codes in category Z37 should not be used on the newborn record.

Z Codes for family planning (contraceptive) or procreative management and counseling should be included on an obstetric record either during the pregnancy or the postpartum stage, if applicable.

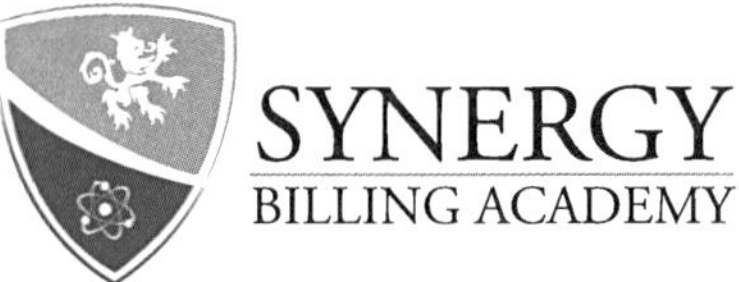

Z Codes/categories for obstetrical and reproductive services are:

- Z30, Encounter for contraceptive management
- Z31, Encounter for procreative management
- Z32.2, Encounter for childbirth instruction
- Z32.3, Encounter for childcare instruction
- Z33, Pregnant state
- Z34, Encounter for supervision of normal pregnancy
- Z36, Encounter for antenatal screening of mother
- Z3A, Weeks of gestation
- Z37, Outcome of delivery
- Z39, Encounter for maternal postpartum care and examination
- Z76.81, Expectant mother prebirth pediatrician visit

12. Newborns and infants

See Section I.C.16. on Newborn (Perinatal) Guidelines for further instruction on the use of these codes.

Newborn Z Codes/categories are:

- Z76.1, Encounter for health supervision and care of foundling
- Z00.1-, Encounter for routine child health examination
- Z38, Liveborn infants according to place of birth and type of delivery

13. Routine and administrative examinations

The Z Codes allow for the description of encounters for routine examinations, such as a general check-up, or examinations for administrative purposes, such as a pre-employment physical. The codes are not to be used if the examination is for diagnosis of a suspected condition or for treatment purposes. In such cases, the diagnosis code is used. Should a disease or condition be discovered during a routine exam and listed with a diagnosis, it should be coded as an additional code. Pre-existing and chronic conditions and history codes may also be included as additional codes as long as the examination is for administrative purposes and not focused on any particular condition.

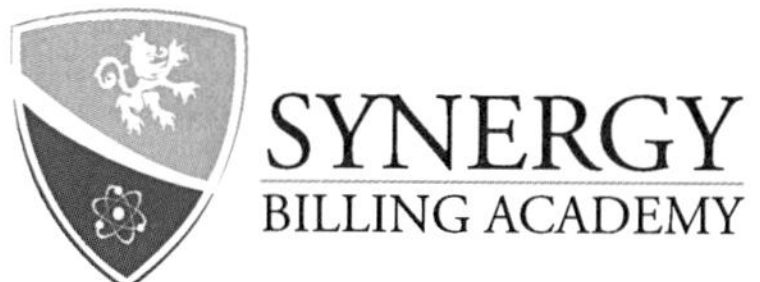

Some of the codes for routine health examinations distinguish between "with" and "without" abnormal findings. Code assignment depends on the information that is known at the time the encounter is being coded. For example, if no abnormal findings were uncovered during the examination but the encounter is being coded before test results are back, it is acceptable to assign the code for "without abnormal findings." When assigning a code for "with abnormal findings," additional code(s) should be assigned to identify the specific abnormal finding(s).

Preoperative examination and pre-procedural laboratory examination Z Codes are for use only in those situations when a patient is being cleared for a procedure or surgery and no treatment is given.

The Z Codes/categories for routine and administrative examinations are:

- Z00, Encounter for general examination without complaint, suspected or reported diagnosis
- Z01, Encounter for other special examination without complaint, suspected or reported diagnosis
- Z02, Encounter for administrative examination
    - — Except: Z02.9, Encounter for administrative examinations, unspecified
- Z32.0-, Encounter for pregnancy test

14. Miscellaneous Z Codes

The miscellaneous Z Codes capture a number of health care encounters that do not fall into one of the other categories. Some of these codes identify the reason for the encounter; others are for use as additional codes that provide useful information on circumstances that may affect a patient's care and treatment.

a. Prophylactic organ removal

For encounters specifically for prophylactic removal of an organ (such as prophylactic removal of breasts due to a genetic susceptibility to cancer or a family history of cancer), the principal or first-listed code should be a code from category Z40, Encounter for prophylactic surgery, followed by the appropriate codes to identify the associated risk factor (such as genetic susceptibility or family history).

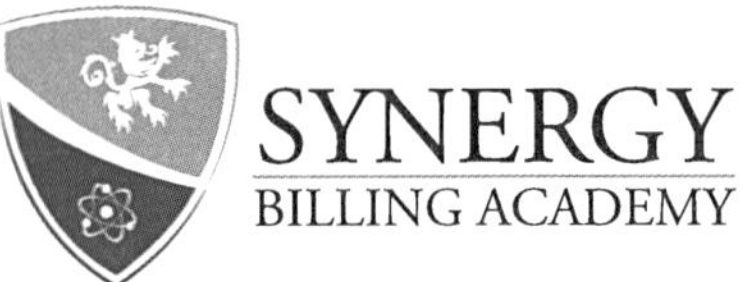

If the patient has a malignancy of one site and is having prophylactic removal at another site to prevent either a new primary malignancy or metastatic disease, a code for the malignancy should also be assigned in addition to a code from subcategory Z40.0, Encounter for prophylactic surgery for risk factors related to malignant neoplasms. A Z40.0 code should not be assigned if the patient is having organ removal for treatment of a malignancy, such as the removal of the testes for the treatment of prostate cancer.

Miscellaneous Z Codes/categories are:

- Z28, Immunization not carried out
  - Except: Z28.3, Underimmunization status
- Z40, Encounter for prophylactic surgery
- Z41, Encounter for procedures for purposes other than remedying health state
  - Except: Z41.9, Encounter for procedure for purposes other than remedying health state, unspecified
- Z53, Persons encountering health services for specific procedures and treatment, not carried out
- Z55, Problems related to education and literacy
- Z56, Problems related to employment and unemployment
- Z57, Occupational exposure to risk factors
- Z58, Problems related to physical environment
- Z59, Problems related to housing and economic circumstances
- Z60, Problems related to social environment
- Z62, Problems related to upbringing
- Z63, Other problems related to primary support group, including family circumstances
- Z64, Problems related to certain psychosocial circumstances
- Z65, Problems related to other psychosocial circumstances
- Z72, Problems related to lifestyle
- Z73, Problems related to life management difficulty
- Z74, Problems related to care provider dependency
  - Except: Z74.01, Bed confinement status
- Z75, Problems related to medical facilities and other health care
- Z76.0, Encounter for issue of repeat prescription
- Z76.3, Healthy person accompanying sick person
- Z76.4, Other boarder to health care facility

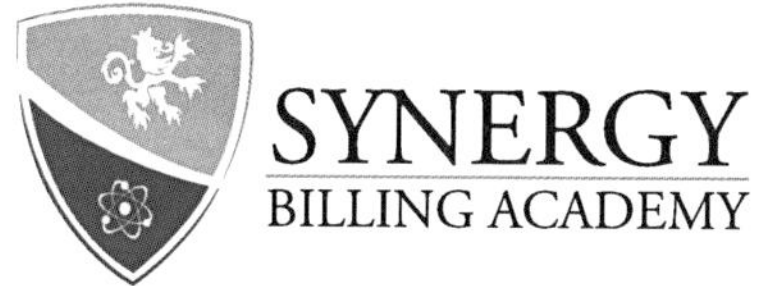

- Z76.5, Malingerer [conscious simulation]
- Z91.1-, Patient's noncompliance with medical treatment and regimen
- Z91.83, Wandering in diseases classified elsewhere
- Z91.89, Other specified personal risk factors, not elsewhere classified

15. Nonspecific Z Codes

Certain Z Codes are so nonspecific, or potentially redundant with other codes in the classification, that there can be little justification for their use in the inpatient setting. Their use in the outpatient setting should be limited to those instances when there is no further documentation to permit more precise coding. Otherwise, any sign or symptom or any other reason for visit that is captured in another code should be used.

Nonspecific Z Codes/categories are:

- Z02.9, Encounter for administrative examinations, unspecified
- Z04.9, Encounter for examination and observation for unspecified reason
- Z13.9, Encounter for screening, unspecified
- Z41.9, Encounter for procedure for purposes other than remedying health state, unspecified
- Z52.9, Donor of unspecified organ or tissue
- Z86.59, Personal history of other mental and behavioral disorders
- Z88.9, Allergy status to unspecified drugs, medicaments, and biological substances status
- Z92.0, Personal history of contraception

16. Z Codes that may only be principal/first-listed diagnosis

The following Z Codes/categories may only be reported as the principal/first-listed diagnosis, except when there are multiple encounters on the same day and the medical records for the encounters are combined:

- Z00, Encounter for general examination without complaint, suspected or reported diagnosis
- Z01, Encounter for other special examination without complaint, suspected or reported diagnosis
- Z02, Encounter for administrative examination
- Z03, Encounter for medical observation for suspected diseases and

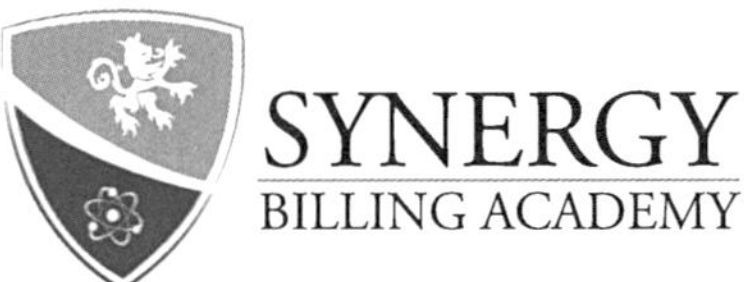

- conditions ruled out
- Z04, Encounter for examination and observation for other reasons
- Z33.2, Encounter for elective termination of pregnancy
- Z31.81, Encounter for male factor infertility in female patient
- Z31.82, Encounter for Rh incompatibility status
- Z31.83, Encounter for assisted reproductive fertility procedure cycle
- Z31.84, Encounter for fertility preservation procedure
- Z34, Encounter for supervision of normal pregnancy
- Z39, Encounter for maternal postpartum care and examination
- Z38, Liveborn infants according to place of birth and type of delivery
- Z42, Encounter for plastic and reconstructive surgery following medical procedure or healed injury
- Z51.0, Encounter for antineoplastic radiation therapy
- Z51.1-, Encounter for antineoplastic chemotherapy and immunotherapy
- Z52, Donors of organs and tissues
  Except: Z52.9, Donor of unspecified organ or tissue
- Z76.1, Encounter for health supervision and care of foundling
- Z76.2, Encounter for health supervision and care of other healthy infant and child
- Z99.12, Encounter for respirator [ventilator] dependence during power failure

Word of Caution [12, 26]

In order to support the depth of ICD-10-CM, physician clinical documentation must, for example, contain details regarding:

- Laterality
- Stages of healing, e.g., routine, delayed, or malunion
- Trimester of pregnancy
- Episode of care, e.g., initial or subsequent encounter, sequela
- Depth, size, and cause of injuries
- Combination codes must reflect the association between conditions
- New clinical concepts such as underdosing

Helpful Tips

- Be specific in describing the patient's condition, illness, or disease.

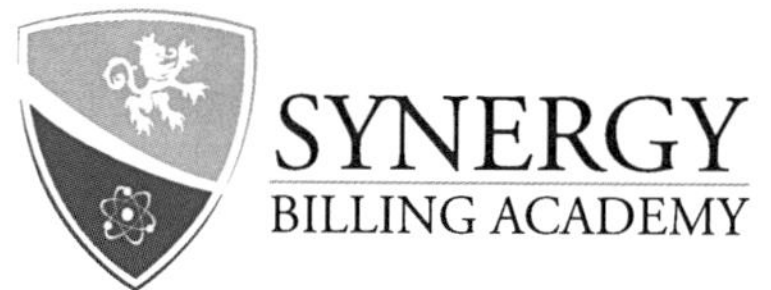

- Distinguish between acute and chronic conditions, when appropriate.
- Identify the acute condition of an emergency situation.
  - Coma, loss of consciousness, hemorrhage, etc.
- Identify chronic complaints or secondary diagnoses.
- Identify how injuries occur.
- Be as granular as possible.
  - Acute, chronic, acute on chronic, recurrent
  - Mild, moderate, severe
  - Site or location
  - Laterality
    - Left, right, bilateral
  - Injury details
    - External cause, activity, place of occurrence

Documentation Requirements

Example 1 – Headache [48]

ICD-10-CM contains many different codes for headaches due to the increased specificity of the new documentation requirements. For example, when a patient presents with a migraine (code G43), physicians must specify whether it is common, hemiplegic, persistent, chronic, ophthalmologic, abdominal, or menstrual.

Cluster headaches and other trigeminal autonomic cephalgias (code G44.0) have been grouped into episodic, chronic, episodic paroxysmal hemicrania, chronic paroxysmal hemicrania, and short-lasting unilateral neuralgiform headache with conjunctival injection and tearing.

There are also codes for vascular headaches (G44.1), tension-type headaches (G44.2), post-traumatic headaches (G44.3), and drug-induced headaches (G44.4), as well as a variety of other headache syndromes.

Many of the codes in the headache section also require the following documentation:

- With or without aura
- Intractable vs. not intractable
- With or without status migrainosus

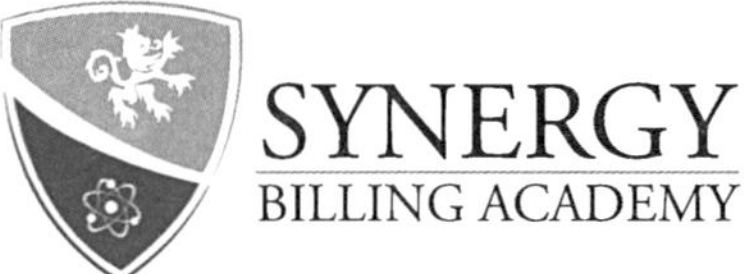

Example 2 – Depression [48]

According to the Centers for Disease Control and Prevention (CDC), an estimated one in every 10 adults reports depression. The section for depression codes has been greatly expanded in ICD-10-CM. When a patient presents with major depression (codes F32-F33), physicians must document the following:

- Single episode vs. recurrent
- Mild, moderate, or severe
- With or without psychotic features
- In partial or full remission

Example 3 – Ear infections [48]

ICD-10-CM includes various codes to denote specific forms of a middle ear infection. These codes are grouped in H65-H67 and distinguish between the following forms of otitis media:

- Serous
- Allergic
- Mucoid
- Nonsuppurative
- Suppurative
- Tubotympanic suppurative
- Atticoantral suppurative

Physicians must also document the following information for many of the codes in this section:

- Acute vs. chronic
- Laterality (left vs. right vs. bilateral)
- Any associated perforated tympanic membrane

Example 4 – Hypertension [48]

ICD-10-CM code I10 denotes essential (primary) hypertension. There are separate codes for hypertension involving vessels of the brain (codes I60-I69) and hypertension involving vessels of the eye (code H35.0).

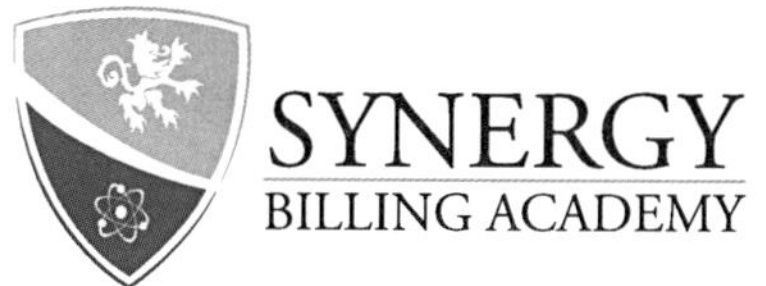

ICD-10-CM also includes codes for hypertensive heart disease with or without heart failure (code I11) and hypertensive chronic kidney disease (code I12). Physicians must also document the stage of the chronic kidney disease, hypertensive heart and chronic kidney disease (code I13), and secondary hypertension (code I15).

Example 5 – Diabetes [48]

Diabetes (codes E08-E13) has also undergone a significant expansion in ICD-10-CM. Physicians must document whether the diabetes is type 1, type 2, drug- or chemical-induced, or due to an underlying condition. They must document the specific underlying condition, the specific drug or toxin, and the use of any insulin. ICD-10-CM requires very specific details regarding any complications or manifestations of the diabetes. For example, code E08.341 denotes diabetes mellitus due to underlying condition with severe nonproliferative diabetic retinopathy with macular edema. A careful review of diabetes codes is required to ensure compliance.

Example 6 – Asthma [48]

Asthma (code J45) is another diagnosis that has been expanded in ICD-10-CM. Physicians must document whether the asthma is:

- Mild intermittent
- Mild persistent
- Moderate persistent
- Severe persistent

They must also specify whether the asthma is uncomplicated, with acute exacerbation, or with status asthmaticus.

Notes to Remember [9, 10]

Chapter 1

We now have a wide range of codes that we can use to identify infections with a predominantly sexual mode of transmission (A50-A64); however, human immunodeficiency virus (HIV) disease was excluded from this new section.

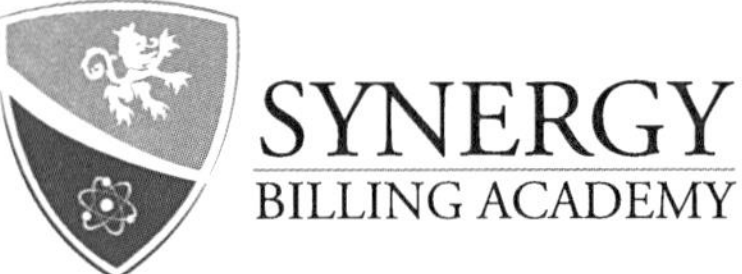

Chapter 4

In the endocrine, nutritional, and metabolic diseases chapter, we need to keep in mind that all codes have been expanded, especially when it comes to diabetes. Remember that more codes means more instructional notes. For example, under category E09 (drug - or chemical-induced diabetes mellitus), we have a note instructing to "code first poisoning due to drug or toxin if applicable;" another note that states to "Use additional code for adverse effect, if applicable," to identify the drug; and a note to "use an additional code to identify any insulin use." After those notes, we also have an Excludes note that we need to pay close attention to.

Chapter 5

In ICD-10-CM, in order to classify that the patient has a history of alcohol and drug abuse, we would identify it as in remission; ICD-10-CM does not have a separate history code section for this. Moreover, we can now specify the level of alcohol in the patient's blood.

Chapter 7

For diseases of the eye and adnexa, we need to specify laterality in our documentation, which is the side that was affected. We now have codes for right, left, bilateral, and unspecified. If we do not have a bilateral code available, we must use two codes, one code for the right side and another code for the left side.

Chapter 8

This chapter details diseases of the ear and mastoid process. Differentiating between the inner, middle, and external ear will help us navigate the arrangement of conditions in this chapter. Several notes under otitis media must be taken into account to allow us to correctly document conditions and code for reimbursement. These notes instruct us to "use additional code for any associated perforated tympanic membrane (H72.-)" and to use additional code(s) to identify any type of exposure such as:

- Exposure to environmental tobacco smoke (Z77.22)
- Exposure to tobacco smoke in the perinatal period (P96.81)
- History of tobacco use (Z87.891)
- Occupational exposure to environmental tobacco smoke (Z57.31)
- Tobacco dependence (F17.-)
- Tobacco use (Z72.0)

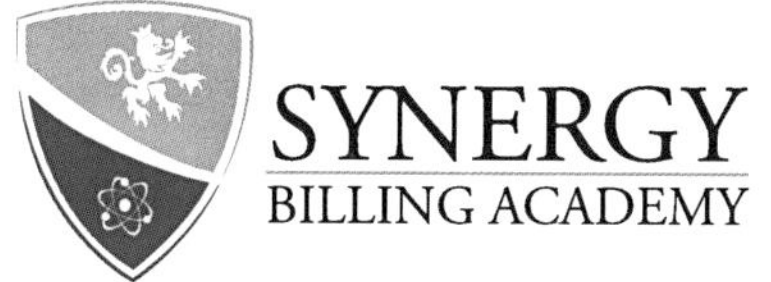

Chapter 9

Hypertension is classified in this chapter of diseases of the circulatory system. In ICD-9-CM, we had a hypertension table; hypertension was classified with category code 401 and we had different types of hypertension such as malignant, benign, and unspecified. Now in ICD-10-CM, that is no longer the case. Hypertension is not classified by type and we no longer have a hypertension table. In this chapter there are also instructional notes that we need to pay close attention to.

Chapter 10

In Chapter 10, Diseases of the Respiratory System, we have new terminology for asthma. Asthma and its stages are classified as intermittent, mild persistent, moderate persistent, or severe persistent. The following table provides shows the difference in stages for children:

Asthma Severity	Frequency of Symptoms (Daytime)
Intermittent	Less than or equal to 2 times per week
Mild Persistent	More than 2 times per week
Moderate Persistent	Daily, may restrict physical activity
Severe Persistent	Throughout the day, frequent severe attacks limiting ability to breathe.

Chapter 11

In Chapter 11, Diseases of the Digestive System, the classification for hernias has changed. Now hernia with gangrene and obstruction is classified as hernia with gangrene. We also have many new combination codes for complications and manifestations of Crohn's disease.

Chapter 13

In Chapter 13, Diseases of the Musculoskeletal System, the 7th character for pathological and stress fractures may be any of the following:

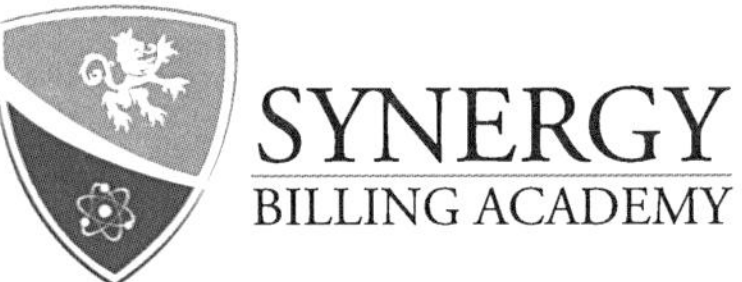

7th character for pathological and stress fractures	
A	Initial Encounter
D	Subsequent - routine healing
G	Subsequent - delayed healing
K	Subsequent - nonunion
P	Subsequent - malunion
S	Sequela

Pathologic fractures can be classified in different categories: pathologic fractures that are due to neoplastic disease, pathologic fractures that are due to osteoporosis, or pathologic fractures that are due to other specified disease. Another classification is the difference between the types of origin, such as spontaneous versus fragility. Spontaneous rupture occurs when normal force is applied to tissues that are inferred to have less than normal strength; fragility fractures are sustained with trauma no more than a fall from a standing height or less occurring under circumstances that would not cause a fracture in a normal, healthy bone. These types of fractures need to be specified in the doctor's documentation; the coder is not able to make such a judgment without specific and clear documentation.

Chapter 14

In Chapter 14, Diseases of the Genitourinary System, we need to carefully identify if extra codes or extra documentation are required. Below are some instructional notes that you will see in the codes in this chapter:

Code	Description
N17	Code also underlying condition
N18	Code first etiology
N30	Additional code infectious agent
N31	Additional code urinary incontinence
N33	Code first underlying disease
N40.1	Additional code for associated symptoms

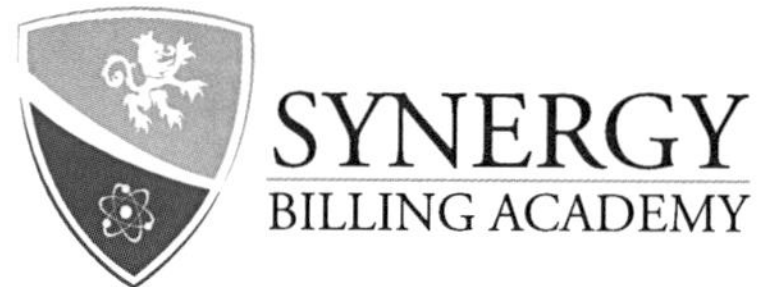

Chapter 15

This chapter can only be used in the mother's record for documentation and coding; Chapter 15 codes are never used in the newborn's because this chapter encompasses the conditions that are related to or aggravated by the pregnancy, childbirth, and the puerperium. For Chapter 15, the trimester is now the measurement of classification. In ICD-9-CM, we used the episode of care, such as delivered, antepartum, intrapartum, and postpartum. We also have to keep in mind that not all codes include the ability to select the trimesters. The trimesters are counted from the first day of the last menstrual period and are classified as follows:

Trimesters	
1st	Less than 14 weeks 0 days
2nd	14 weeks to less than 28 weeks 0 days
3rd	28 weeks 0 days until delivery

We must also specify the week of gestation. We are now required to code this using category code Z3A. In Chapter 15, we have a combination code that incorporates obstructed labor with the reason for the obstruction into one code. We also have some definitions we need to keep in mind, such as: the timeline for abortion versus fetal death is now 20 weeks instead of 22; early versus late vomiting is now 20 weeks instead of 22; and preterm labor still happens before completing a full 37 weeks of gestation.

For certain conditions, we need to specify the fetus that is being affected. For a single pregnancy, the 7th character will be "0;" this is also the case for multiple gestations where the fetus is unspecified. 7th characters of 1 through 9 are used for cases of multiple gestations to identify the fetus for which the code applies. Below are the 7th characters for fetus identification:

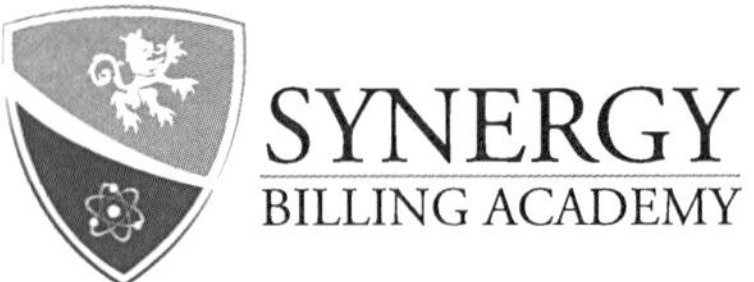

Fetus Identification	
0	Not applicable or unspecified
1	Fetus 1
2	Fetus 2
3	Fetus 3
4	Fetus 4
5	Fetus 5
9	Other fetus

Chapter 16

Codes from this chapter are for use on newborn records only, never on maternal records. The codes in this chapter, Certain Conditions Originating in the Perinatal Period, include conditions that have their origin in the fetal or perinatal period (before birth through the first 28 days after birth) even if morbidity occurs later.

The codes in block P00-P04 (Newborn affected by maternal factors and by complication of pregnancy, labor, and delivery) are for use when the listed maternal conditions are specified as the cause of confirmed morbidity or potential morbidity that have their origin in the perinatal period, which is before birth through the first 28 days after birth. These codes can be used for newborns who are suspected of having an abnormal condition resulting from exposure from the mother or the birth process, but without signs or symptoms, and which, after examination and observation, is found not to exist. These codes may be used even if treatment is begun for a suspected condition that is ruled out.

When using codes from this chapter, we need to pay close attention to instructional notes throughout the chapter and in several of the classifications. For deliveries, we need to make sure that we use category Z38 (liveborn infants according to place of birth and type of delivery), which indicates the following:

Category Z38	
Classifies Liveborn	• Place of birth • Type of delivery
Principal Code	• Initial record • Newborn
Not Used	Mother's record

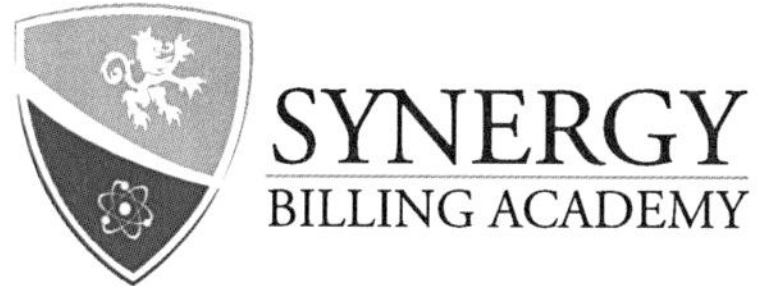

Chapter 17

We can use the codes from Chapter 17, Congenital Malformations, Deformations, and Chromosomal Abnormalities, when a malformation/deformation or chromosomal abnormality is actually documented by the physician. When no unique code is available, assign additional code(s) for any manifestations. When a malformation/deformation or chromosomal abnormality does not have a unique code assignment, assign additional code(s) for any manifestations that may be present.

When the code assignment specifically identifies the malformation/deformation or chromosomal abnormality, manifestations that are inherent components of the anomaly should not be coded separately. Additional codes should be assigned for manifestations that are not inherent components. These codes are to be used throughout the life of the patient. Although present at birth, malformation/deformation or chromosomal abnormality may not be identified until later in life. Whenever the condition is diagnosed by the physician, it is appropriate to assign a code from codes Q00-Q99.

Chapter 18

Codes in this chapter were added to classify symptoms, signs, and abnormal clinical and laboratory findings that are not elsewhere classified. The uses for these codes are as follows:

Code	Description
A	No more specific diagnosis can be made even after all facts have been investigated
B	Signs or symptoms existing at time of initial encounter are transient and causes not determined
C	Provisional diagnosis in patient failing to return
D	Referred elsewhere before diagnosis made
E	More precise diagnosis not available
F	Certain symptoms, for which supplementary information is provided, that represent important problems in medical care in their own right

Another addition to this chapter is the Glasgow Coma Scale. This scale is used along with traumatic brain injury, acute cerebrovascular disease, or sequelae of cerebrovascular disease codes. These are primarily used by trauma registries and in research, but may be used in any other setting. These codes have to be sequenced after the diagnosis code. These codes help

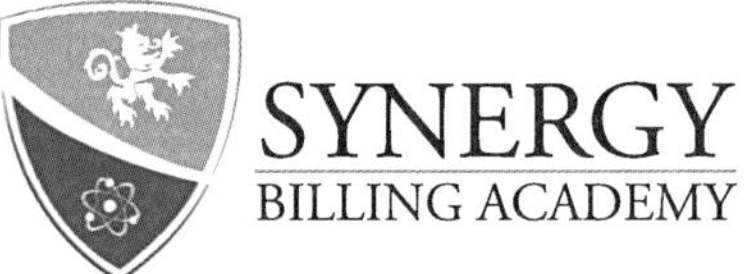

identify the patient's eye response, verbal response, and motor response, as well as where and when these elements were recorded, such as:

7th Character	Meaning
0	Unspecified time
1	In field (EMT or ambulance)
2	At arrival to ER
3	At hospital admission
4	24 hours after admission

Chapter 19

Chapter 19 is the chapter where injuries, poisoning, and certain other consequences of external causes have been classified. This chapter has a total of two letters, "S" for injuries that are related to a body region and "T" for injuries to unspecified regions as well as poisoning and external causes. Here you will find the classification for injuries, which is different from ICD-9-CM. In ICD-9-CM, injuries were grouped by the type of injury, such as fracture, strain, sprain, etc. In ICD-10-CM, injuries are now grouped by body part, then by type of injury. An example of the classification is as follows:

Body Part	Code Range
Head	S00 - S09
Neck	S10 - S19
Thorax	S20 - S29

Many elements must be taken into consideration when dealing with fractures. If a fracture is not indicated as open or closed, we would code it as closed. If a fracture is not indicated as displaced or nondisplaced, we would code it as displaced. Some other elements that need to be included in the documentation are the type of fracture, the specific anatomical site, displaced vs. nondisplaced, laterality, routine vs. delayed healing, nonunion, malunion, and the type of encounter (initial, subsequent, sequela). Depending on the fracture, the following shows what the 7th character might be:

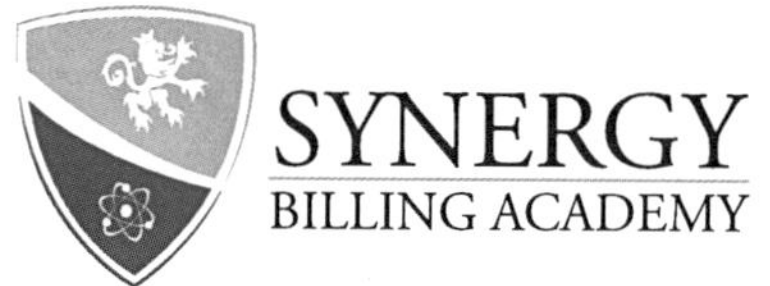

7th Character Stress Fractures	
A	Initial closed
B	Initial open
D	Subsequent - routine
G	Subsequent - delayed
K	Subsequent - nonunion
P	Subsequent - malunion
S	Sequela

Initial encounter is used when the patient is receiving active treatment for the condition, such as surgical treatment, an emergency department encounter, or an evaluation and treatment by a new physician. A subsequent encounter is used after the patient has received active treatment for the condition and is now receiving routine care during the healing or recovery phase, such as a cast change or removal, a removal of external or internal fixation device, a medication adjustment, or other aftercare and follow-up visits following injury treatment. Sequela is used when complications or conditions that arise as a direct result of a condition, such as scar formation after a burn.

We must understand the difference between poisoning, adverse effect, and underdosing, as all of these terms are used in this chapter.

Term	Definition
Poisoning	Overdose of substances; wrong substance given or taken in error
Adverse effect	"Hypersensitivity," "reaction," or correct substance properly administered
Underdosing	Taking less of a medication than is prescribed or instructed by manufacturer, either inadvertently or deliberately

Gustilo Anderson Classification

ICD-10-CM uses the Gustilo Anderson system to identify the severity of soft tissue damage for open fractures. Only three categories of codes in ICD-10-CM require the Gustilo Anderson classifications: S52, Fracture of forearm; S72, Fracture of femur; and S82, Fracture of lower leg, including ankle. For open fractures, the 7th characters from the Gustilo classification are B, C, E, F, H, J, M, N, Q, or R. The classification is arranged as follows:

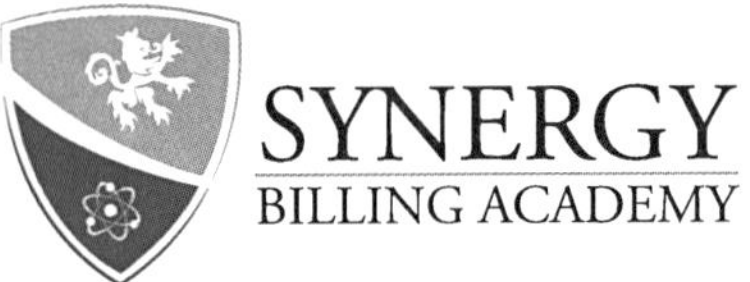

Classification	Definition
I	Low energy wound less than 1 cm
II	Greater than 1 cm with moderate soft tissue damage
III	High energy wound greater than 1 cm with extensive soft tissue damage
IIIA	Adequate soft tissue cover
IIIB	Inadequate soft tissue cover
IIIC	Associated with arterial injury

Chapter 20

Chapter 20, External Causes of Morbidity, allows for the classification of environmental events and circumstances as the cause of injury, and other adverse effects. These codes are to never be used as the primary code on a medical claim. The chapter has blocks from letters V to Y. With these codes, we also need to specify the type of encounter, whether initial, subsequent encounter, or sequela.

In this chapter are the codes for transport accidents, place of occurrence, and the activity the patient was involved when he or she suffered the injury. A transport accident is defined as one in which a vehicle is moving or running or in use for transport purposes at the time of the accident. Below is a note directing us to use an additional code to identify other elements of these accidents.

Use additional code(s) to identify:

- Airbag injury (W22.1)
- Type of street or road (Y92.4-)
- Use of cellular telephone at time of transport accident (Y93.C-)

The place of occurrence is classified in category Y92; this is to be used with the activity code and only recorded on the initial encounter. The category use for the activity is Y93; as with Y92, this can only be added on the record once at the initial encounter, and this code is also not to be used with poisoning, adverse effects, misadventures, or late effects.

Another classification in this chapter is category Y99; this is used as the external cause status to indicate work status. This is used to indicate whether the incident was part of military

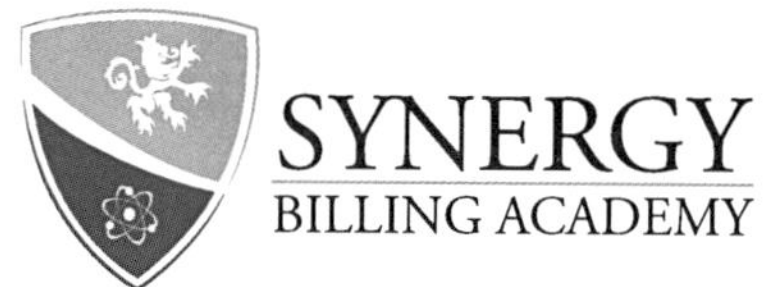

activity, while a non-military person was at work, or when an individual including a student or volunteer was involved in a non-work activity. These codes are to be assigned with other external cause codes, such as transport accidents and falls; they are not to be used with poisonings, adverse effects, misadventures, or late effects.

Everyone needs to understand the classification of burns, the calculation of total body surface area (TBSA) and the rule of nines when assessing the total percentage of area burned for each major section of the body. We also need to keep in mind that there are differences between adults and children in the classification of total body surface area. Clear documentation of burns is required.

Chapter 21

Chapter 21 contains the codes for factors that influence health status and contact with health services; these codes are the equivalent of V Codes. Z Codes represent the reason for the encounter. They are used when a person who may or may not be sick encounters health services for some specific purpose, such as to receive limited care or service for a current condition, to donate an organ or tissue, to receive prophylactic vaccination, or to discuss a problem. These codes are used when some circumstance or problem is present which influences person's health status but is not a current illness or injury.

Most Used Codes

ICD-10-CM and ICD-9-CM – Chapter 1

ICD-9-CM		ICD-10-CM	
034.0	Streptococcal sore throat	J02.0	Streptococcal pharyngitis
		J03.00	Acute streptococcal tonsillitis, unspecified
041.00	Streptococcus, unspecified	B95.5	Unspecified streptococcus as the cause of diseases classified elsewhere
042	HIV disease	B20	Human immunodeficiency virus [HIV] disease

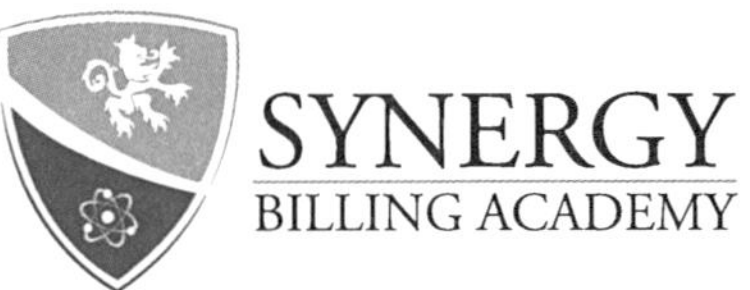

052.9	Varicella without mention of complication	B01.9	Varicella without complication
054.10	Genital herpes, unspecified	A60.9	Anogenital herpesviral infection, unspecified
070.53	Hepatitis e without mention of hepatic coma	B17.2	Acute hepatitis E
078.10	Viral warts, unspecified	B07.9	Viral wart, unspecified
079.4	Human papillomavirus	B97.7	Papillomavirus as the cause of diseases classified elsewhere
099.41	Chlamydia trachomatis	N34.1	Nonspecific urethritis
110.1	Dermatophytosis of nail	B35.1	Tinea unguium
112.1	Candidiasis of vulva and vagina	B37.3	Candidiasis of vulva an vagina

ICD-10-CM Chapter 4 – ICD-9-CM Chapter 3

ICD-9-CM		ICD-10-CM	
244.9	Unspecified hypothyroidism	E03.9	Hypothyroidism, unspecified
250.00	Diabetes mellitus without mention of complication,Type II or unspecified type, not stated as uncontrolled	E11.9	Type 2 diabetes mellitus without complications
250.01	Diabetes mellitus without mention of complication,Type I [juvenile type], not stated as uncontrolled	E10.9	Type 1 diabetes mellitus without complications
250.02	Diabetes mellitus without mention of complication, Type II or unspecified type, uncontrolled	E11.65	Type 2 diabetes mellitus with hyperglycemia
250.21	Diabetes w/hyperosmolarity Type I	E10.69	Type 1 diabetes mellitus with other specified complication
250.62	Diabetes Type II uncontrolled with neurological manifestations	E11.40 E11.65	Type 2 diabetes mellitus with diabetic neuropathy, unspecified Type 2 diabetes mellitus with hyperglycemia
257.2	Other testicular hypofunction	E29.1	Testicular hypofunction
266.2	Other B-complex deficiencies	E53.8	Deficiency of other specified B group vitamins

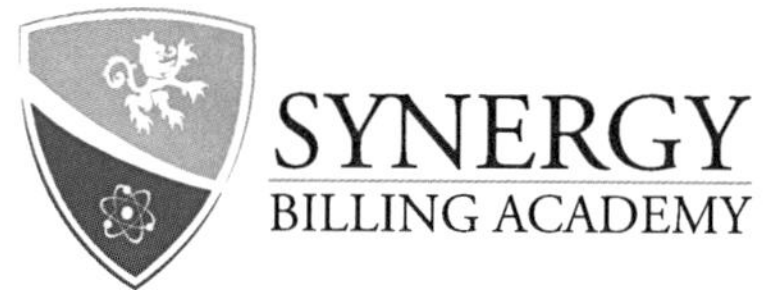

272.0	Pure hypercholesterolemia	E78.0	Pure hypercholesterolemia
272.2	Mixed hyperlipidemia	E78.2	Mixed hyperlipidemia
272.4	Other and unspecified hyperlipidemia	E78.4 E78.5	Other hyperlipidemia Hyperlipidemia, unspecified
274.10	Gouty arthropathy, unspecified	M10.30	Gout due to renal impairment, unspecified site
277.7	Dysmetabolic Syndrome X	E88.81	Metabolic syndrome
278.00	Obesity, unspecified	E66.9	Obesity, unspecified
278.01	Morbid obesity	E66.01	Morbid (severe) obesity due to excess calories

ICD-10-CM and ICD-9-CM – Chapter 5

ICD-9-CM		ICD-10-CM	
293.81	Psychotic disorder with delusions in conditions classified elsewhere	F06.2	Psychotic disorder with delusions due to known physiological condition
293.83	Mood disorder in conditions classified elsewhere	F06.30	Mood disorder due to known physiological condition, unspecified
293.84	Anxiety disorder in conditions classfied elsewhere	F06.4	Anxiety disorder due to known physiological condition
295.60	Schizophrenic disorders - residual type - unspecified	F20.5	Residual schizophrenia
296.21	Majors depressive disorder, mild single episode	F32.0	Major depressive disorder, single episode, mild
296.32	Moderate recurrent major depression	F33.1	Major depressive disorder, recurrent, moderate
297.9	Unspecified paranoid state	F23	Brief psychotic disorder
300.00	Anxiety, dissociative, and somatoform disorders - anxiety state, unspecified	F41.9	Anxiety disorder, unspecified
302.70	Psychosexual dysfunction, unspecified	R37	Sexual dysfunction, unspecified

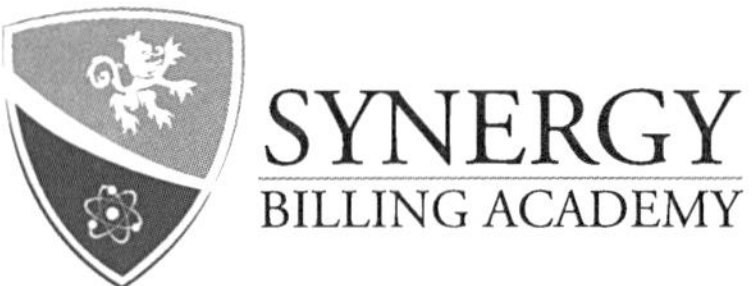

302.85	Gender identity disorder in adolescents or adults	F64.1	Gender identity disorder in adolescence and adulthood
304.90	Unspecified drug dependence – unspecified	F19.20	Other psychoactive substance dependence, uncomplicated
305.1	Nondependent tobacco use disorder	F17.200	Nicotine dependence, unspecified, uncomplicated

ICD-10-CM Chapter 6, 7, 8 – ICD-9-CM Chapter 6

ICD-9-CM		ICD-10-CM	
338.4	Chronic pain syndrome	G89.4	Chronic pain syndrome
367.1	Myopia	H52.13	Myopia, bilateral
372.00	Acute disorders of conjunctiva unspecified	H10.33	Unspecified acute conjunctivitis, bilateral
381.02	Acute mucoid otitis media	H65.119	Acute and subacute allergic otitis media (mucoid) (sanguinous) (serous), unspecified ear
382.9	Unspecified otitis media	H66.90	Otitis media, unspecified, unspecified ear

ICD-10-CM Chapter 9 – ICD-9-CM Chapter 7

ICD-9-CM		ICD-10-CM	
401.0	Essential hypertension, malignant	I10	Essential (primary) hypertension
401.1	Essential hypertension, benign	I10	Essential (primary) hypertension
401.9	Essential hypertension, unspecified	I10	Essential (primary) hypertension
415.19	Pulmonary embolism and infarction, other	I26.99	Other pulmonary embolism without acute cor pulmonale
428.0	Congestive heart failure, unspecified	I50.9	Heart failure, unspecified
429.2	Unspecified cardiovascular disease	I25.10	Atherosclerotic heart disease of native coronary artery without angina pectoris

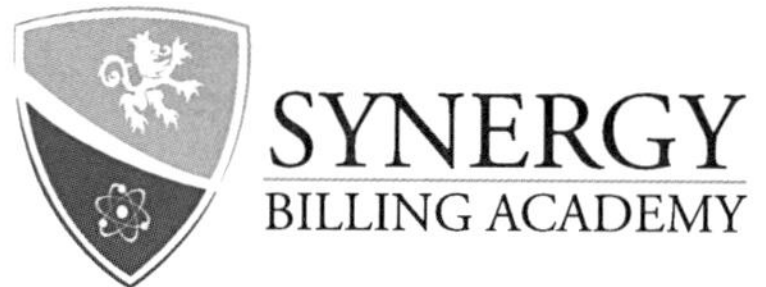

ICD-10-CM Chapter 10 – ICD-9-CM Chapter 8

ICD-9-CM		ICD-10-CM	
460	Acute nasopharyngitis	J00	Acute nasopharyngitis [common cold]
461.9	Acute sinusitis, unspecified	J01.90	Acute sinusitis, unspecified
462	Acute pharyngitis	J02.9	Acute pharyngitis, unspecified
465.9	Acute upper respiratory infection unspecified site NOS	J06.9	Acute upper respiratory infection, unspecified
466.0	Acute bronchitis	J20.9	Acute bronchitis, unspecified
466.19	Acute bronchiolitis due to other infections organisms	J21.8	Acute bronchiolitis due to other specified organisms
472.0	Chronic rhinitis	J31.0	Chronic rhinitis
472.1	Chronic pharyngitis	J31.2	Chronic pharyngitis
472.2	Chronic nasopharyngitis	J31.1	Chronic nasopharyngitis
473.9	Unspecified sinusitis	J32.9	Chronic sinusitis, unspecified
477.0	Allergic rhinitis due to pollen	J30.1	Allergic rhinitis due to pollen
477.9	Allergic rhinitis, cause unspecified	J30.0 J30.9	Vasomotor rhinitis Allergic rhinitis, unspecified
486	Pneumonia, organism unspecified	J18.9	Pneumonia, unspecified organism
490	Bronchitis, not specified as acute or chronic	J40	Bronchitis, not specified as acute or chronic
491.20	Obstructive chronic bronchitis, without exacerbation	J44.9	Chronic obstructive pulmonary disease, unspecified
493.00	Extrinsic asthma, unspecified	J45.20	Mild intermittent asthma, uncomplicated
493.90	Asthma NOS	J45.909 J45.998	Unspecified asthma, uncomplicated Other asthma
496	(Chronic airway obstruction, not elsewhere classified)	J44.9	Chronic obstructive pulmonary disease, unspecified

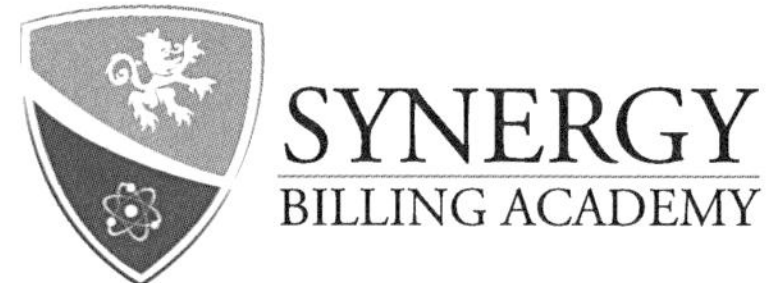

ICD-10-CM Chapter 11 – ICD-9-CM Chapter 9

ICD-9-CM		ICD-10-CM	
521.00	Unspecified dental caries	K02.9	Dental caries, unspecified
525.9	Toothache	K08.9	Disorder of teeth and supporting structures, unspecified
530.11	Reflux esophagitis	K21.0	Gastro-esophageal reflux disease with esophagitis
530.81	Esophageal reflux	K21.9	Gastro-esophageal reflux disease without esophagitis
564.00	Unspecified constipation	K59.00	Constipation, unspecified

ICD-10-CM Chapter 13 – ICD-9-CM Chapter 6

ICD-9-CM		ICD-10-CM	
714.0	Rheumatoid arthritis	M06.9	Rheumatoid arthritis, unspecified
715.90	Osteoarthritis unspecified, site unspecified	M15.9 M19.90	Polyosteoarthritis, unspecified Unspecified osteoarthritis, unspecified site
716.90	Unspecified arthropathy, site unspecified	M12.9	Arthropathy
719.41	Pain in joint, shoulder region	M25.519	Pain in unspecified shoulder
719.44	Pain in joint, hand	M79.643 M79.646	Pain in unspecified hand Pain in unspecified finger(s)
719.46	Pain in joint, lower leg	M25.569	Pain in unspecified knee
719.47	Pain in joint, ankle and foot	M25.579	Pain in unspecified ankle and joints of unspecified foot
719.48	Pain in joint, other specified sites	M25.50	Pain in unspecified joint
719.49	Pain in joint, multiple sites	M25.50	Pain in unspecified joint
723.1	Cervicalgia	M54.2	Cervicalgia
724.2	Lumbago	M54.5	Low back pain

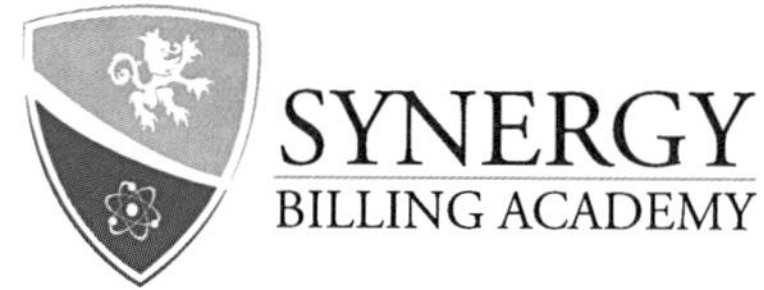

724.4	Thoracic or lumbosacral neuritis or radiculitis, unspecified	M54.14 M54.15 M54.16 M54.17	Radiculopathy, thoracic region Radiculopathy, thoracolumbar region Radiculopathy, lumbar region Radiculopathy, lumbosacral region
724.5	Back pain	M54.89 M54.9	Other dorsalgia Dorsalgia, unspecified
728.85	Spasm of muscle	M62.40 M62.838	Contracture of muscle, unspecified site Other muscle spasm
729.1	Unspecified myalgia and myositis	M60.9 M79.1 M79.7	Myositis, unspecified Myalgia Fibromyalgia

ICD-10-CM Chapter 14 – ICD-9-CM Chapter 10

ICD-9-CM		ICD-10-CM	
599.0	Urinary tract infection, site not specified	N39.0	Urinary tract infection, site not specified
616.10	Vaginitis	N76.0 N76.1 N76.2 N76.3	Acute vaginitis Subacute and chronic vaginitis Acute vulvitis Subacute and chronic vulvitis
616.11	Vaginitis and vulvovaginitis in diseases classified elsewhere	N77.1	Vaginitis, vulvitis, and vulvovaginitis in diseases classified elsewhere
623.5	Vaginal discharge (unspecified)	N89.8	Other specified noninflammatory disorders of vagina
626.2	Excessive or frequent menstruation	N92.0	Excessive and frequent menstruation with regular cycle

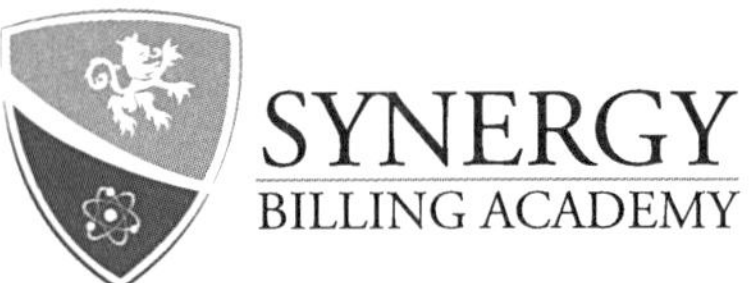

ICD-10-CM Chapter 15 – ICD-9-CM Chapter 11

ICD-9-CM		ICD-10-CM	
654.23	Previous c-section delivery antepartum condition	O34.21	Maternal care for scar from previous cesarean delivery

ICD-10-CM Chapter 16 – ICD-9-CM Chapter 15

ICD-9-CM	ICD-10-CM
Certain Conditions Originating in the Perinatal Period (760-779)	Certain Conditions Originating in the Perinatal Period (P00-P96)

ICD-10-CM Chapter 17 – ICD-9-CM Chapter 14

ICD-9-CM	ICD-10-CM
Congenital Anomalies (740-759)	Congenital Malformations, Deformations, and Chromosomal Abnormalities (Q00-Q99)

ICD-10-CM Chapter 18 – ICD-9-CM Chapter 16

ICD-9-CM		ICD-10-CM	
780.52	Insomnia, unspecified	G47.00	Insomnia, unspecified
780.60	Fever, unspecified	R50.2 R50.9	Drug-induced fever Fever, unspecified
780.79	Other malaise and fatigue	G93.3 R53.1 R53.81 R53.83	Postviral fatigue syndrome Weakness Other malaise Other fatigue
782.1	Rash and other nonspecific skin erupt	R21	Rash and other nonspecific skin eruption

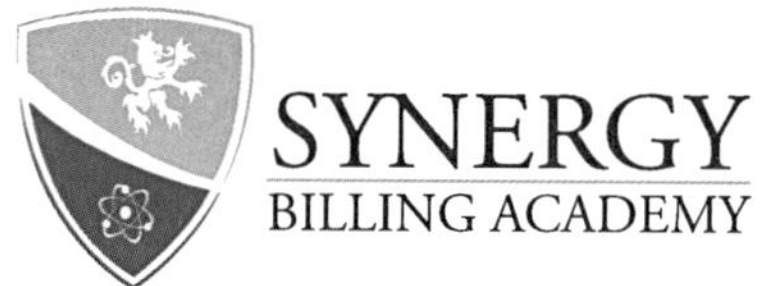

ICD-9-CM		ICD-10-CM	
782.3	Edema	R60.0 R60.1 R60.9	Localized edema Generalized edema Edema, unspecified
784.0	Headache	G44.1 R51	Vascular headache, not elsewhere classified Headache
786.05	Shortness of breath	R06.02	Shortness of breath
786.2	Cough	R05	Cough
786.50	Chest pain, unspecified	R07.9	Chest pain, unspecified
788.1	Dysuria	R30.0 R30.9	Dysuria Painful micturition, unspecified
789.00	Abdominal pain, unspecified site	R10.9	Unspecified abdominal pain
789.01	Abdominal pain, right upper quadrant	R10.11	Right upper quadrant pain

ICD-10-CM Chapter 19 – ICD-9-CM Chapter 17

ICD-9-CM	ICD-10-CM
Injury and Poisoning (800-999)	Injury, Poisoning, and Certain Other Consequences of External Causes (S00-T88) T = Toxicity

ICD-10-CM Chapter 20 – ICD-9-CM E Codes

ICD-9-CM	ICD-10-CM
Supplemental Classification of External Causes of Injury and Poisoning (E800-E99)	Injury, Poisoning, and Certain Other Consequences of External Causes (S00-T88) T = Toxicity; External Causes of Morbidity (V01-Y99); Y = Why did it happen?

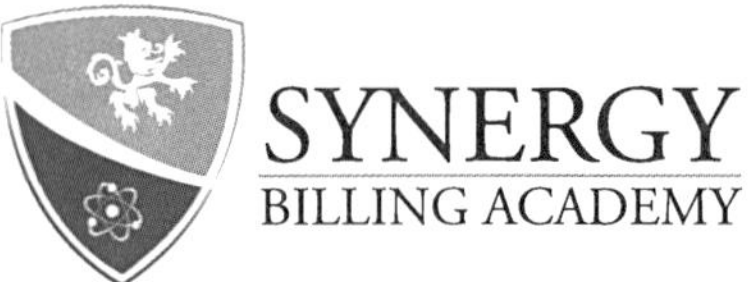

ICD-10-CM Chapter 21/Z Codes – ICD-9-CM V Codes

ICD-9-CM		ICD-10-CM	
V01.6	Contact with or exposure to venereal disease	Z20.2	Contact with and (suspected) exposure to infections with a predominantly sexual mode of transmission
V03.81	Hemophilus influenza, type B vaccine	Z23	Encounter for immunization
V03.82	Pneumococcal vaccine	Z23	Encounter for immunization
V03.89	Other specified vaccination	Z23	Encounter for immunization
V03.9	Vaccine for bacterial disease	Z23	Encounter for immunization
V04.81	Need for prophylactic vaccination and inoculation, influenza	Z23	Encounter for immunization
V04.89	Vaccine for viral disease	Z23	Encounter for immunization
V05.3	Viral hepatitis	Z23	Encounter for immunization
V05.8	Need for prophylactic vaccine and inoculation against other specified	Z23	Encounter for immunization
V05.9	Need for prophylactic vaccine and inoculation against unspecified	Z23	Encounter for immunization
V06.1	Diphtheria-tetanus-pertussis	Z23	Encounter for immunization
V06.4	Measles-mumps-rubella	Z23	Encounter for immunization
V06.8	Other combination	Z23	Encounter for immunization
V06.9	Unspecified combination vaccine	Z23	Encounter for immunization
V07.8	Need for other specified prophylactic or treatment	Z41.8	Encounter for other procedures for purposes other than remedying health state
V15.81	Noncompliance with medical treatment	Z91.19	Patient's noncompliance with other medical treatment and regimen
V15.82	Personal history of tobacco use, presenting hazards to health	Z87.891	Personal history of nicotine dependence
V20.0	Health supervision of infant or child – foundling	Z76.1	Encounter for health supervision and care of foundling

Primary Care Providers

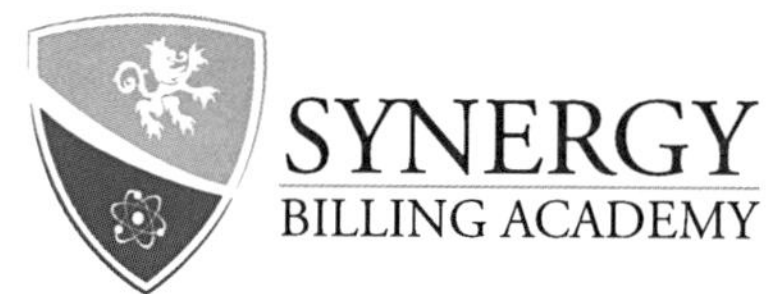

ICD-9	Description	ICD-10	Description
V20.1	Health supervision – healthy infant/ child receiving care	Z76.2	Encounter for health supervision and care of other healthy infant and child
V20.2	Routine infant/child check-up	Z00.129	Encounter for routine child health examination without abnormal findings
V22.0	Supervision of normal first pregnancy	Z34.00	Encounter for supervision of normal first pregnancy, unspecified trimester
V22.1	Supervision of other normal pregnancy	Z34.80	Encounter for supervision of other normal pregnancy, unspecified trimester
		Z34.90	Encounter for supervision of normal pregnancy, unspecified, unspecified trimester
V22.2	Pregnant state, incidental	Z33.1	Pregnant state, incidental
V24.2	Routine postpartum follow-up	Z39.2	Encounter for routine postpartum follow-up
V25.02	General counseling for initiation of other contraceptive measures	Z30.018	Encounter for initial prescription of other contraceptives
V25.09	Other general counseling and advice on contraceptive management	Z30.09	Encounter for other general counseling and advice on contraception
V25.40	Contraception maintenance	Z30.40	Encounter for surveillance of contraceptives, unspecified
V25.49	Surveillance other previous contraceptive method	Z30.49	Encounter for surveillance of other contraceptives
V27.0	Outcome of delivery single live born	Z37.0	Single live birth
V29.0	Observation and evaluation newborn and infants suspected infectious condition	P00.2	Newborn (suspected to be) affected by maternal infectious and parasitic diseases
V52.3	Fitting and adjustment of dental prosthetic device	Z46.3	Encounter for fitting and adjustment of dental prosthetic device
V62.3	Educational circumstance	Z55.9	Problems related to education and literacy, unspecified

Primary Care Providers

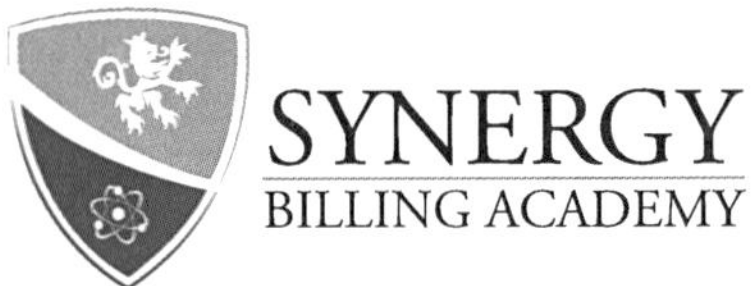

V65.40	Counseling NOS	Z71.9	Counseling, unspecified
V65.49	Other specified counseling	Z71.89	Other specified counseling
V68.01	Disability examination	Z02.71	Encounter for disability determination
V68.1	Issue of repeat prescriptions	Z76.0	Encounter for issue of repeat prescription
V69.2	Problems related to high-risk sexual behavior	Z72.51	High-risk heterosexual behavior
V70.0	Exam, general adult medical	Z00.00	Encounter for general adult medical examination without abnormal findings
V70.3	Exam, marriage/camp/school/ sports	Z02.89	Encounter for other administrative examinations
V70.5	Health examination of defined subpopulation	Z02.1 Z02.3 Z02.89	Encounter for pre-employment examination Encounter for examination for recruitment to armed forces Encounter for other administrative examinations
V72.2	Dental examination	Z01.20 Z01.21	Encounter for dental examination and cleaning without abnormal findings Encounter for dental examination and cleaning with abnormal findings
V72.31	Exam, gynecological	Z01.411 Z01.419	Encounter for gynecological examination (general) (routine) with abnormal findings Encounter for gynecological examination (general) (routine) without abnormal findings
V72.32	Encounter for pap cervical smear to confirm findings of recent normal smear following initial abnormal smear	Z01.42	Encounter for cervical smear to confirm findings of recent normal smear following initial abnormal smear

Primary Care Providers

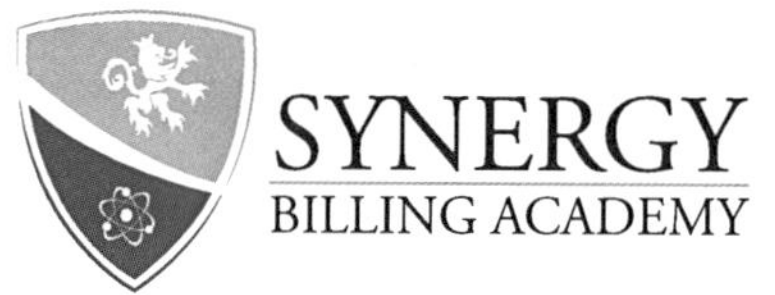

V72.41	Pregnancy examination or test negative	Z32.02	Encounter for pregnancy test, result negative
V72.85	Other specified examination	Z01.89	Encounter for other specified special examinations
V74.1	Screening examination for pulmonary tuberculosis	Z11.1	Encounter for screening for respiratory tuberculosis
V74.5	Screen for venereal disease STI	Z11.3	Encounter for screening for infections with a predominantly sexual mode of transmission
V76.2	Screen malignant neoplasm-cervix	Z12.4	Encounter for screening for malignant neoplasm of cervix
V76.44	Special screening for malignant neoplasm of prostate	Z12.5	Encounter for screening for malignant neoplasm of prostate
V77.91	Screening for lipoid disorders	Z13.220	Encounter for screening for lipoid disorders
V78.0	Screening for iron deficiency or anemia	Z13.0	Encounter for screening for diseases of the blood and blood-forming organs and certain disorders involving the immune mechanism

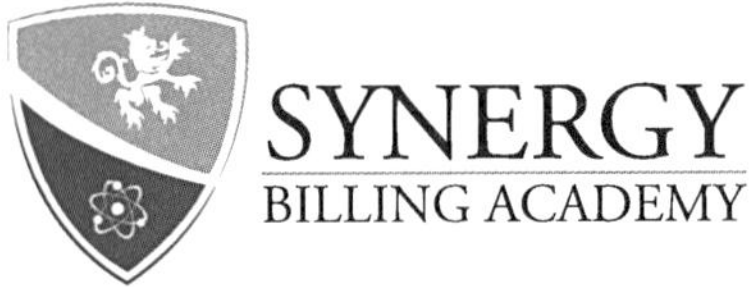

Check Your Understanding

1. For otitis media, we need to document exposure to tobacco smoke, if any, as well as how the patient was exposed to it.

   a. True
   b. False

2. We now have new terminology to help us with asthma and its severity.

   a. True
   b. False

3. Combination codes make it more difficult to classify diseases, complications, and manifestations.

   a. True
   b. False

4. A spontaneous rupture and a fragility fracture are the same thing.

   a. True
   b. False

5. Injuries were grouped by type of injury rather than the body part affected.

   a. True
   b. False

6. ICD-10-CM provides for greater specificity and detail.

   a. True
   b. False

7. Laterality indicates the side of the body that has been affected.

   a. True
   b. False

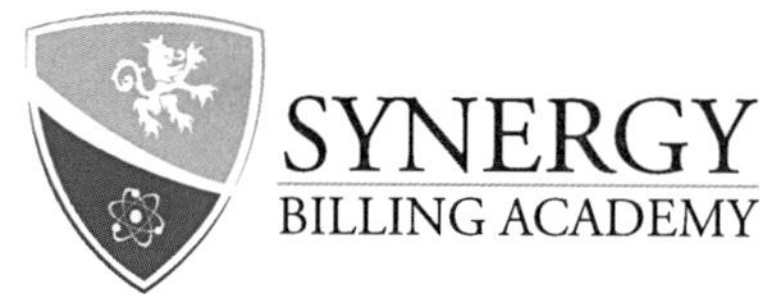

8. Z Codes are what we knew as V Codes in ICD-9-CM.

   a. True
   b. False

9. It is not necessary to indicate the weeks of gestation on the patient's chart.

   a. True
   b. False

10. All chronic conditions need to be added on the patient's records.

   a. True
   b. False

ICD-10-CM International Classification of Diseases 10th Revision Clinical Modification

Obstetrics & Gynecology

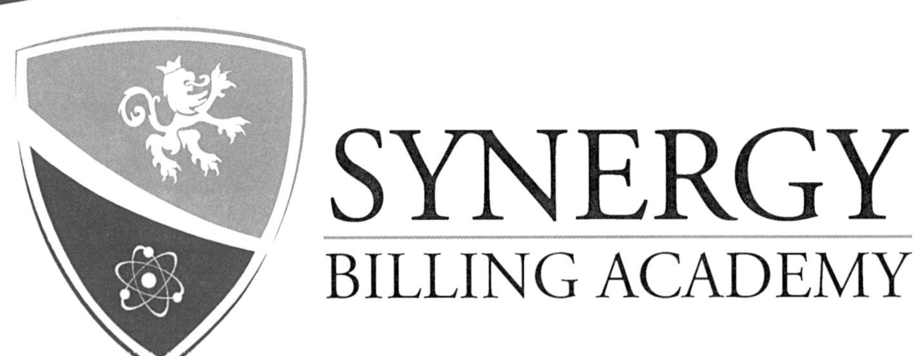

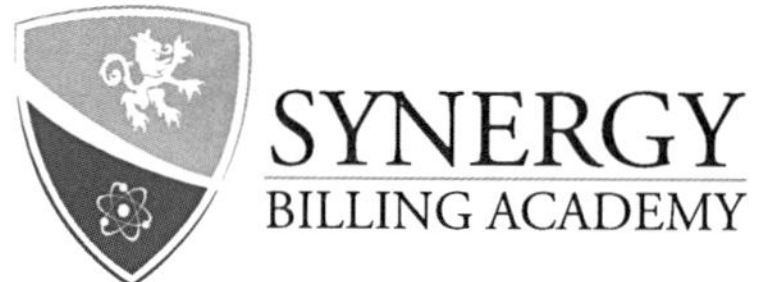

Obstetrics and Gynecology Background and Practice [25]

Obstetrics and gynecology is a discipline dedicated to the broad, integrated medical and surgical care of women's health throughout their lifespan. The combined discipline of obstetrics and gynecology requires extensive study and understanding of reproductive physiology, including the physiologic, social, cultural, environmental, and genetic factors that influence disease in women. This study and understanding of the reproductive physiology of women gives obstetricians and gynecologists a unique perspective in addressing gender-specific health care issues.

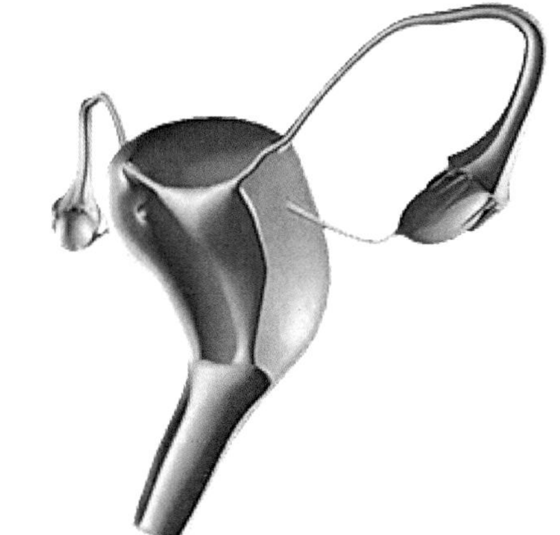

Preventive counseling and health education are essential and integral parts of the practice of obstetricians and gynecologists as they advance the individual and community-based health of women of all ages.

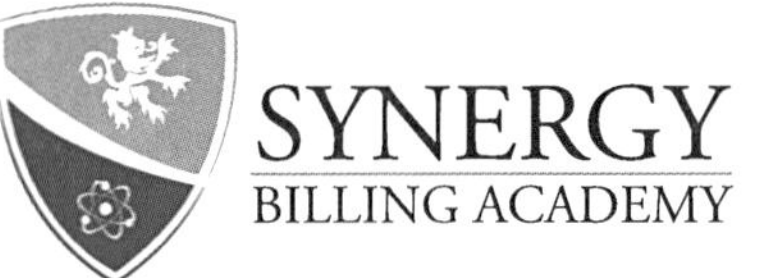

OB/GYN Claims and Coding Manuals

In 2003, it was mandated that all HIPAA-covered entities use diagnostic codes. In other words, even dentists are required to use ICD-9-CM to report a patient's diagnosis and the reason for his or her visit.

On October 1, 2015, the ICD-10-CM (International Classification of Diseases 10th Revision Clinical Modification) will be released, marking the replacement of ICD-9-CM, which is what all OB/GYN providers have been using to add the diagnosis or reason for visit to their patients' claims. ICD-9-CM codes do not have sufficient coverage due to lack of specificity for many diagnoses. Below is a short list of some of the codes that we are currently using:

Categories	ICD-9-CM
Well Care/Preventive	• V70.0 Routine physical (12+) • V70.5 Health exam
Counseling	• V65.44 HIV counseling • V65.45 STD counseling
Other Preventive	• V76.2 Routine pap smear • V22.2 Pregnant state, incidental
Contraception	• V25.01 Rx oral contraceptive • V25.09 Management, contraceptive, other
Pregnancy Postpartum	• 650 Delivery, normal • 648.8 Gestational diabetes
Menstruation	• 626.0 Amenorrhea • 626.4 Irregular menstrual cycle
GYN	• 789.00 Abdominal pain • 620.2 Ovarian cyst

ICD-10-CM will not have any effects in Current Procedural Terminology (CPT) codes.

ICD-10-CM Diseases and Disorders

Transitioning to ICD-10-CM will completely change the codes used in obstetrics and gynecology. Each and every one of the codes and their descriptions will be more specific to the patient's condition. Overall, ICD-9-CM codes are vague and not very descriptive, whereas ICD-10-CM

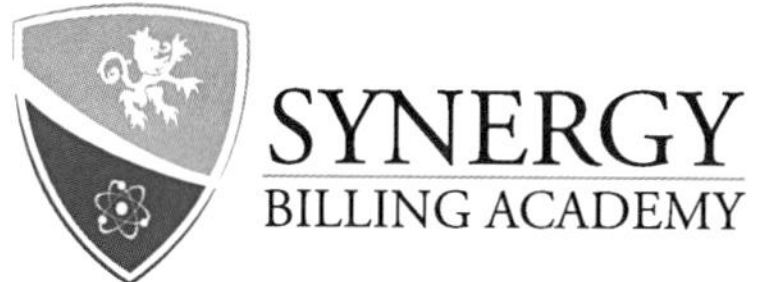

codes are more descriptive. Obstetrics and gynecology encompasses several parts of ICD-10-CM. Below is a list of where all the OB/GYN conditions will be found.

Chapters	Title
Chapter 1	Certain Infectious and Parasitic Diseases (A00-B99)
Chapter 14	Diseases of the Genitourinary System (N00-N99)
Chapter 15	Pregnancy, Childbirth, and the Puerperium (O00-O9A)
Chapter 21	Factors Influencing Health Status and Contact with Health Services (Z00-Z99)

ICD-9-CM and ICD-10-CM – Chapter 1 [9, 20, 24]

Chapter 1 is indexed very similarly in both coding manuals, even though some category and subcategory titles have been changed.

Examples

ICD-9-CM		ICD-10-CM	
008	Intestinal infections due to other organisms	A08	Viral and other specified intestinal infections
024 025	Glanders Melioidosis	A24	Glanders and melioidosis
036.4	Meningococcal carditis	A39.5	Meningococcal heart disease

ICD-9-CM and ICD-10-CM – Chapter 14 [9, 20, 24]

In ICD-9-CM, genitourinary disorders in diseases classified elsewhere are classified within different subcategories. In ICD-10-CM, they are placed in their own category at the end of each block of this chapter.

Since the terminology in ICD-9-CM is outdated, changes were necessary in some sections.

Because of new discoveries on male erectile dysfunction since the last revision of ICD-9-CM, ICD-10-CM now includes category N52 for this condition, with subcategories to identify the

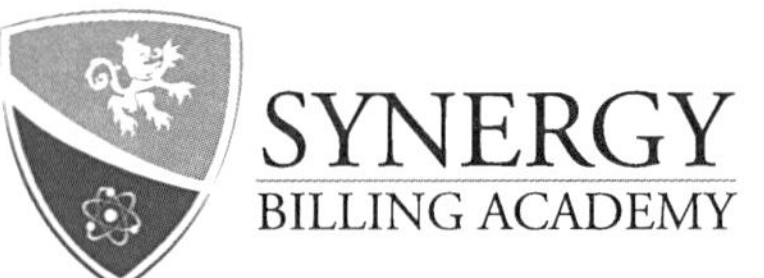

different causes of the dysfunction. ICD-9-CM has a single code, 607.84, Impotence of organic origin.

To code to the highest level of specificity for post-traumatic urethral stricture, professionals will need to identify the patient's gender. This is not necessary for ICD-9-CM code selection for this disorder.

ICD-9-CM and ICD-10-CM – Chapter 15 [9, 20, 24]

Just as in ICD-9-CM, codes from Chapter 15 are to be used only on the maternal record and never on the newborn record.

ICD-9-CM		ICD-10-CM	
654	Abnormality of organs and soft tissues of pelvis	O34	Maternal care for abnormality of pelvic organs
664	Trauma to perineum and vulva during delivery	O70	Perineal laceration during delivery

ICD-9-CM to ICD-10-CM – Chapter 21 [9, 20, 24]

Professionals will find the listing of codes for factors influencing health status and contact with health services somewhat different in ICD-10-CM than in ICD-9-CM.

What were formerly V Codes are now Z Codes–this is a huge difference.

Certain codes have been moved from other chapters in ICD-9-CM to Chapter 21.

Elective, legal, or therapeutic abortions have been moved from ICD-9-CM Chapter 11, Complications of Pregnancy, Childbirth, and the Puerperium, to ICD-10-CM Chapter 21.

ICD-10-CM Chapter Categories

Professionals will find the listing of obstetrics and gynecological codes a little different in ICD-10-CM than what is currently found in ICD-9-CM. The following tables will show you all of the different sections related to OB/GYN and the code representations for them:

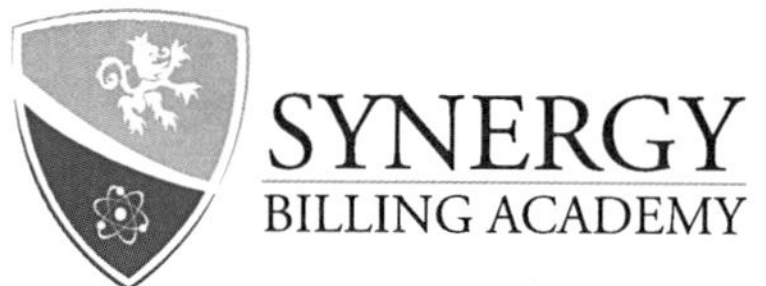

Chapter 1: Classification of Diseases and Disorders	
A00-A09	Intestinal infectious diseases
A15-A19	Tuberculosis
A20-A28	Certain zoonotic bacterial diseases
A30-A49	Other bacterial diseases
A50-A64	***Infections with a predominantly sexual mode of transmission***
A65-A69	Other spirochetal diseases
A70-A74	***Other diseases caused by chlamydia***
A75-A79	Rickettsioses
A80-A89	Viral and prion infections of the central nervous system
A90-A99	Arthropod-borne viral fevers and viral hemorrhagic fevers
B00-B09	Viral infections characterized by skin and mucous membrane lesions
B10	***Other human herpes viruses***
B15-B19	Viral hepatitis
B20	***Human immunodeficiency virus (HIV) disease***
B25-B34	Other viral diseases
B35-B49	Mycoses
B50-B64	Protozoal diseases
B65-B83	Helminthiasis
B85-B89	Pediculosis, acariasis, and other infestations
B90-B94	Sequelae or infectious and parasitic diseases
B95-B97	***Bacterial and viral infectious agents***
B99	***Other infectious diseases***
Chapter 14: Classification of Diseases and Disorders	
N00-N08	Glomerular diseases
N10-N16	Renal tubulo-interstitial diseases
N17-N19	Acute kidney failure and chronic kidney diseases
N20-N23	Urolithiasis
N25-N29	Other disorders of kidney and ureter
N30-N39	***Other diseases of the urinary system***
N40-N53	Diseases of male genital organs

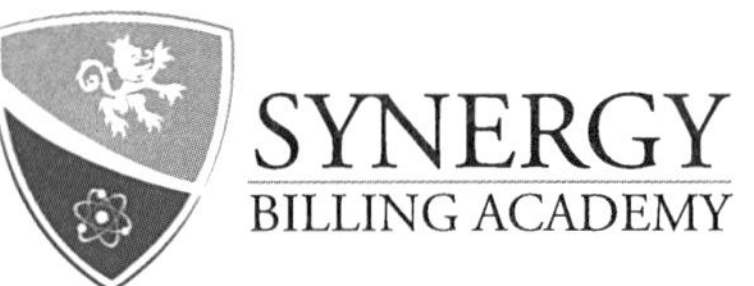

N60-N65	***Disorders of breast***
N70-N77	***Inflammatory diseases of female pelvic organs***
N80-N98	***Noninflammatory disorders of female genital tract***
N99	Intraoperative and postprocedural complications and disorders of genitourinary system, not elsewhere classified
Chapter 15: Classification of Diseases and Disorders	
O00-O08	Pregnancy with abortive outcome
O09	Supervision of high-risk pregnancy
O10-O16	Edema, proteinuria, and hypertensive disorders in pregnancy, childbirth, and the puerperium
O20-O29	Other maternal disorders predominantly related to pregnancy
O30-O48	Maternal care related to the fetus and amniotic cavity and possible delivery problems
O60-O77	Complications of labor and delivery
O80, O82	Encounter for delivery
O85-O92	Complications predominantly related to the puerperium
O94-O9A	Other obstetric conditions, not elsewhere classified
Chapter 21: Classification of Diseases and Disorders	
Z00-Z13	***Persons encountering health services for examinations***
Z14-Z15	Genetic carrier and genetic susceptibility to disease
Z16	Resistance to antimicrobial drugs
Z17	Estrogen receptor status
Z18	Retained foreign body fragment
Z20-Z28	***Persons with potential health hazards related to communicable diseases***
Z30-Z39	***Persons encountering health services in circumstances related to reproduction***
Z40-Z53	Encounters for other specific health care
Z55-Z65	Persons with potential health hazards related to socioeconomic and psychosocial circumstances
Z66	Do not resuscitate status
Z67	Blood type
Z68	Body mass index (BMI)

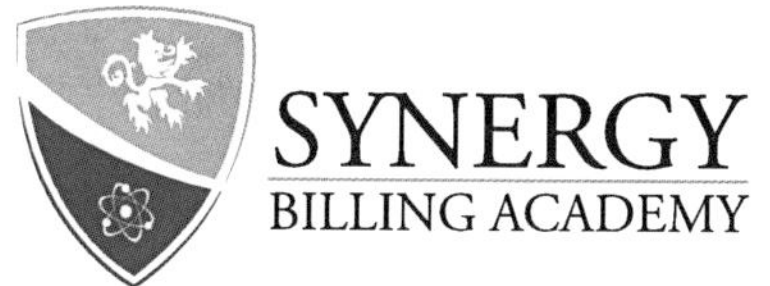

Z69-Z76	*Persons encountering health services in other circumstances*
Z77-Z99	*Persons with potential health hazards related to family and personal history and certain conditions influencing health status*

ICD-10-CM Diseases and Disorders [9, 20, 24]

Many medical specialties have undergone a significant amount of changes with ICD-10-CM. OB/GYN has also been affected. In the transition to ICD-10-CM, all of the chapters that make up OB/GYN include a variety of changes related to diagnosis codes. The following is a detailed list of all the changes in the organization of diseases and disorders per chapter.

Chapter 1: Certain Infectious and Parasitic Diseases

- Includes diseases generally recognized as communicable or transmissible.
- Use additional code to identify resistance to antimicrobial drugs (Z16).
- Categories B90-B94 are to be used to indicate conditions in categories A00-B89 as the cause of sequelae, which are themselves classified elsewhere.
- Code first condition resulting from the infectious or parasitic disease (sequela).
- Bacterial and viral infectious agents (B95-B97) are provided for use as supplementary or additional codes to identify the infectious agent(s) in diseases classified elsewhere
    - Index
        - Infection
        - Organism (Streptococcus)
- Certain diseases have also been rearranged in this chapter. We now have separate subchapters, or blocks, and appropriate conditions have been grouped together for infections with a predominantly sexual mode of transmission.
- A new section called infections with a predominantly sexual mode of transmission (A50–A64) has been added.
- Some terminology changes and revisions to the classification of specific infectious and parasitic disease in ICD-10-CM have been made.
- The term "sepsis" has replaced "septicemia" throughout this chapter.
- Many of the codes in this chapter have been expanded to reflect manifestations of the disease with the use of 4th or 5th characters, allowing the infectious disease and manifestation to be captured in one code instead of two.

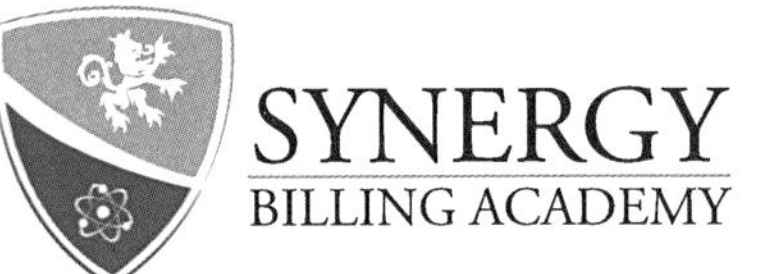

Chapter 14: Diseases of the Genitourinary System

Throughout this chapter, there are new "includes notes" that help clarify the types of disorders that are classified to the various categories.

A similar change has occurred to the instruction for menopausal and other perimenopausal disorders. In ICD-9-CM, there is no guideline under category 627 to help coding professionals select a code for these disorders. However, ICD-10-CM includes a note stating that menopausal and other perimenopausal disorders due to naturally occurring (age-related) menopause and perimenopause are classified to category N95.

Several blocks and category title changes have been made in this particular chapter. An example of this is subsection 617-629 in ICD-9-CM, Other disorders of female genital tract; the corresponding section in ICD-10-CM is N80-N98, Noninflammatory disorders of the female genital tract.

Codes have also moved to this chapter from other chapters. An example of this is code 099.40 from Chapter 1, which is now found in this chapter as the new ICD-10-CM code N34.1.

Chapter 15: Pregnancy, Childbirth, and the Puerperium

The ICD-10-CM manual also requires that we use a 7th character for extensions. In this chapter, the 7th character helps us identify the fetus to which certain complication codes apply. These are the applicable 7th characters:

0 = not applicable or unspecified
1 = fetus 1
2 = fetus 2
3 = fetus 3
4 = fetus 4
5 = fetus 5
9 = other fetus

The 7th character 0 is for single and multiple gestations where the affected fetus is unspecified. 7th characters 1 through 9 are for cases of multiple gestations to identify the fetus for which the code applies. A code from category O30 "multiple gestation" must also be assigned when assigning these codes.

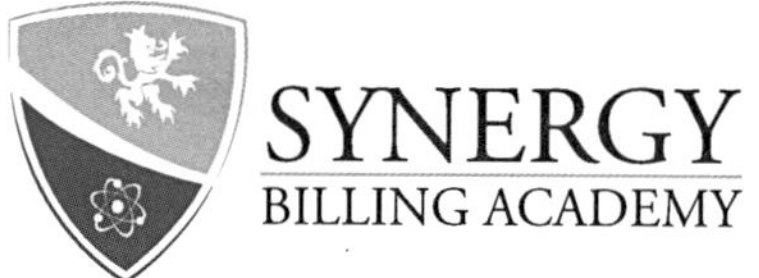

In ICD-9-CM, the codes for elective (legal or therapeutic) abortion are classified with the abortion codes. Now, the elective abortion (without complication) has been moved to code Z33.2, Encounter for elective termination of pregnancy, and O04 is now used for "elective abortion with complication."

The time frame for differentiating the abortion and fetal death codes has changed from 22 to 20 weeks. The time frame for differentiating early and late vomiting in pregnancy has changed from 22 to 20 weeks. Preterm labor is now defined as before 37 completed weeks of gestation.

For ICD-10-CM, code titles were revised in various places within this chapter. An example of this is in code 653.2 of ICD-9-CM; its terminology states the indication for care, such as inlet contraction of pelvis, but its equivalent ICD-10-CM code, O33.2, is much more descriptive. This code actually represents maternal care for disproportion due to inlet contractions of pelvis.

The secondary axis is no longer the episode of care for most conditions that are classified in this particular chapter. ICD-10-CM uses the trimester in which the condition occurred at the 5th and 6th character level. This is because certain conditions or complications occur during certain trimesters. Not all conditions include codes for all three trimesters. Some codes do not include the trimester classification at all because the condition always occurs in a specific trimester, or the concept of trimester of pregnancy is not applicable.

Trimesters are counted from the first day of the last menstrual period:

- 1st trimester = less than 14 weeks 0 days
- 2nd trimester = 14 weeks 0 days to less than 28 weeks 0 days
- 3rd trimester = 28 weeks 0 days until delivery

A code from category Z3A, Weeks of gestation, should be coded to identify the specific week of the pregnancy. The date of admission should be used to determine weeks of gestation for inpatient admissions that encompass more than one gestational week.

One of the blocks in Chapter 21, Factors Influencing Health Status and Contact with Health Services, is Z30-Z39, Persons encountering health services in circumstances related to reproduction. Several categories relate to the pregnant female. They are:

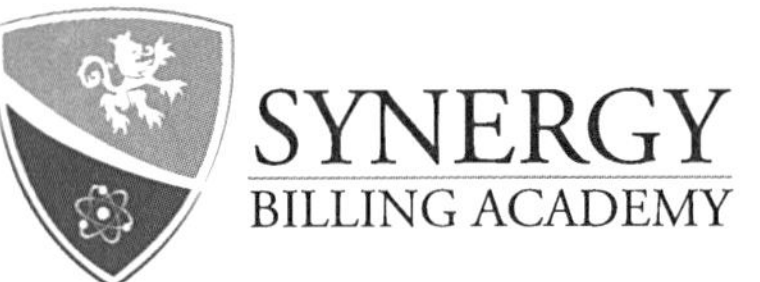

Persons Encountering Health Services in Circumstances Related to Reproduction	
Z32	Encounter for pregnancy test and childbirth and childcare instruction
Z33	Pregnant state
Z34	Encounter for supervision of normal pregnancy
Z36	Encounter for antenatal screening of mother
Z3A	Weeks of gestation
Z37	Outcome of delivery
Z39	Encounter for maternal postpartum care and examination

Outcome of delivery codes (Z37.0-Z37.9) are intended for use as an additional code to identify the outcome of delivery on the mother's record. It is not for use on the newborn record. These codes exclude stillbirth (P95).

Chapter 21: Factors Influencing Health Status and Contact with Health Services

Some category titles have been rephrased to better reflect the situations the codes classify.

The description for Z08 is "encounter for follow-up examination after completed treatment for malignant neoplasm," compared to the ICD-9-CM code title for V67.2, "Follow-up examination following chemotherapy."

An example of decreased specificiity in ICD-10-CM is code Z23, Encounter for immunization. This code is not further classified. In ICD-9-CM, category codes V03, V04, V05, and V06 are used to identify the types of immunizations.

Several codes have been expanded, such as personal and family history.

- Codes have been added for concepts that do not exist in ICD-9-CM.
- Category Z67 identifies the patient's blood type.
- Category Z68, Body Mass Index (BMI), is divided into adult and pediatric codes.
  - The adult BMI codes are for use for persons 21 years of age or older.
  - Pediatric BMI codes are for use for persons 2–20 years of age.
  - The percentiles listed with the codes are based on the growth charts published by the Centers for Disease Control and Prevention (CDC)
- Instructional notes have been added to different categories to explain how codes

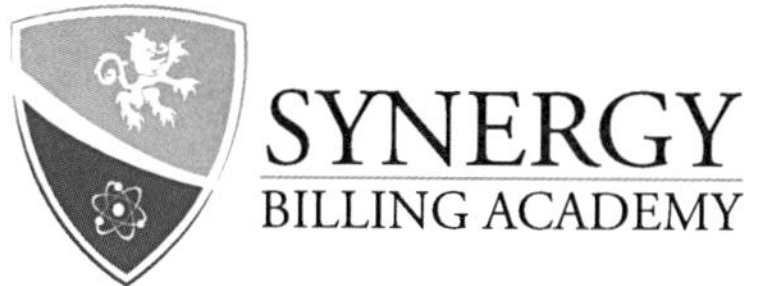

should be assigned.

Under category Z01, Encounter for other special examination without complaint, suspected or reported diagnosis, is the following note: "Codes from category Z01 represent the reason for the encounter. A separate procedure code is required to identify any examination or procedure performed."

Under category Z85, Personal history of malignant neoplasm, is the following note: "Code first any follow-up examination after treatment of malignant neoplasm (Z08)."

Guidelines [9]

As mentioned before, the National Center of Health Statistics (NCHS) along with the American Hospital Association (AHA), the American Health Information Management Association (AHIMA), and the Centers for Medicare and Medicaid Services (CMS) developed and approved coding and reporting guidelines for ICD-10-CM; these organizations also maintain the manual.

Below are the official guidelines published by the NCHS in 2014 as they relate to the OB/GYN chapters:

Chapter 1: Guidelines List

The NCHS has published the following guidelines:

A. Human Immunodeficiency Virus (HIV) Infections
    1. Code only confirmed cases
    2. Selection and sequencing of HIV codes
        a. Patient admitted for HIV-related condition
        b. Patient with HIV disease admitted for unrelated condition
        c. Whether the patient is newly diagnosed
        d. Asymptomatic human immunodeficiency virus
        e. Patients with inconclusive HIV serology
        f. Previously diagnosed HIV-related illness
        g. HIV infection in pregnancy, childbirth, and the puerperium
        h. Encounters for testing for HIV

B. Infectious Agents as the Cause of Diseases Classified to Other Chapters

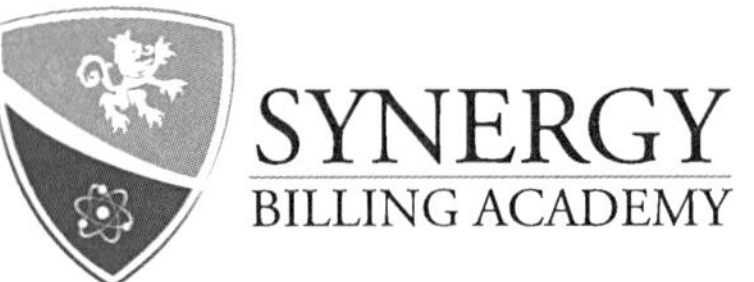

C. Infections Resistant to Antibiotics

D. Sepsis, Severe Sepsis, Septic Shock
   1. Coding of sepsis and severe sepsis
      a. Sepsis
         i. Negative or inconclusive blood cultures and sepsis
         ii. Urosepsis
         iii. Sepsis with organ dysfunction
         iv. Acute organ dysfunction that is not clearly associated with the sepsis
      b. Severe sepsis
   2. Septic shock
   3. Sequencing of severe sepsis
   4. Sepsis and severe sepsis with a localized infection
   5. Sepsis due to a postprocedural infection
      a. Documentation of causal relationship
      b. Sepsis due to a postprocedural infection
      c. Postprocedural infection and postprocedural septic shock
   6. Sepsis and severe sepsis associated with a noninfectious process (condition)
   7. Sepsis and septic shock complicating abortion, pregnancy, childbirth, and the puerperium
   8. Newborn sepsis

E. Methicillin Resistant Staphylococcus Aureus (MRSA) Conditions
   1. Selection and sequencing of MRSA codes
      a. Combination codes for MRSA infection
      b. Other codes for MRSA infection
      c. Methicillin susceptible Staphylococcus aureus (MSSA) and MRSA colonization
      d. MRSA colonization and infection

Chapter 1: Detailed Guidelines

A. Human Immunodeficiency Virus (HIV) Infections

1. Code only confirmed cases
2. Selection and sequencing of HIV codes

   a. Patient admitted for HIV-related condition

   If a patient is admitted for an HIV-related condition, the principal diagnosis should be B20, Human immunodeficiency virus [HIV] disease, followed by additional diagnosis codes for all reported HIV-related conditions.

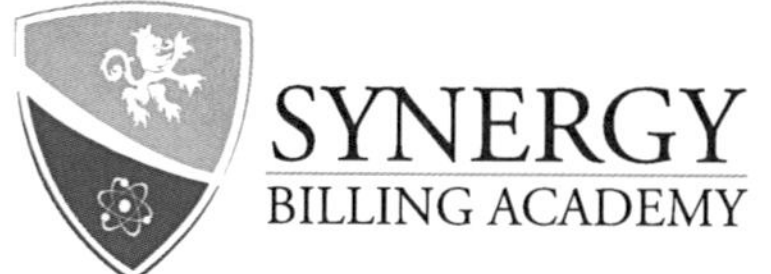

b. **Patient with HIV disease admitted for unrelated condition**

If a patient with HIV disease is admitted for an unrelated condition (such as a traumatic injury), the code for the unrelated condition (e.g., the nature of injury code) should be the principal diagnosis. Other diagnoses would be B20, followed by additional diagnosis codes for all reported HIV-related conditions.

c. **Whether the patient is newly diagnosed**

Whether the patient is newly diagnosed or has had previous admissions/ encounters for HIV conditions is irrelevant to the sequencing decision.

d. **Asymptomatic human immunodeficiency virus**

Z21, Asymptomatic human immunodeficiency virus [HIV] infection status, is to be applied when the patient without any documentation of symptoms is listed as being "HIV positive," "known HIV," "HIV test positive," or similar terminology. Do not use this code if the term "AIDS" is used or if the patient is treated for any HIV-related illness or is described as having any condition(s) resulting from his/ her HIV positive status; use B20 in these cases.

e. **Patients with inconclusive HIV serology**

Patients with inconclusive HIV serology but no definitive diagnosis or manifestations of the illness may be assigned code R75, Inconclusive laboratory evidence of human immunodeficiency virus [HIV].

f. **Previously diagnosed HIV-related illness**

Patients with any known prior diagnosis of an HIV-related illness should be coded to B20. Once a patient has developed an HIV-related illness, the patient should always be assigned code B20 on every subsequent admission/ encounter. Patients previously diagnosed with any HIV illness (B20) should never be assigned to R75 or Z21, Asymptomatic human immunodeficiency virus [HIV] infection status.

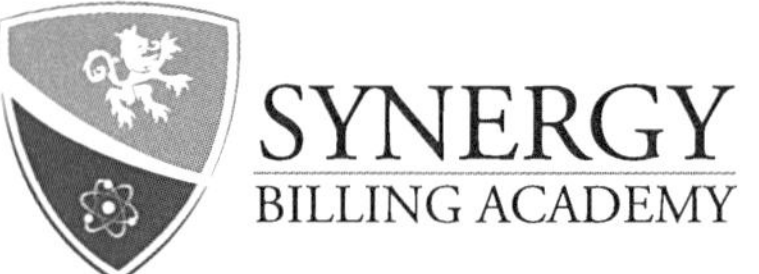

g. **HIV infection in pregnancy, childbirth and the puerperium**

During pregnancy, childbirth, or the puerperium, a patient admitted (or presenting for a health care encounter) because of an HIV-related illness should receive a principal diagnosis code of O98.7-, Human immunodeficiency [HIV] disease complicating pregnancy, childbirth, and the puerperium, followed by B20 and the code(s) for the HIV-related illness(es). Codes from Chapter 15 always take sequencing priority.

Patients with asymptomatic HIV infection status admitted (or presenting for a health care encounter) during pregnancy, childbirth, or the puerperium should receive codes of O98.7- and Z21.

h. **Encounters for testing for HIV**

If a patient is being seen to determine his/her HIV status, use code Z11.4, Encounter for screening for human immunodeficiency virus [HIV]. Use additional codes for any associated high-risk behavior.

If a patient with signs or symptoms is being seen for HIV testing, code the signs and symptoms. An additional counseling code Z71.7, Human immunodeficiency virus [HIV] counseling, may be used if counseling is provided during the encounter for the test.

When a patient returns to be informed of his/her HIV test results and the test result is negative, use code Z71.7, Human immunodeficiency virus [HIV] counseling.

If the results are positive, see previous guidelines and assign codes as appropriate.

B. Infectious Agents as the Cause of Diseases Classified to Other Chapters

Certain infections are classified in chapters other than Chapter 1 and no organism is identified as part of the infection code. In these instances, it is necessary to use an additional code from Chapter 1 to identify the organism. A code from category B95, Streptococcus, Staphylococcus, and Enterococcus as the cause of diseases classified to other chapters; B96, Other bacterial agents as the cause of diseases classified to other chapters; or B97, Viral agents as the cause

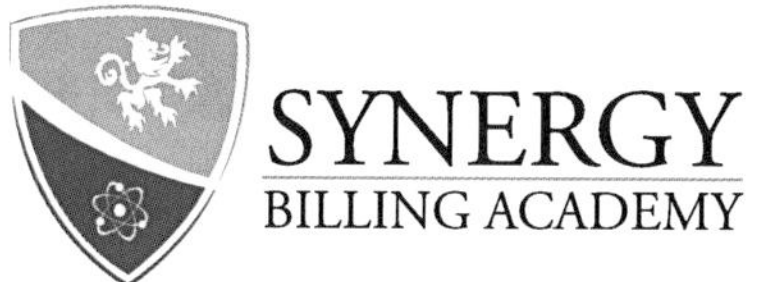

of diseases classified to other chapters, is to be used as an additional code to identify the organism. An instructional note will be found at the infection code advising that an additional organism code is required.

C. Infections Resistant to Antibiotics

Many bacterial infections are resistant to current antibiotics. It is necessary to identify all infections documented as antibiotic resistant. Assign a code from category Z16, Resistance to antimicrobial drugs, following the infection code only if the infection code does not identify drug resistance.

D. Sepsis, Severe Sepsis, and Septic Shock

1. Coding of sepsis and severe sepsis

a. Sepsis

For a diagnosis of sepsis, assign the appropriate code for the underlying systemic infection. If the type of infection or causal organism is not further specified, assign code A41.9, Sepsis, unspecified organism.

A code from subcategory R65.2, Severe sepsis, should not be assigned unless severe sepsis or an associated acute organ dysfunction is documented.

i. Negative or inconclusive blood cultures and sepsis

Negative or inconclusive blood cultures do not preclude a diagnosis of sepsis in patients with clinical evidence of the condition; however, the provider should be queried.

ii. Urosepsis

The term urosepsis is a nonspecific term. It is not to be considered synonymous with sepsis. It has no default code in the Alphabetic Index. Should a provider use this term, he/she must be queried for clarification.

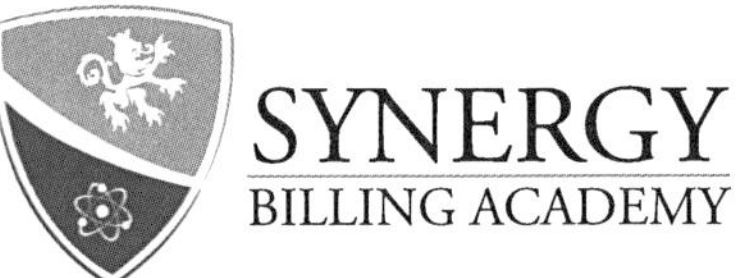

iii. Sepsis with organ dysfunction

If a patient has sepsis and associated acute organ dysfunction or multiple organ dysfunction (MOD), follow the instructions for coding severe sepsis.

iv. Acute organ dysfunction that is not clearly associated with the sepsis

If a patient has sepsis and an acute organ dysfunction, but the medical record documentation indicates that the acute organ dysfunction is related to a medical condition other than the sepsis, do not assign a code from subcategory R65.2, Severe sepsis. An acute organ dysfunction must be associated with the sepsis in order to assign the severe sepsis code. If the documentation is not clear as to whether an acute organ dysfunction is related to the sepsis or another medical condition, query the provider.

b. Severe sepsis

The coding of severe sepsis requires a minimum of two codes: first a code for the underlying systemic infection, then a code from subcategory R65.2, Severe sepsis. If the causal organism is not documented, assign code A41.9, Sepsis, unspecified organism, for the infection. Additional code(s) for the associated acute organ dysfunction are also required.

Due to the complex nature of severe sepsis, some cases may require querying the provider prior to assignment of the codes.

2. Septic shock

a. Septic shock generally refers to circulatory failure associated with severe sepsis, and therefore, it represents a type of acute organ dysfunction.

For cases of septic shock, the code for the systemic infection should be sequenced first, followed by code R65.21, Severe sepsis with septic shock or code T81.12, Postprocedural septic shock. Any additional codes for the other acute organ dysfunctions should also be assigned. As noted in the sequencing instructions in the Tabular List, the code for septic shock cannot be assigned as a principal diagnosis.

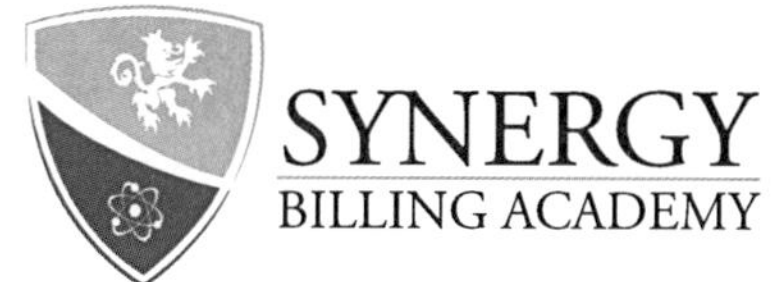

3. **Sequencing of severe sepsis**

   If severe sepsis is present on admission and meets the definition of principal diagnosis, the underlying systemic infection should be assigned as principal diagnosis followed by the appropriate code from subcategory R65.2 as required by the sequencing rules in the Tabular List. A code from subcategory R65.2 can never be assigned as a principal diagnosis.

   When severe sepsis develops during an encounter (it was not present on admission) the underlying systemic infection and the appropriate code from subcategory R65.2 should be assigned as secondary diagnoses.

   Severe sepsis may be present on admission but the diagnosis may not be confirmed until sometime after admission. If the documentation is not clear whether severe sepsis was present on admission, the provider should be queried.

4. **Sepsis and severe sepsis with a localized infection**

   If the reason for admission is both sepsis or severe sepsis and a localized infection, such as pneumonia or cellulitis, a code(s) for the underlying systemic infection should be assigned first and the code for the localized infection should be assigned as a secondary diagnosis. If the patient has severe sepsis, a code from subcategory R65.2 should also be assigned as a secondary diagnosis. If the patient is admitted with a localized infection such as pneumonia and sepsis/severe sepsis doesn't develop until after admission, the localized infection should be assigned first, followed by the appropriate sepsis/severe sepsis codes.

5. **Sepsis due to a postprocedural infection**

   a. **Documentation of causal relationship**

      As with all postprocedural complications, code assignment is based on the provider's documentation of the relationship between the infection and the procedure.

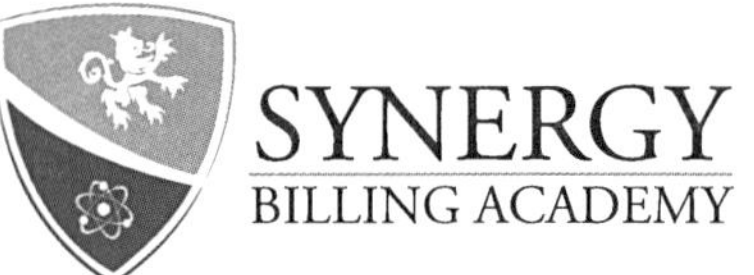

b. **Sepsis due to a postprocedural infection**

For such cases, the postprocedural infection code, such as T80.2, Infections following infusion, transfusion, and therapeutic injection; T81.4, Infection following a procedure; T88.0, Infection following immunization; or O86.0, Infection of obstetric surgical wound, should be coded first, followed by the code for the specific infection. If the patient has severe sepsis, the appropriate code from subcategory R65.2 should also be assigned with the additional code(s) for any acute organ dysfunction.

c. **Postprocedural infection and postprocedural septic shock**

In cases where a postprocedural infection has occurred and has resulted in severe sepsis and postprocedural septic shock, the code for the precipitating complication, such as code T81.4, Infection following a procedure; or O86.0, Infection of obstetrical surgical wound, should be coded first, followed by code R65.21, Severe sepsis with septic shock and a code for the systemic infection.

6. **Sepsis and severe sepsis associated with a noninfectious process (condition)**

In some cases, a noninfectious process (condition) such as trauma may lead to an infection which can result in sepsis or severe sepsis. If sepsis or severe sepsis is documented as associated with a noninfectious condition such as a burn or serious injury and this condition meets the definition for principal diagnosis, the code for the noninfectious condition should be sequenced first, followed by the code for the resulting infection. If severe sepsis is present, a code from subcategory R65.2 should also be assigned with any associated organ dysfunction(s) codes. It is not necessary to assign a code from subcategory R65.1, Systemic inflammatory response syndrome (SIRS) of noninfectious origin, for these cases.

If the infection meets the definition of principal diagnosis, it should be sequenced before the noninfectious condition. When both the associated noninfectious condition and the infection meet the definition of principal diagnosis, either may be assigned as principal diagnosis.

Only one code from category R65, Symptoms and signs specifically associated with systemic inflammation and infection, should be assigned. Therefore, when a noninfectious condition leads to an infection resulting in severe sepsis, assign the

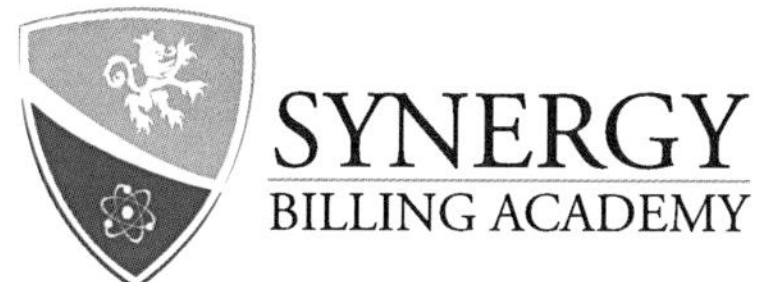

appropriate code from subcategory R65.2, Severe sepsis. Do not additionally assign a code from subcategory R65.1, Systemic inflammatory response syndrome (SIRS) of noninfectious origin.

See Section I.C.18. SIRS due to noninfectious process.

7. **Sepsis and septic shock complicating abortion, pregnancy, childbirth, and the puerperium**

   See Section I.C.15. Sepsis and septic shock complicating abortion, pregnancy, childbirth, and the puerperium.

8. **Newborn sepsis**

   See Section I.C.16. f. Bacterial sepsis of newborn.

E. Methicillin Resistant Staphylococcus Aureus (MRSA) Conditions

1. Selection and sequencing of MRSA codes

a. Combination codes for MRSA infection

When a patient is diagnosed with an infection that is due to methicillin resistant Staphylococcus aureus (MRSA) and that infection has a combination code that includes the causal organism (e.g., sepsis, pneumonia), assign the appropriate combination code for the condition (e.g., code A41.02, Sepsis due to methicillin resistant Staphylococcus aureus, or code J15.212, Pneumonia due to methicillin resistant Staphylococcus aureus). Do not assign code B95.62, Methicillin resistant Staphylococcus aureus infection as the cause of diseases classified elsewhere, as an additional code because the combination code includes the type of infection and the MRSA organism. Do not assign a code from subcategory Z16.11, Resistance to penicillins, as an additional diagnosis.

See Section C.1. for instructions on coding and sequencing of sepsis and severe sepsis.

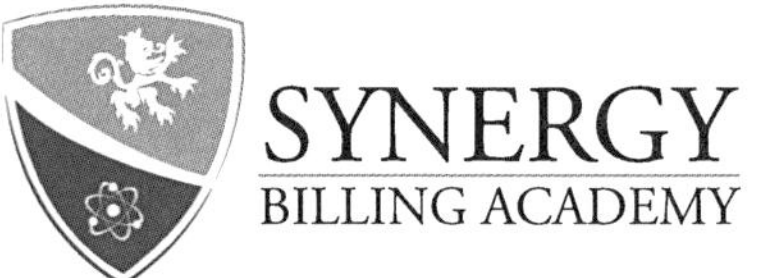

b. Other codes for MRSA infection

When there is documentation of a current infection (e.g., wound infection, stitch abscess, urinary tract infection) due to MRSA and that infection does not have a combination code that includes the causal organism, assign the appropriate code to identify the condition along with code B95.62, Methicillin resistant Staphylococcus aureus infection as the cause of diseases classified elsewhere, for the MRSA infection. Do not assign a code from subcategory Z16.11, Resistance to penicillins.

c. Methicillin susceptible Staphylococcus aureus (MSSA) and MRSA colonization

The condition or state of being colonized by or carrying MSSA or MRSA is called colonization or carriage, while an individual person is described as being colonized or being a carrier. Colonization means that MSSA or MSRA is present on or in the body without necessarily causing illness. A positive MRSA colonization test might be documented by the provider as "MRSA screen positive" or "MRSA nasal swab positive."

Assign code Z22.322, Carrier or suspected carrier of Methicillin resistant Staphylococcus aureus, for patients documented as having MRSA colonization. Assign code Z22.321, Carrier or suspected carrier of Methicillin susceptible Staphylococcus aureus, for patient documented as having MSSA colonization. Colonization is not necessarily indicative of a disease process or as the cause of a specific condition the patient may have unless documented as such by the provider.

d. MRSA colonization and infection

If a patient is documented as having both MRSA colonization and infection during a hospital admission, code Z22.322, Carrier or suspected carrier of methicillin resistant Staphylococcus aureus, and a code for the MRSA infection may both be assigned.

Chapter 14: Guidelines List

Several notes have been made available to indicate that additional codes are needed and should be used.

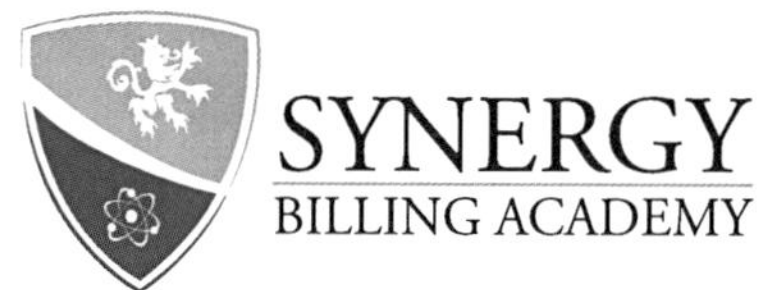

- N17, Acute kidney failure – Code also associated underlying condition
- N18, Chronic kidney disease (CKD) – Code first any associated:
    - Diabetic chronic kidney disease (E08.22, E09.22, E10.22, E11.22, E13.22)
    - Hypertensive chronic kidney disease (I12.-, I13.-)
    - Use additional code to identify kidney transplant status, if applicable (Z94.0)
- N30, Cystitis – Use additional code to identify infectious agents (B95-B97)
- N31, Neuromuscular dysfunction of bladder, NEC – Use additional code to identify any associated urinary incontinence (N39.3-N39.4-)
- N33, Bladder disorders in diseases classified elsewhere – Code first underlying disease, such as schistosomiasis (B65.0-B6.9)
- N40.1, Enlarged prostate with lower urinary tract symptoms (LUTS) – Use additional code for associated symptoms, when specified:
    - Incomplete bladder emptying (R39.14)
    - Nocturia (R35.1)
    - Straining on urination (R39.16)
    - Urinary frequency (R35.0)
    - Urinary hesitancy (R39.11)
    - Urinary incontinence (N39.1-)
    - Urinary obstruction (N13.8)
    - Urinary retention (R33.8)
    - Urinary urgency (R39.15)
    - Weak urinary stream (R39.12)

Chapter 14: Detailed Guidelines

Chronic Kidney Disease

1. **Stages of chronic kidney disease (CKD)**

   The ICD-10-CM classifies CKD based on severity. The severity of CKD is designated by stages 1-5. Stage 2, code N18.2, equates to mild CKD; stage 3, code N18.3, equates to moderate CKD; and stage 4, code N18.4, equates to severe CKD. Code N18.6, End-stage renal disease (ESRD), is assigned when the provider has documented end-stage renal disease (ESRD).

   If both a stage of CKD and ESRD are documented, assign code N18.6 only.

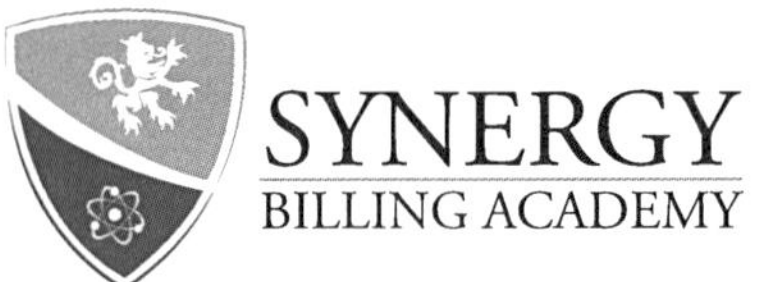

2. **Chronic kidney disease and kidney transplant status**

   Patients who have undergone a kidney transplant may still have some form of chronic kidney disease (CKD) because the kidney transplant may not fully restore kidney function. Therefore, the presence of CKD alone does not constitute a transplant complication. Assign the appropriate N18 code for the patient's stage of CKD and code Z94.0, Kidney transplant status. If a transplant complication such as failure or rejection or other transplant complication is documented, see section I.C.19.g for information on coding complications of a kidney transplant. If the documentation is unclear as to whether the patient has a complication of the transplant, query the provider.

3. **Chronic kidney disease with other conditions**

   Patients with CKD may also suffer from other serious conditions, most commonly diabetes mellitus and hypertension. The sequencing of the CKD code in relationship to codes for other contributing conditions is based on the conventions in the Tabular List.

Chapter 15: Guidelines List

The NCHS has published chapter-specific guidelines for this chapter:

A. General Rules for Obstetric Cases
B. Selection of OB Principal or First-Listed Diagnosis
C. Pre-Existing Conditions Versus Conditions Due to the Pregnancy
D. Pre-Existing Hypertension in Pregnancy
E. Fetal Conditions Affecting the Management of the Mother
F. HIV Infection in Pregnancy, Childbirth, and the Puerperium
G. Diabetes Mellitus in Pregnancy
H. Long-Term Use of Insulin
I. Gestational (Pregnancy-induced) Diabetes
J. Sepsis and Septic Shock Complicating Abortion, Pregnancy, Childbirth, and the Puerperium
K. Puerperal Sepsis
L. Alcohol and Tobacco Use During Pregnancy, Childbirth, and the Puerperium
M. Poisoning, toxic Effects, Adverse Effects, and Underdosing in a Pregnant Patient
N. Code O80, Normal Delivery
O. The Peripartum and Postpartum Periods
P. Code O94, Sequelae of Complication Of Pregnancy, Childbirth, and the Puerperium
Q. Termination of Pregnancy and Spontaneous Abortions
R. Abuse in a Pregnant Patient

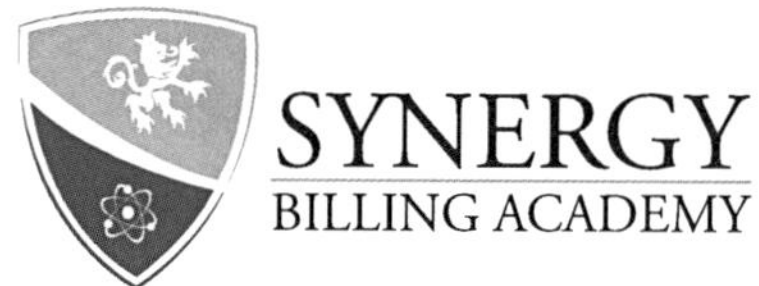

Chapter 15: Detailed Guidelines

A. General Rules for Obstetric Cases

1. **Codes from Chapter 15 and sequencing priority**
   Obstetric cases require codes from Chapter 15, codes in the range O00-O9A, Pregnancy, Childbirth, and the Puerperium. Chapter 15 codes have sequencing priority over codes from other chapters. Additional codes from other chapters may be used in conjunction with Chapter 15 codes to further specify conditions. Should the provider document that the pregnancy is incidental to the encounter, then code Z33.1, Pregnant state, incidental, should be used in place of any Chapter 15 codes. It is the provider's responsibility to state that the condition being treated is not affecting the pregnancy.

2. **Chapter 15 codes used only on the maternal record**

   Chapter 15 codes are to be used only on the maternal record, never on the record of the newborn.

3. **Final character for trimester**

   The majority of codes in Chapter 15 have a final character indicating the trimester of pregnancy. The time frames for the trimesters are indicated at the beginning of the chapter. If trimester is not a component of a code, it is because the condition always occurs in a specific trimester, or the concept of trimester of pregnancy is not applicable. Certain codes have characters for only certain trimesters because the condition does not occur in all trimesters, but it may occur in more than just one.

   Assignment of the final character for trimester should be based on the provider's documentation of the trimester (or number of weeks) for the current admission/encounter. This applies to the assignment of trimester for pre-existing conditions as well as those that develop during or are due to the pregnancy. The provider's documentation of the number of weeks may be used to assign the appropriate code identifying the trimester.

   Whenever delivery occurs during the current admission and there is an "in childbirth" option for the obstetric complication being coded, the "in childbirth" code should be assigned.

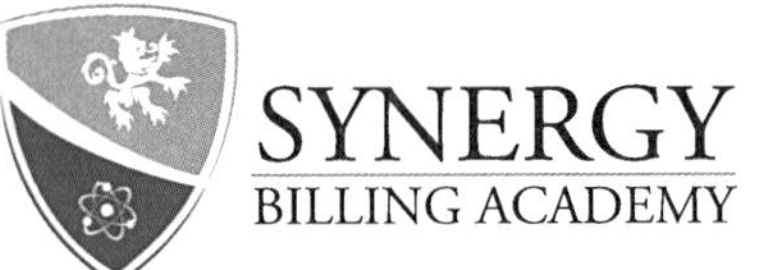

4. **Selection of trimester for inpatient admissions that encompass more than one trimester**

   In instances when a patient is admitted to a hospital for complications of pregnancy during one trimester and remains in the hospital into a subsequent trimester, the trimester character for the antepartum complication code should be assigned based on the trimester when the complication developed, not the trimester of the discharge. If the condition developed prior to the current admission/encounter or represents a pre-existing condition, the trimester character for the trimester at the time of the admission/encounter should be assigned.

5. **Unspecified trimester**

   Each category that includes codes for trimester has a code for "unspecified trimester." The "unspecified trimester" code should rarely be used, such as when the documentation in the record is insufficient to determine the trimester and it is not possible to obtain clarification.

6. **7th character for fetus identification**

   Where applicable, a 7th character is to be assigned for certain categories (O31, O32, O33.3 - O33.6, O35, O36, O40, O41, O60.1, O60.2, O64, and O69) to identify the fetus for which the complication code applies.

   Assign 7th character "0":

   - For single gestations
   - When the documentation in the record is insufficient to determine the fetus affected and it is not possible to obtain clarification
   - When it is not possible to clinically determine which fetus is affected

B. Selection of OB Principal or First-Listed Diagnosis

1. **Routine outpatient prenatal visits**

   For routine outpatient prenatal visits when no complications are present, a code from category Z34, Encounter for supervision of normal pregnancy, should be used as the first-listed diagnosis. These codes should not be used in conjunction with Chapter 15 codes.

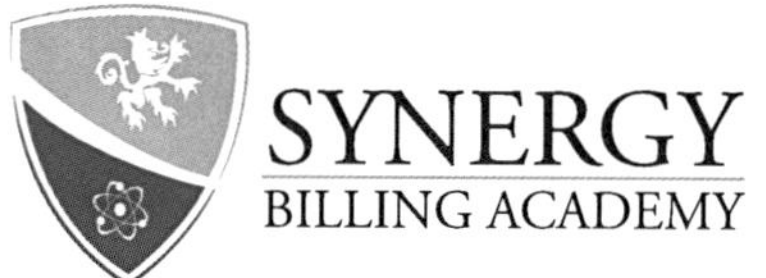

2. **Prenatal outpatient visits for high-risk patients**

   For routine prenatal outpatient visits for patients with high-risk pregnancies, a code from category O09, Supervision of high-risk pregnancy, should be used as the first-listed diagnosis. Secondary Chapter 15 codes may be used in conjunction with these codes if appropriate.

3. **Episodes when no delivery occurs**

   In episodes when no delivery occurs, the principal diagnosis should correspond to the principal complication of the pregnancy which necessitated the encounter. Should more than one complication exist, all of which are treated or monitored, any of the complications codes may be sequenced first.

4. **When a delivery occurs**

   When a delivery occurs, the principal diagnosis should correspond to the main circumstances or complication of the delivery. In cases of cesarean delivery, the selection of the principal diagnosis should be the condition established after study that was responsible for the patient's admission. If the patient was admitted with a condition that resulted in the performance of a cesarean procedure, that condition should be selected as the principal diagnosis. If the reason for the admission/encounter was unrelated to the condition resulting in the cesarean delivery, the condition related to the reason for the admission/encounter should be selected as the principal diagnosis

5. **Outcome of delivery**

   A code from category Z37, Outcome of delivery, should be included on every maternal record when a delivery has occurred. These codes are not to be used on subsequent records or on the newborn record.

C. **Pre-Existing Conditions Versus Conditions Due to the Pregnancy**

Certain categories in Chapter 15 distinguish between conditions of the mother that existed prior to pregnancy (pre-existing) and those that are a direct result of pregnancy. When assigning codes from Chapter 15, it is important to assess if a condition was pre-existing prior to pregnancy or developed during or due to the pregnancy in order to assign the correct code.

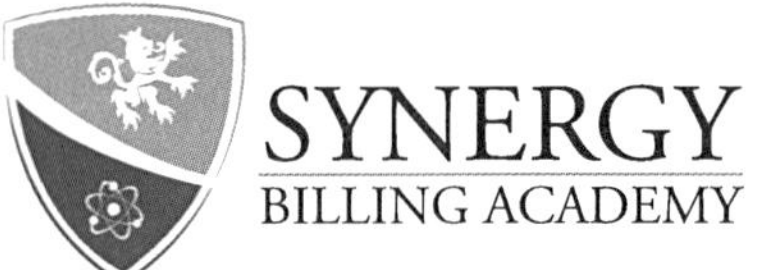

D. Pre-Existing Hypertension in Pregnancy

Category O10, Pre-existing hypertension complicating pregnancy, childbirth, and the puerperium, includes codes for hypertensive heart and hypertensive chronic kidney disease. When assigning one of the O10 codes that includes hypertensive heart disease or hypertensive chronic kidney disease, it is necessary to add a secondary code from the appropriate hypertension category to specify the type of heart failure or chronic kidney disease.

E. Fetal Conditions Affecting the Management of the Mother

1. Codes from categories O35 and O36

Codes from categories O35, Maternal care for known or suspected fetal abnormality and damage, and O36, Maternal care for other fetal problems, are assigned only when the fetal condition is actually responsible for modifying the management of the mother, e.g., by requiring diagnostic studies, additional observation, special care, or termination of pregnancy. The fact that the fetal condition exists does not justify assigning a code from this series to the mother's record.

2. In utero surgery

In cases when surgery is performed on the fetus, a diagnosis code from category O35, Maternal care for known or suspected fetal abnormality and damage should be assigned identifying the fetal condition. Assign the appropriate procedure code for the procedure performed.

No code from Chapter 16, or the perinatal codes, should be used on the mother's record to identify fetal conditions. Surgery performed in utero on a fetus is still to be coded as an obstetric encounter.

F. HIV Infection in Pregnancy, Childbirth, and the Puerperium

During pregnancy, childbirth, or the puerperium, a patient admitted because of an HIV-related illness should receive a principal diagnosis from subcategory O98.7-, Human immunodeficiency [HIV] disease complicating pregnancy, childbirth, and the puerperium, followed by the code(s) for the HIV-related illness(es).

Patients with asymptomatic HIV infection status admitted during pregnancy, childbirth, or the puerperium should receive codes of O98.7- and Z21, Asymptomatic human immunodeficiency virus [HIV] infection status.

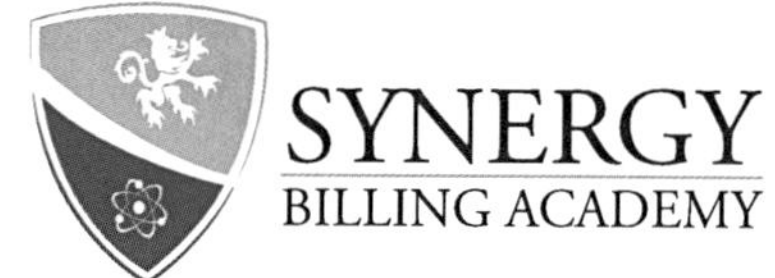

G. Diabetes Mellitus in Pregnancy

Diabetes mellitus is a significant complicating factor in pregnancy. Pregnant women who are diabetic should be assigned a code from category O24, Diabetes mellitus in pregnancy, childbirth, and the puerperium, first followed by the appropriate diabetes code(s) (E08-E13) from Chapter 4.

H. Long-Term Use of Insulin

Code Z79.4, Long-term (current) use of insulin, should also be assigned if the diabetes mellitus is being treated with insulin.

I. Gestational (Pregnancy-Induced) Diabetes

Gestational (pregnancy induced) diabetes can occur during the second and third trimester of pregnancy in women who were not diabetic prior to pregnancy. Gestational diabetes can cause complications in the pregnancy similar to those of pre-existing diabetes mellitus. It also puts the woman at greater risk of developing diabetes after the pregnancy. Codes for gestational diabetes are in subcategory O24.4, Gestational diabetes mellitus. No other code from category O24, Diabetes mellitus in pregnancy, childbirth, and the puerperium, should be used with a code from O24.4.

The codes under subcategory O24.4 include diet-controlled and insulin-controlled. If a patient with gestational diabetes is treated with both diet and insulin, only the code for insulin-controlled is required.

Code Z79.4, Long-term (current) use of insulin, should not be assigned with codes from subcategory O24.4.

An abnormal glucose tolerance in pregnancy is assigned a code from subcategory O99.81, Abnormal glucose complicating pregnancy, childbirth, and the puerperium.

J. Sepsis and Septic Shock Complicating Abortion, Pregnancy, Childbirth, and the Puerperium

When assigning a Chapter 15 code for sepsis complicating abortion, pregnancy, childbirth, and the puerperium, a code for the specific type of infection should be assigned as an additional diagnosis. If severe sepsis is present, a code from subcategory R65.2, Severe sepsis, and code(s) for associated organ dysfunction(s) should also be assigned as additional diagnoses.

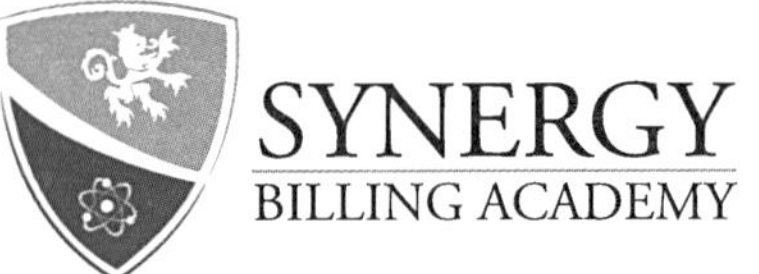

K. Puerperal Sepsis

Code O85, Puerperal sepsis, should be assigned with a secondary code to identify the causal organism (e.g., for a bacterial infection, assign a code from category B95-B96, Bacterial infections in conditions classified elsewhere). A code from category A40, Streptococcal sepsis, or A41, Other sepsis, should not be used for puerperal sepsis. If applicable, use additional codes to identify severe sepsis (R65.2-) and any associated acute organ dysfunction.

L. Alcohol and Tobacco Use During Pregnancy, Childbirth, and the Puerperium

1. Alcohol use during pregnancy, childbirth, and the puerperium

Codes under subcategory O99.31, Alcohol use complicating pregnancy, childbirth, and the puerperium, should be assigned for any pregnancy case when a mother uses alcohol during the pregnancy or postpartum. A secondary code from category F10, Alcohol related disorders, should also be assigned to identify manifestations of the alcohol use.

2. Tobacco use during pregnancy, childbirth, and the puerperium

Codes under subcategory O99.33, Smoking (tobacco) complicating pregnancy, childbirth, and the puerperium, should be assigned for any pregnancy case when a mother uses any type of tobacco product during the pregnancy or postpartum. A secondary code from category F17, Nicotine dependence, should also be assigned to identify the type of nicotine dependence.

M. Poisoning, Toxic Effects, Adverse Effects, and Underdosing in a Pregnant Patient

A code from subcategory O9A.2, Injury, poisoning, and certain other consequences of external causes complicating pregnancy, childbirth, and the puerperium, should be sequenced first, followed by the appropriate injury, poisoning, toxic effect, adverse effect, or underdosing code, and then the additional code(s) that specifies the condition caused by the poisoning, toxic effect, adverse effect, or underdosing.

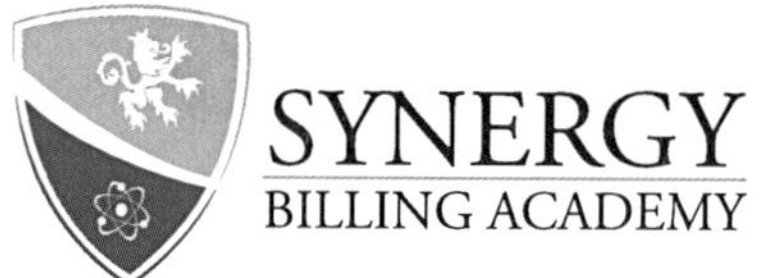

N. Code O80, Normal Delivery

1. Encounter for full-term uncomplicated delivery

Code O80 should be assigned when a woman is admitted for a full-term normal delivery and delivers a single, healthy infant without any complications antepartum, during the delivery, or postpartum during the delivery episode. Code O80 is always a principal diagnosis. It is not to be used if any other code from Chapter 15 is needed to describe a current complication of the antenatal, delivery, or perinatal period. Additional codes from other chapters may be used with code O80 if they are not related to or are in any way complicating the pregnancy.

2. Uncomplicated delivery with resolved antepartum complication

Code O80 may be used if the patient had a complication at some point during the pregnancy, but the complication is not present at the time of the admission for delivery.

3. Outcome of delivery for O80

Z37.0, Single live birth, is the only outcome of delivery code appropriate for use with O80.

O. The Peripartum and Postpartum Periods

1. Peripartum and postpartum periods

The postpartum period begins immediately after delivery and continues for six weeks following delivery. The peripartum period is defined as the last month of pregnancy to five months postpartum.

2. Peripartum and postpartum complication

A postpartum complication is any complication occurring within the six-week period.

3. Pregnancy-related complications after six-week period

Chapter 15 codes may also be used to describe pregnancy-related complications after the peripartum or postpartum period if the provider documents that a condition is pregnancy related.

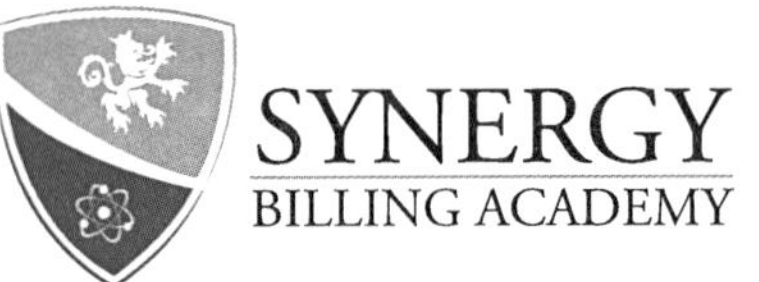

4. **Admission for routine postpartum care following delivery outside hospital**

   When the mother delivers outside the hospital prior to admission and is admitted for routine postpartum care and no complications are noted, code Z39.0, Encounter for care and examination of mother immediately after delivery, should be assigned as the principal diagnosis.

5. **Pregnancy-associated cardiomyopathy**

   Pregnancy-associated cardiomyopathy, code O90.3, is unique in that it may be diagnosed in the third trimester of pregnancy but may continue to progress months after delivery. For this reason, it is referred to as peripartum cardiomyopathy. Code O90.3 is only for use when the cardiomyopathy develops as a result of pregnancy in a woman who did not have pre-existing heart disease.

P. Code 094, Sequelae of Complication of Pregnancy, Childbirth, and the Puerperium

1. **Code O94**

   Code O94, Sequelae of complication of pregnancy, childbirth, and the puerperium, is for use in those cases when an initial complication of a pregnancy develops a sequelae requiring care or treatment at a future date.

2. **After the initial postpartum period**

   This code may be used at any time after the initial postpartum period.

3. **Sequencing of code O94**

   This code, like all sequela codes, is to be sequenced following the code describing the sequelae of the complication.

Q. Termination of pregnancy and spontaneous abortions

1. **Abortion with liveborn fetus**

   When an attempted termination of pregnancy results in a liveborn fetus, assign code Z33.2, Encounter for elective termination of pregnancy, and a code from category Z37, Outcome of Delivery.

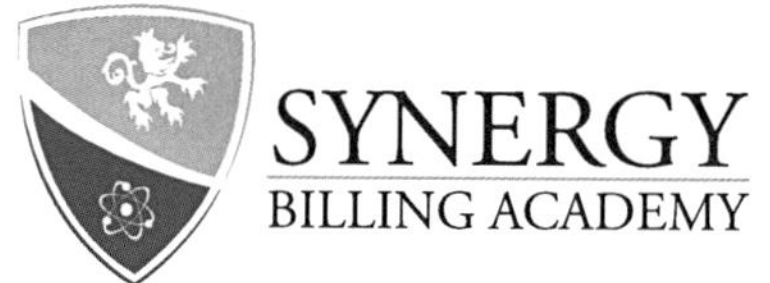

2. **Retained products of conception following an abortion**

   Subsequent encounters for retained products of conception following a spontaneous abortion or elective termination of pregnancy are assigned the appropriate code from category O03, Spontaneous abortion, or codes O07.4, Failed attempted termination of pregnancy without complication, and Z33.2, Encounter for elective termination of pregnancy. This advice is appropriate even when the patient was discharged previously with a discharge diagnosis of complete abortion.

3. **Complications leading to abortion**

   Codes from Chapter 15 may be used as additional codes to identify any documented complications of the pregnancy in conjunction with codes in categories in O07 and O08.

R. Abuse in a Pregnant Patient

For suspected or confirmed cases of abuse of a pregnant patient, a code(s) from subcategories O9A.3, Physical abuse complicating pregnancy, childbirth, and the puerperium; O9A.4, Sexual abuse complicating pregnancy, childbirth, and the puerperium; or O9A.5, Psychological abuse complicating pregnancy, childbirth, and the puerperium, should be sequenced first, followed by the appropriate codes (if applicable) to identify any associated current injury due to physical abuse, sexual abuse, as well as the perpetrator of abuse.

Chapter 21: Guidelines List

The chapter-specific guidelines provide additional information about the use of Z Codes for specified encounters.

The NCHS has published the following guidelines:

A. Use of Z Codes in any Health Care Setting
B. Z Codes Indicate a Reason for an Encounter
C. Categories of Z Codes
   1. Contact/Exposure
   2. Inoculations and Vaccinations
   3. Status
   4. **History (Of)**

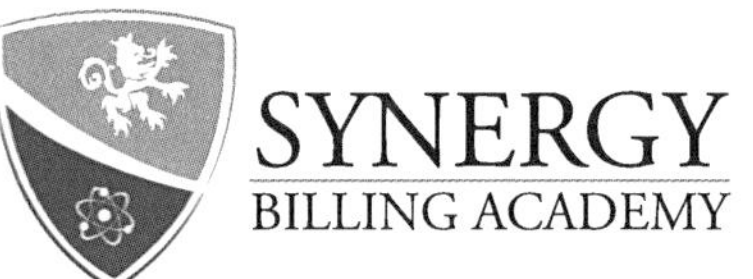

5. **Screening**
6. Observation
7. Aftercare
8. **Follow-Up**
9 Donor
10. **Counseling**
11. **Encounters for Obstetrical and Reproductive Services**
12. Newborns and Infants
13. **Routine and Administrative Examinations**
14. Miscellaneous Z Codes
    I. Prophylactic Organ Removal
15. Nonspecific Z Codes
16. Z Codes That May Only Be Principal/First-Listed Diagnosis

Chapter 21: Detailed Guidelines

A. Use of Z Codes in any Health Care Setting

Z Codes are for use in any health care setting. Z Codes may be used as either a first-listed (principal diagnosis code in the inpatient setting) or secondary code, depending on the circumstances of the encounter. Certain Z Codes may only be used as first-listed or principal diagnosis.

B. Z Codes Indicate a Reason for an Encounter

Z Codes are not procedure codes. A corresponding procedure code must accompany a Z Code to describe any procedure performed.

C. Categories of Z Codes

4. History (of)

There are two types of history Z Codes, personal and family. Personal history codes explain a patient's past medical condition that no longer exists and is not currently being treated, but that has the potential for recurrence and therefore may require continued monitoring.

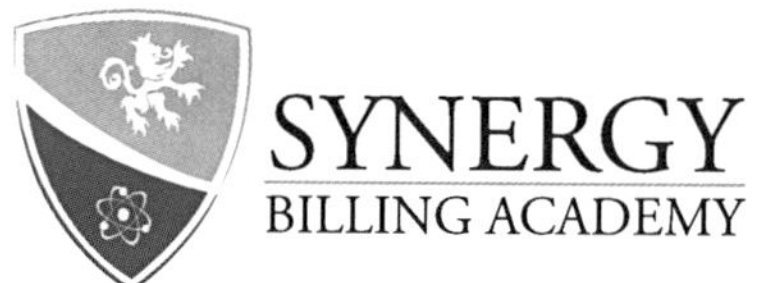

Family history codes are for use when a patient has a family member(s) who has had a particular disease that causes the patient to be at higher risk of also developing the disease.

Personal history codes may be used in conjunction with follow-up codes and family history codes may be used in conjunction with screening codes to explain the need for a test or procedure. History codes are also acceptable on any medical record regardless of the reason for visit. A history of an illness, even if no longer present, is important information that may alter the type of treatment ordered.

The history Z Code categories are:

Code	Description
Z80	Family history of primary malignant neoplasm
Z81	Family history of mental and behavioral disorders
Z82	Family history of certain disabilities and chronic diseases (leading to disablement)
Z83	Family history of other specific disorders
Z84	Family history of other conditions
Z85	Personal history of malignant neoplasm
Z86	Personal history of certain other diseases
Z87	Personal history of other diseases and conditions
Z91.4	Personal history of psychological trauma, not elsewhere classified
Z91.5	Personal history of self-harm
Z91.8	Other specified personal risk factors, not elsewhere classified • Except: Z91.83, Wandering in diseases classified elsewhere
Z92	Personal history of medical treatment • Except: Z92.0, Personal history of contraception • Except: Z92.82, Status post administration of tPA (rtPA) in a different facility within the last 24 hours prior to admission to a current facility

5. **Screening**

Screening is the testing for disease or disease precursors in seemingly well individuals so that early detection and treatment can be provided for those who test positive for the disease (e.g., screening mammogram).

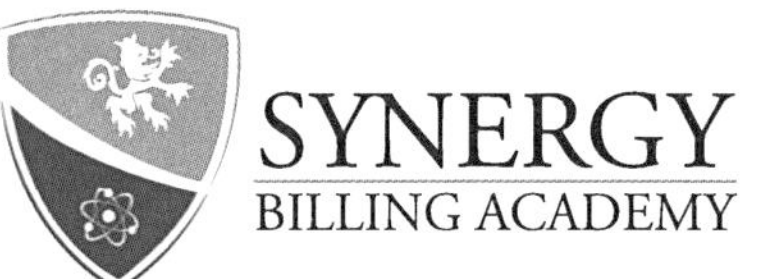

The testing of a person to rule out or confirm a suspected diagnosis because the patient has some sign or symptom is a diagnostic examination, not a screening. In these cases, the sign or symptom is used to explain the reason for the test.

A screening code may be a first-listed code if the reason for the visit is specifically the screening exam. It may also be used as an additional code if the screening is done during an office visit for other health problems. A screening code is not necessary if the screening is inherent to a routine examination, such as a pap smear done during a routine pelvic examination.

Should a condition be discovered during the screening, then the code for the condition may be assigned as an additional diagnosis.

The Z Code indicates that a screening exam is planned. A procedure code is required to confirm that the screening was performed.

The screening Z Codes/categories are:

Code	Description
Z11	Encounter for screening for infectious and parasitic diseases
Z12	Encounter for screening for malignant neoplasms
Z13	Encounter for screening for other diseases and disorders Except: Z13.9, Encounter for screening, unspecified
Z36	Encounter for antenatal screening for mother

10. Counseling

Counseling Z Codes are used when a patient or family member receives assistance in the aftermath of an illness or injury, or when support is required in coping with family or social problems. They are not used in conjunction with a diagnosis code when the counseling component of care is considered integral to standard treatment.

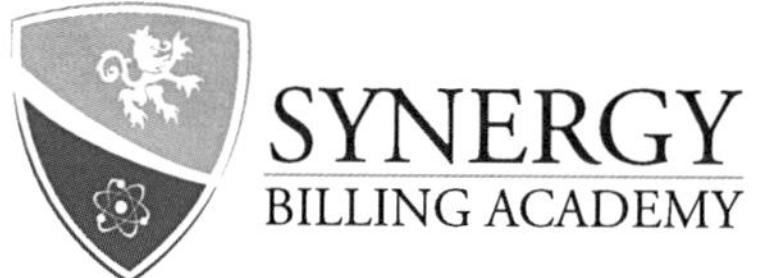

The counseling Z Codes/categories are:

Code	Description
Z30.0	Encounter for general counseling and advice on contraception
Z31.5	Encounter for genetic counseling
Z31.6	Encounter for general counseling and advice on procreation
Z32.2	Encounter for childbirth instruction
Z32.3	Encounter for childcare instruction
Z69	Encounter for mental health services for victim and perpetrator of abuse
Z70	Counseling related to sexual attitude, behavior, and orientation
Z71	Persons encountering health services for other counseling and medical advice, not elsewhere classified
Z76.81	Expectant mother prebirth pediatrician visit

11. Encounters for Obstetrical and Reproductive Services

Z Codes for pregnancy are for use in those circumstances when none of the problems or complications included in the codes from the Obstetrics chapter exist (a routine prenatal visit or postpartum care). Codes in category Z34, Encounter for supervision of normal pregnancy, are always first-listed and are not to be used with any other code from the OB chapter.

Codes in category Z3A, Weeks of gestation, may be assigned to provide additional information about the pregnancy. The date of the admission should be used to determine weeks of gestation for inpatient admissions that encompass more than one gestational week.

The outcome of delivery, category Z37, should be included on all maternal delivery records. It is always a secondary code. Codes in category Z37 should not be used on the newborn record.

Z Codes for family planning (contraceptive) or procreative management and counseling should be included on an obstetric record either during the pregnancy or the postpartum stage, if applicable.

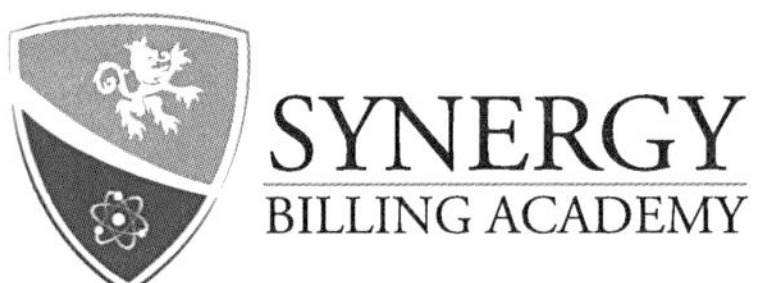

The Z Codes/categories for obstetrical and reproductive services are:

Code	Description
Z30	Encounter for contraceptive management
Z31	Encounter for procreative management
Z32.2	Encounter for childbirth instruction
Z32.3	Encounter for childcare instruction
Z33	Pregnant state
Z34	Encounter for supervision of normal pregnancy
Z36	Encounter for antenatal screening of mother
Z3A	Weeks of gestation
Z37	Outcome of delivery
Z39	Encounter for maternal postpartum care and examination
Z76.81	Expectant mother prebirth pediatrician visit

12. Newborns and infants

The newborn Z Codes/categories are:

Code	Description
Z76.1	Encounter for health supervision and care of foundling
Z00.1	Encounter for routine child health examination
Z38	Liveborn infants according to place of birth and type of delivery

13. Routine and administrative examinations

The Z Codes allow for the description of encounters for routine examinations, such as a general check-up, or examinations for administrative purposes, such as a pre-employment physical. The codes are not to be used if the examination is for diagnosis of a suspected condition or for treatment purposes. In such cases, the diagnosis code is used. Should a disease or condition be discovered during a routine exam and listed

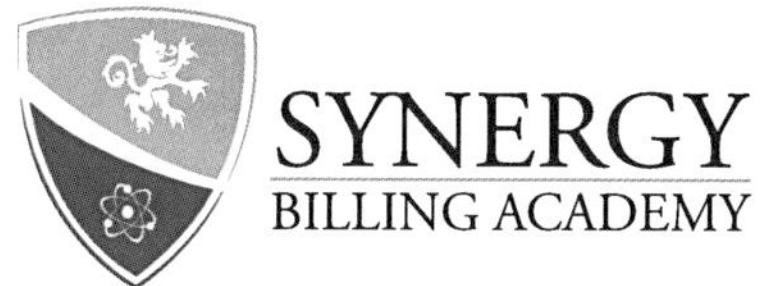

with a diagnosis, it should be coded as an additional code. Pre-existing and chronic conditions and history codes may also be included as additional codes as long as the examination is for administrative purposes and not focused on any particular condition.

Some of the codes for routine health examinations distinguish between "with" and "without" abnormal findings. Code assignment depends on the information that is known at the time the encounter is being coded. For example, if no abnormal findings were uncovered during the examination but the encounter is being coded before test results are back, it is acceptable to assign the code for "without abnormal findings." When assigning a code for "with abnormal findings," additional code(s) should be assigned to identify the specific abnormal finding(s).

Preoperative examination and pre-procedural laboratory examination Z Codes are for use only in those situations when a patient is being cleared for a procedure or surgery and no treatment is given.

The Z Codes/categories for routine and administrative examinations are:

Code	Description
Z00	Encounter for general examination without complaint, suspected or reported diagnosis
Z01	Encounter for other special examination without complaint, suspected or reported diagnosis
Z02	Encounter for administrative examination Except: Z02.9, Encounter for administrative examinations, unspecified
Z32.0	Encounter for pregnancy test

15. Nonspecific Z Codes

Certain Z Codes are so nonspecific, or potentially redundant with other codes in the classification, that there can be little justification for their use in the inpatient setting Their use in the outpatient setting should be limited to those instances when there is no further documentation to permit more precise coding. Otherwise, any sign or symptom or any other reason for visit that is captured in another code should be used.

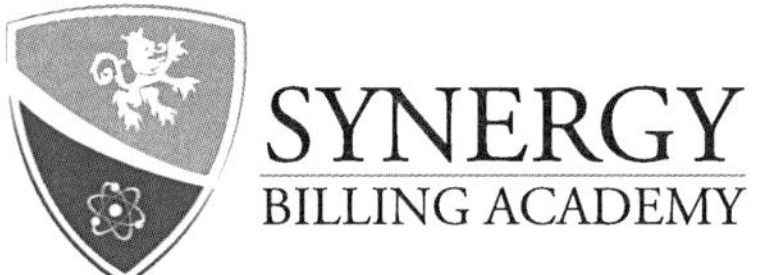

The nonspecific Z Codes/categories are:

Code	Description
Z02.9	Encounter for administrative examinations, unspecified
Z04.9	Encounter for examination and observation for unspecified reason
Z13.9	Encounter for screening, unspecified
Z41.9	Encounter for procedure for purposes other than remedying health state, unspecified
Z52.9	Donor of unspecified organ or tissue
Z86.59	Personal history of other mental and behavioral disorders
Z88.9	Allergy status to unspecified drugs, medicaments, and biological substances status
Z92.0	Personal history of contraception

Z. Codes That May Only be Principal/First-Listed Diagnosis

The following Z Codes/categories may only be reported as the principal/first-listed diagnosis, except when there are multiple encounters on the same day and the medical records for the encounters are combined:

Code	Description
Z00	Encounter for general examination without complaint, suspected or reported diagnosis
Z01	Encounter for other special examination without complaint, suspected or reported diagnosis
Z02	Encounter for administrative examination
Z03	Encounter for medical observation for suspected diseases and conditions ruled out
Z04	Encounter for examination and observation for other reasons
Z33.2	Encounter for elective termination of pregnancy
Z31.81	Encounter for male factor infertility in female patient
Z31.82	Encounter for Rh incompatibility status
Z31.83	Encounter for assisted reproductive fertility procedure cycle

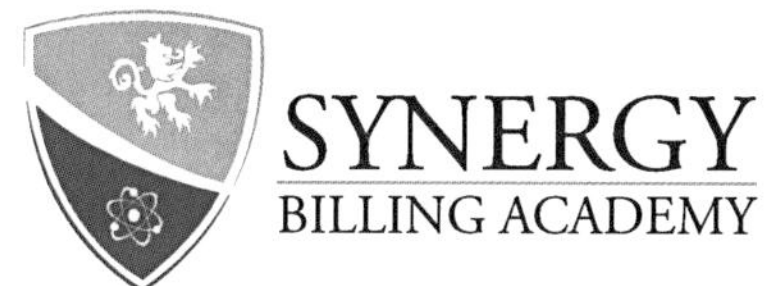

Code	Description
Z31.84	Encounter for fertility preservation procedure
Z34	Encounter for supervision of normal pregnancy
Z39	Encounter for maternal postpartum care and examination
Z38	Liveborn infants according to place of birth and type of delivery
Z42	Encounter for plastic and reconstructive surgery following medical procedure or healed injury
Z51.0	Encounter for antineoplastic radiation therapy
Z51.1	Encounter for antineoplastic chemotherapy and immunotherapy
Z52	Donors of organs and tissues Except: Z52.9, Donor of unspecified organ or tissue
Z76.1	Encounter for health supervision and care of foundling
Z76.2	Encounter for health supervision and care of other healthy infant and child
Z99.12	Encounter for respirator [ventilator] dependence during power failure

Word of Caution [12, 26]

In order to support the depth of ICD-10-CM, physician clinical documentation must, for example, contain details regarding:

- Laterality
- Stages of healing, e.g., routine, delayed, or malunion
- Trimester of pregnancy
- Episode of care, e.g., initial or subsequent encounter, sequela
- Depth, size, and cause of injuries
- Combination codes must reflect the association between conditions
- New clinical concepts such as underdosing

Helpful Tips

- Be specific in describing the patient's condition, illness, or disease.
- Distinguish between acute and chronic conditions, when appropriate.
- Identify the acute condition of an emergency situation.
    - Coma, loss of consciousness, hemorrhage, etc.
- Identify chronic complaints or secondary diagnoses.
- Identify how injuries occur.
- Be as granular as possible.

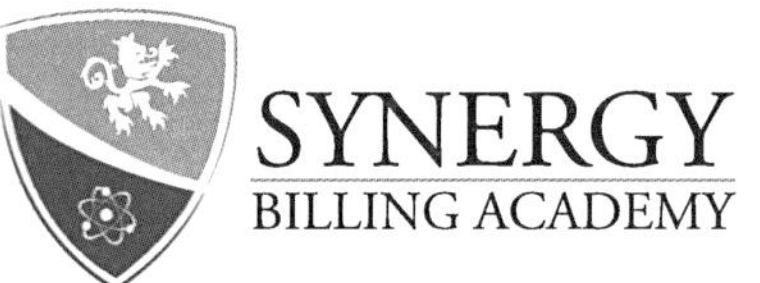

- Acute, chronic, acute on chronic, recurrent
- Mild, moderate, severe
- Site or location
- Laterality
  - Left, right, bilateral
    - Injury details
    - External cause, activity, place of occurrence

Documentation Requirements

- Document the specific trimester. [27]
  - Many of the codes in Chapter 15 of the ICD-10-CM require coders to report the specific trimester of the patient's pregnancy. For example, ICD-10-CM code O09.01 denotes supervision of pregnancy with history of infertility, first trimester. ICD-10-CM code O60.02 denotes preterm labor without delivery, second trimester. Trimesters are counted from the first day of the last menstrual period and are defined as follows:
    - 1st trimester: Fewer than 14 weeks 0 days
    - 2nd trimester: 14 weeks 0 days to fewer than 28 weeks 0 days
    - 3rd trimester: 28 weeks 0 days until delivery
  - Physicians can also simply document the specific number of weeks and days (rather than the trimester). Even this information is helpful because coders can calculate the trimester themselves. What physicians do not want to do is force coders to report an unspecified trimester. This reflects poorly on the physician and his or her attention to detail and clinical care.
- Be careful when reporting an annual GYN exam [27]
  - In ICD-10-CM, the code for an annual GYN exam is not included in Chapter 15. Instead, it is located in Chapter 21. Code Z01.4- denotes an encounter for a routine GYN exam, including the following:
    - Encounter for general GYN exam with or without cervical smear
    - Encounter for GYN exam (general) (routine), not otherwise specified
    - Encounter for pelvic exam (annual) (periodic)

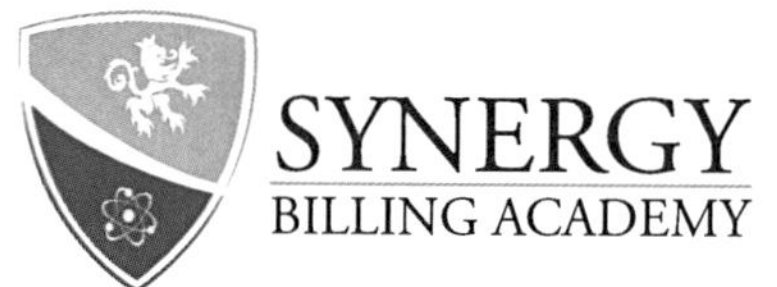

- Physicians must document whether the exam is with or without abnormal findings, as this affects code assignment. Physicians can bill an E/M code in conjunction with the appropriate ICD-10-CM code for this visit; however, only the lab can bill for the cervical smear test itself.

• Document the cause of pelvic pain, if known. [27]

- As in ICD-9-CM, if OB/GYN specialists can identify the cause of any abdominal and pelvic pain associated with menstruation, they should document this information. Causes of pain include—but are not limited to—adhesions, a history of endometriosis, cystic ovaries, or menorrhagia. It is important to paint the most comprehensive picture of the patient's clinical presentation so coders can capture all of the appropriate codes in addition to the code for pelvic and abdominal pain (ICD-10-CM code I10.-).

• Pay attention to detail when documenting migraines. [27]

- When a patient presents complaining of chronic migraines related to menstrual cramps, be sure to specify that the patient has menstrual migraines. ICD-10-CM includes codes for a variety of migraines, including those that are neurologic, abdominal, and ophthalmologic. Also specify whether the menstrual migraine (ICD-10-CM codes G43.82- and G43.83-) is intractable vs. not intractable as well as whether it is with or without status migrainosus.

• Document the reason for any fetus viability scans performed. [27]

- Is the scan performed for routine screening for viability, or are there signs and symptoms (e.g., decreased fetal movement or fetal anemia and thrombocytopenia) that indicate that the patient may have a miscarriage? This information affects code assignment.

• Specify whether advanced maternal age (elderly primigravida) complicates a patient's pregnancy. [27]

- If a patient is over the age of 35, specify whether her advanced maternal age is a factor in the delivery and, if so, what specific problem it caused. For example, during delivery, these patients may have pre/post eclampsia, an increased likelihood of postpartum hemorrhage, or placenta accretes. During antepartum care, they may have an increased genetic risk factor for fetal abnormalities.

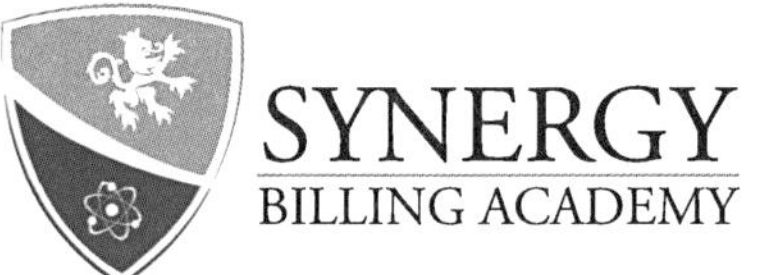

Changes Relevant to OB/GYN [28]

There are twice as many obstetrical codes in ICD-10-CM (2,155) as in ICD-9 (1,104). These new codes add specificity to the characterization of obstetrical conditions. The ICD-10-CM obstetric codes are listed in Chapter 15. These codes have sequencing priority over those from other chapters and start with the letter "O," not the number zero.

Unlike the ICD-9 codes, ICD-10-CM obstetrical codes are not divided by antepartum, delivery, and postpartum status, but most new codes indicate the trimester of pregnancy in their final character. An additional code from category Z3A should be used to define specific weeks of gestation (e.g., Z3A.42 would indicate 42 weeks' gestation). The Z Codes report reasons for encounters in the ICD-10 system.

There are now more codes to describe the nature of medical complications in pregnancy. For example, when diabetes complicates pregnancy, it can be further classified as pre-existing (type 1 or 2) and by the trimester in which the encounter occurred (e.g., O24.011 reports "Pre-existing diabetes mellitus, type 1, in pregnancy, first trimester"). Alternatively, gestational diabetes can be described along with its treatment (O24.011 reports "Gestational diabetes mellitus in pregnancy, diet-controlled").

Conversely, routine office visits during uncomplicated pregnancies require a code from category Z34 ("Encounter for supervision of normal pregnancy") as the first-listed diagnosis, but no codes from Chapter 15. When a patient has had a full-term uncomplicated delivery of a healthy singleton fetus following an uncomplicated pregnancy and postpartum course, code O80 is used and no others from Chapter 15. This code should be accompanied by Z37.0 (Single live birth) as the only outcome of delivery code.

The ICD-10-CM codes for elective abortion are contained in Chapter 21 (Factors Influencing Health Status and Contact with Health Services). As noted, Chapter 14 (N00-N99) itemizes diseases of the genitourinary system, which include diagnoses related to the female reproductive and urinary tracts.

Notes to Remember [9, 10 24]

Chapter 1

We now have a wide range of codes that we can use to identify infections with a predominantly

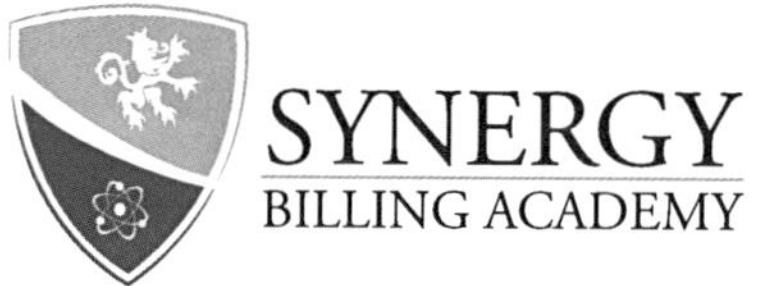

sexual mode of transmission (A50-A64), although human immunodeficiency virus (HIV) disease is actually excluded from this section.

Chapter 14

In Chapter 14, or diseases of the genitourinary system, we need to carefully identify if extra codes or extra documentation are required. Below are some instructional notes that you will see in the codes in this chapter:

Category Code	Instructional Note
N17	Code also underlying condition
N18	Code first etiology
N30	Additional code infectious agent
N31	Additional code urinary incontinence
N33	Code first underlying disease
N40.1	Additional code for associated symptoms

Chapter 15

This chapter can only be used in the mother's record for documentation and coding; Chapter 15 codes are never used in the newborn's because this chapter encompasses the conditions that are related to or aggravated by the pregnancy, childbirth, and the puerperium. For Chapter 15, the trimester is now the measurement of classification. In ICD-9-CM, we used the episode of care, such as delivered, antepartum, intrapartum, and postpartum. We also have to keep in mind that not all codes include the ability to select the trimesters. The trimesters are counted from the first day of the last menstrual period and are classified as follows:

Trimesters	
1st	Less than 14 weeks 0 days
2nd	14 weeks 0 days to less than 28 weeks 0 days
3rd	28 weeks 0 days until delivery

We must also specify the week of gestation. We are now required to code this using category code Z3A. In Chapter 15, we have a combination code that incorporates obstructed labor with

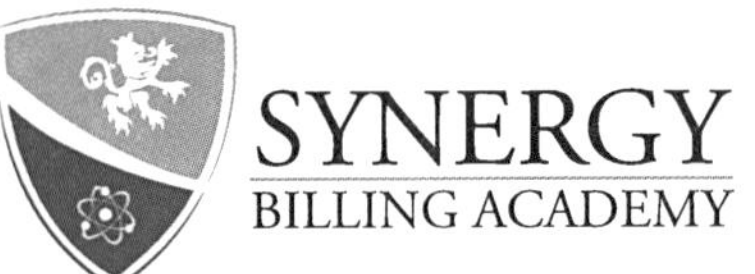

the reason for the obstruction into one code. We also have some definitions we need to keep in mind, such as: the timeline for abortion versus fetal death is now 20 weeks instead of 22; early versus late vomiting is now 20 weeks instead of 22; and preterm labor still happens before completing a full 37 weeks of gestation.

For certain conditions, we need to specify the fetus that is being affected. For a single pregnancy, the 7th character will be "0;" this is also the case for multiple gestations where the fetus is unspecified. 7th characters of 1 through 9 are used for cases of multiple gestations to identify the fetus for which the code applies. Below are the 7th characters for fetus identification:

Seventh Character for Fetus	
0	Not applicable or unspecified
1	Fetus 1
2	Fetus 2
3	Fetus 3
4	Fetus 4
5	Fetus 5
9	Other Fetus

ICD-10-CM provides a combination code for obstructed labor, incorporating the obstructed labor with the reason for the obstruction into one code.

Categories O03-O07 include spontaneous abortions with and without complications. Also included here are complications following (induced) termination of pregnancy, while an uncomplicated encounter for elective termination of pregnancy is coded Z33.2.

Chapter 21

Use a Z Code when a person who may or may not be sick encounters health services for some specific purpose, such as to receive limited care or service for current condition, donate an organ or tissue, receive prophylactic vaccination, or discuss a problem.

Use a Z Code when some circumstance or problem is present which influences a person's health status but is not a current illness or injury.

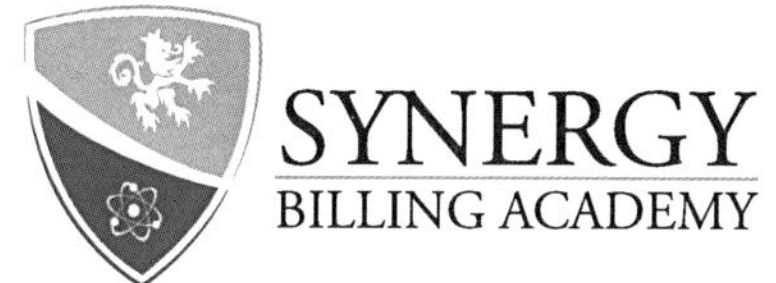

Documentation Requirements [29]

Obstetric cases require codes from Chapter 15, Pregnancy, Childbirth, and the Puerperium (O00-O9A). These codes have sequencing priority over codes from other chapters. Additional codes from other chapters may be used in conjunction with Chapter 15 codes to further specify conditions. Should the provider document that the pregnancy is incidental to the encounter, then code Z33.1, Pregnant state, incidental, should be used in place of any Chapter 15 codes. It is the provider's responsibility to state that the condition being treated is not affecting the pregnancy. Codes from Chapter 15 should only be used on the maternal record, never on the newborn's record.

The majority of codes in Chapter 15 have a final character indicating the trimester of pregnancy.

Additionally, a code from category Z3A, Weeks of gestation, should also be reported to identify the specific week of the pregnancy.

Where applicable, a 7th character is to be assigned for certain categories to identify the fetus for which the complication code applies.

Trimester Designation

Trimesters are counted from the first day of the last menstrual period. They are defined as follows:

- First trimester - Less than 14 weeks 0 days
- Second trimester - 14 weeks 0 days to less than 28 weeks 0 days
- Third trimester - 28 weeks 0 days until delivery

7th Character Extender Designation

One of the following 7th characters is to be assigned to each code under the stated category. 7th character 0 is for single gestations and multiple gestations where the fetus is unspecified. 7th characters 1 through 9 are for cases of multiple gestations to identify the fetus for which the code applies. The appropriate code from the stated category must also be assigned when assigning a code from stated category that has a 7th character 1 through 9.

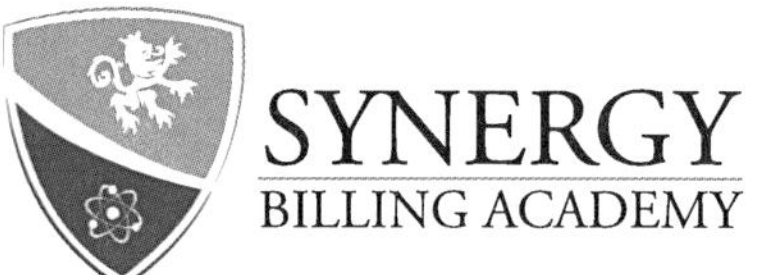

Weeks of Gestation Designation			
Code	**Description**	**Code**	**Description**
Z3A.OO	Weeks of gestation of pregnancy not specified	Z3A.25	25 weeks gestation of pregnancy
Z3A.01	Less than 8 weeks gestation of pregnancy	Z3A.26	26 weeks gestation of pregnancy
Z3A.08	8 weeks gestation of pregnancy	Z3A.27	27 weeks gestation of pregnancy
Z3A.09	9 weeks gestation of pregnancy	Z3A.28	28 weeks gestation of pregnancy
Z3A.10	10 weeks gestation of pregnancy	Z3A.29	29 weeks gestation of pregnancy
Z3A.11	11 weeks gestation of pregnancy	Z3A.30	30 weeks gestation of pregnancy
Z3A.12	12 weeks gestation of pregnancy	Z3A.31	31 weeks gestation of pregnancy
Z3A.13	13 weeks gestation of pregnancy	Z3A.32	32 weeks gestation of pregnancy
Z3A.14	14 weeks gestation of pregnancy	Z3A.33	33 weeks gestation of pregnancy
Z3A.15	15 weeks gestation of pregnancy	Z3A.34	34 weeks gestation of pregnancy
Z3A.16	16 weeks gestation of pregnancy	Z3A.35	35 weeks gestation of pregnancy
Z3A.17	17 weeks gestation of pregnancy	Z3A.36	36 weeks gestation of pregnancy
Z3A.18	18 weeks gestation of pregnancy	Z3A.37	37 weeks gestation of pregnancy
Z3A.19	19 weeks gestation of pregnancy	Z3A.38	38 weeks gestation of pregnancy
Z3A.20	20 weeks gestation of pregnancy	Z3A.39	39 weeks gestation of pregnancy
Z3A.21	21 weeks gestation of pregnancy	Z3A.40	40 weeks gestation of pregnancy
Z3A.22	22 weeks gestation of pregnancy	Z3A.41	41 weeks gestation of pregnancy
Z3A.23	23 weeks gestation of pregnancy	Z3A.42	42 weeks gestation of pregnancy
Z3A.24	24 weeks gestation of pregnancy	Z3A.49	Greater than 42 weeks gestation of pregnancy

For most codes in category Z3A (Z3A.08-Z3A.42), the last two characters correlate to the weeks of gestation.

Examples

EXAMPLE 1:

Patient is a type 1 diabetic. She is 16 weeks pregnant.

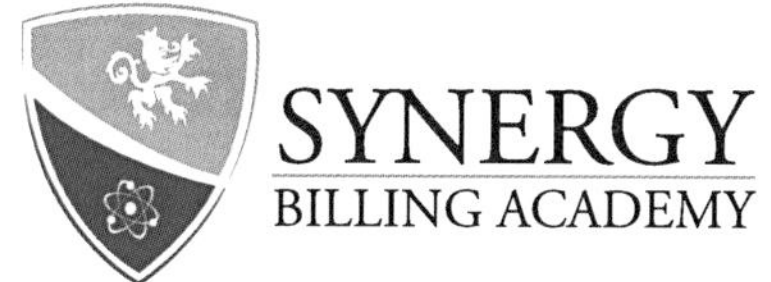

- O24.012, Pre-existing diabetes mellitus, type 1, in pregnancy, second trimester
- Z3A.16, 16 weeks gestation of pregnancy

EXAMPLE 2:

Patient with monochorionic twin gestations presents with ultrasound indicating polyhydramnios of twin A (fetus 1). She is 30 weeks gestation.

- O40.3XX1, Polyhydramnios, third trimester, fetus 1
- Z3A.30, 30 weeks gestation of pregnancy

Note the use of the placeholders "XX" in order to maintain the integrity of the 7th character extender in the code for polyhydramnios.

Routine GYN Encounters [30]

- Z01.411, General, routine, GYN exam with abnormality
- Z01.419, General, routine, GYN exam without abnormality
- Z34.01, Supervision normal 1st pregnancy, 1st trimester
- Z34.02, Supervision normal 1st pregnancy, 2nd trimester
- SZ34.03, Supervision normal 1st pregnancy, 3rd trimester
- O09.611, Supervision of young primigravida, first trimester

Pregnancy Guideline [9, 10, 31]

In order to code pregnancy supervision, the documentation should indicate the trimester of the patient. The trimester in ICD-10-CM has been defined in Chapter 15, Pregnancy, Childbirth, and the Puerperium, as follows: 1st trimester – less than 14 weeks 0 days; 2nd trimester – 14 weeks 0 days to less than 28 weeks 0 days; 3rd trimester – 28 weeks 0 days until delivery. Trimesters are counted from the first day of the last menstrual period.

Pregnancy has many code selections for the supervision of pregnancy, including normal first pregnancy, other pregnancy, unspecified pregnancy, and high-risk pregnancy. Each code set also has a code for first, second, and third or unspecified trimester. There is also a secondary code that specifies the weeks of pregnancy.

Code: Z34.90, Supervision of normal pregnancy, unspecified, unspecified trimester

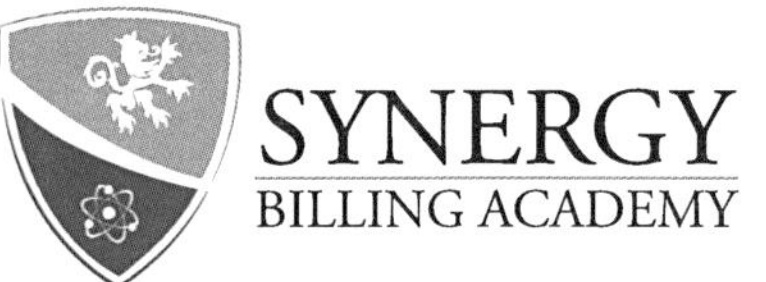

Ovarian Cysts Guideline [9, 10, 31]

In order to code ovarian cysts to the correct level of specificity, documentation should indicate the type of cyst (follicular, corpus luteum, etc.).

Codes: Z01.411, Encounter for gynecological examination (general) (routine) with abnormal findings; N83.20, Ovarian cyst; unspecified; and Z12.72, Encounter for screening for malignant neoplasm of vagina

Poor Fetal Growth – Maternal Record [32]

It is important for providers to understand the elements necessary for the documentation of poor fetal growth for the maternal record in ICD-10-CM. Please make sure to document the following key pieces of information:

- Maternal care for known or suspected poor fetal growth
  - Due to known or suspected
    - Placental insufficiency
    - Other poor fetal growth
      - Light-for-dates NOS
      - Small-for-dates NOS
- Trimester
  - First (less than 14 weeks 0 days)
  - Second (14 weeks 0 days to less than 28 weeks 0 days)
  - Third (28 weeks 0 days until delivery)
  - Unspecified
- Fetus affected by complication
  - Multiple gestation pregnancy
    - Fetus 1
    - Fetus 2
    - Fetus 3
    - Fetus 4
    - Fetus 5
    - Other
  - Unspecified or not applicable (i.e., single fetus)

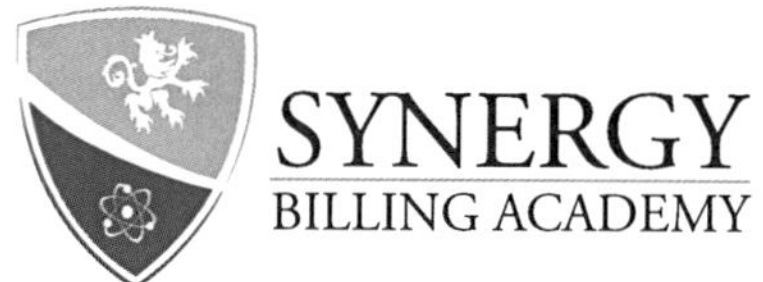

ICD-9-CM Conversion to ICD-10-CM:

Diseases of the Genitourinary System

ICD-9-CM Chapter 10		ICD-10-CM Chapter 14	
599.0	Urinary tract infection, site not specified	N39.0	Urinary tract infection, site not specified
616.10	Vaginitis	N76.0 N76.1 N76.2 N76.3	Acute vaginitis Subacute and chronic vaginitis Acute vulvitis Subacute and chronic vulvitis
616.11	Vaginitis and vulvovaginitis in diseases classified elsewhere	N77.1	Vaginitis, vulvitis and vulvovaginitis in diseases classified elsewhere
623.5	Vaginal discharge (unspecified)	N89.8	Other specified noninflammatory disorders of vagina
626.2	Excessive or frequent menstruation	N92.0	Excessive and frequent menstruation with regular cycle

Pregnancy, Childbirth, and the Puerperium

ICD-9-CM Chapter 11		ICD-10-CM Chapter 15	
654.23	Previous c-section delivery antepartum condition	O34.21	Maternal care for scar from previous cesarean delivery

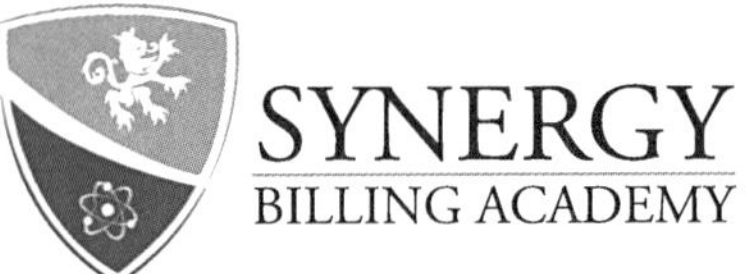

Factors Influencing Health Status and Contact with Health Services

ICD-9-CM V Codes		ICD-10-CM Chapter 21 (Z Codes)	
V01.6	Contact with or exposure to venereal disease	Z20.2	Contact with and (suspected) exposure to infections with a predominantly sexual mode of transmission
V03.89	Other specified vaccination	Z23	Encounter for immunization
V15.81	Noncompliance with medical treatment	Z91.19	Patient's noncompliance with other medical treatment and regimen
V15.82	Personal history of tobacco use, presenting hazards to health	Z87.891	Personal history of nicotine dependence
V22.0	Supervision of normal first pregnancy	Z34.00	Encounter for supervision of normal first pregnancy, unspecified trimester
V22.1	Supervision of other normal pregnancy	Z34.80	Encounter for supervision of other normal pregnancy, unspecified trimester
		Z34.90	Encounter for supervision of normal pregnancy, unspecified, unspecified trimester
V22.2	Pregnant state, incidental	Z33.1	Pregnant state, incidental
V24.2	Routine postpartum follow-up	Z39.2	Encounter for routine postpartum follow-up
V25.02	General counseling for initiation of other contraceptive measures	Z30.018	Encounter for initial prescription of other contraceptives
V25.09	Other general counseling and advice, contraceptive management	Z30.09	Encounter for other general counseling and advice on contraception
V25.40	Contraception maintenance	Z30.40	Encounter for surveillance of contraceptives, unspecified
V25.49	Surveillance other previous contraceptive method	Z30.49	Encounter for surveillance of other contraceptives

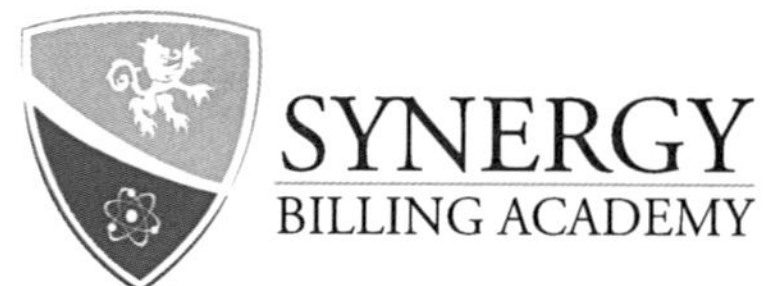

V27.0	Outcome of delivery single live born	Z37.0	Single live birth
V65.40	Counseling NOS	Z71.9	Counseling, unspecified
V65.49	Other specified counseling	Z71.89	Other specified counseling
V68.01	Disability examination	Z02.71	Encounter for disability determination
V68.1	Issue of repeat prescriptions	Z76.0	Encounter for issue of repeat prescription
V69.2	Problems related to high-risk sexual behavior	Z72.51	High-risk heterosexual behavior
V70.0	Exam, general adult medical	Z00.00	Encounter for general adult medical examination without abnormal findings
V70.3	Exam, marriage/camp/school/ sports	Z02.89	Encounter for other administrative examinations
V70.5	Health examination of defined subpopulation	Z02.1 Z02.3 Z02.89	Encounter for pre-employment examination Encounter for examination for recruitment to armed forces Encounter for other administrative examinations
V72.31	Exam, gynecological	Z01.411 Z01.419	Encounter for gynecological examination (general) (routine) with abnormal findings Encounter for gynecological examination (general) (routine) without abnormal findings
V72.32	Encounter for pap cervical smear, confirm findings of recent normal smear following initial abnormal smear	Z01.42	Encounter for cervical smear to confirm findings of recent normal smear following initial abnormal smear
V72.41	Pregnancy examination or test negative	Z32.02	Encounter for pregnancy test, result negative
V72.85	Other specified examination	Z01.89	Encounter for other specified special examinations

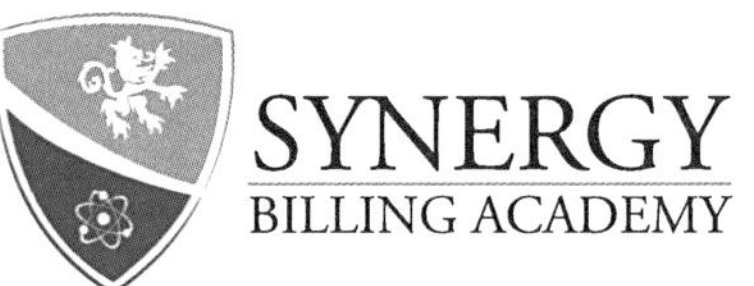

V74.1	Screening examination for pulmonary tuberculosis	Z11.1	Encounter for screening for respiratory tuberculosis
V74.5	Screen for venereal disease STI	Z11.3	Encounter for screening for infections with a predominantly sexual mode of transmission
V76.2	Screen malignant neoplasm, cervix	Z12.4	Encounter for screening for malignant neoplasm of cervix

Certain Infectious and Parasitic Diseases

ICD-9-CM		ICD-10-CM	
034.0	Streptococcal sore throat	J02.0	Streptococcal pharyngitis
		J03.00	Acute streptococcal tonsillitis, unspecified
041.00	Streptococcus, unspecified	B95.5	Unspecified streptococcus as the cause of diseases classified elsewhere
042	HIV disease	B20	Human immunodeficiency virus [HIV] disease
052.9	Varicella without mention of complication	B01.9	Varicella without complication
054.10	Genital herpes, unspecified	A60.9	Anogenital herpesviral infection, unspecified
070.53	Hepatitis E without mention of hepatic coma	B17.2	Acute hepatitis E
078.10	Viral warts, unspecified	B07.9	Viral wart, unspecified
079.4	Human papillomavirus	B97.7	Papillomavirus as the cause of diseases classified elsewhere
099.41	Chlamydia trachomatis	N34.1	Nonspecific urethritis
110.1	Dermatophytosis of nail	B35.1	Tinea unguium
112.1	Candidiasis of vulva and vagina	B37.3	Candidiasis of vulva and vagina

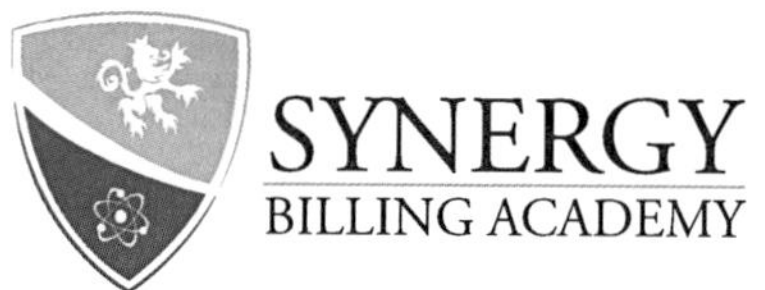

Check Your Understanding

True and False

1. Some of the new codes for OB/GYN will be found under categories N, O, and Z.

   a. True
   b. False

2. OB/GYN providers will be required to use both ICD-9-CM codes and ICD-10-CM codes.

   a. True
   b. False

3. OB/GYN providers have specific Z Codes for screening and counseling.

   a. True
   b. False

4. The 3rd trimester is defined as 28 weeks to zero days until delivery.

   a. True
   b. False

5. Chapter 16 was designed to be used on the mother's record.

   a. True
   b. False

6. The final character in codes from Chapter 15 will indicate the trimester.

   a. True
   b. False

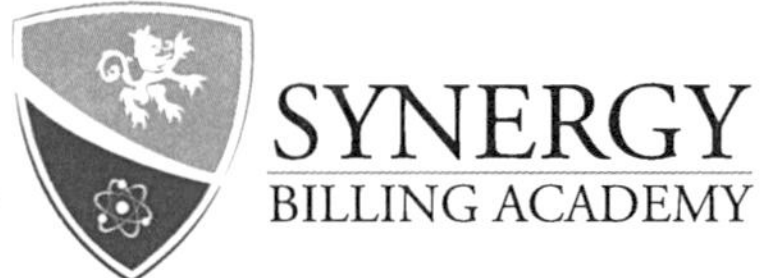

7. It is not necessary to indicate the weeks of gestation on the patient's charts.

    a. True
    b. False

8. ICD-10-CM codes are less descriptive than ICD-9-CM codes.

    a. True
    b. False

9. OB/GYN practictioners will need to use Z Codes, as they are the replacement for V Codes.

    a. True
    b. False

10. Complete and accurate medical records are needed to ensure the proper treatment of patients.

    a. True
    b. False

ICD-10-CM International Classification of Diseases 10th Revision Clinical Modification

Behavioral Health

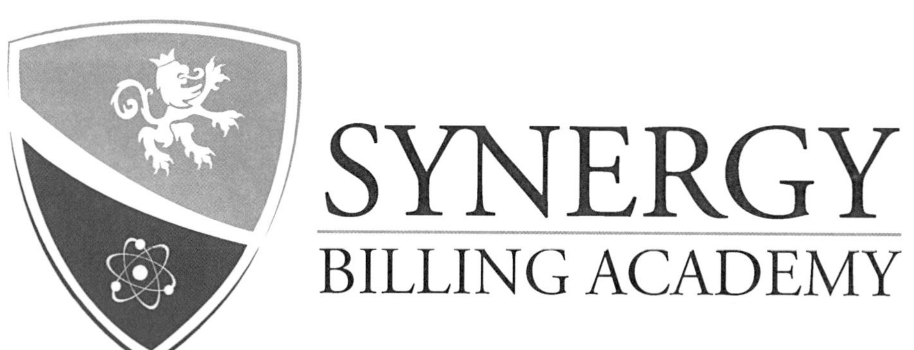

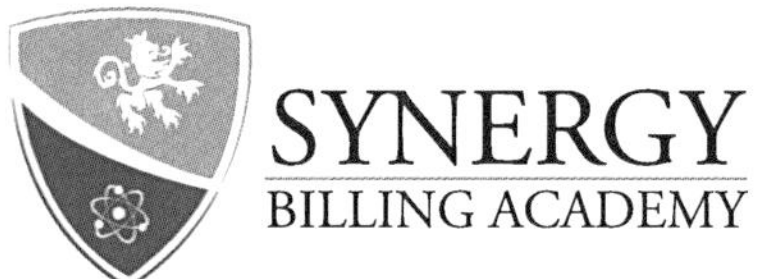

Behavioral Background and Practice

The term "behavioral" refers to overt actions; to underlying psychological processes such as cognition, emotion, temperament, and motivation; and to bio-behavioral interactions. The term "social" encompasses sociocultural, socioeconomic, and sociodemographic status; bio-social interactions; and the various levels of social context from small groups to complex cultural systems and societal influences. [33]

Behavioral health services are services for any mental health diagnosis, any substance abuse diagnosis, or any combination thereof. Substance abuse includes drug and alcohol abuse and the detoxification and withdrawal treatment that may be required. [33]

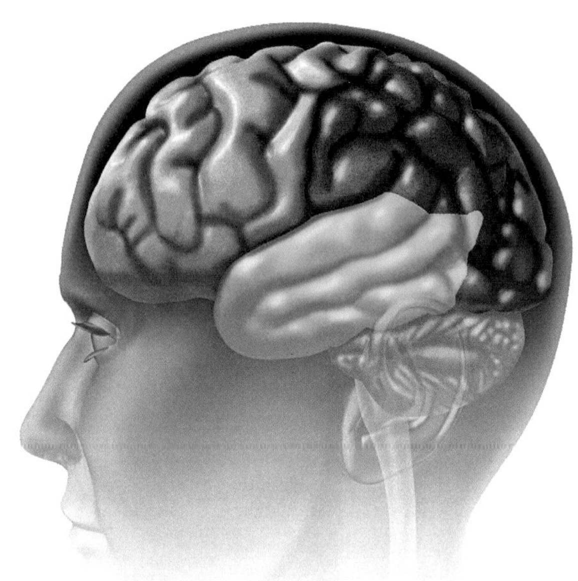

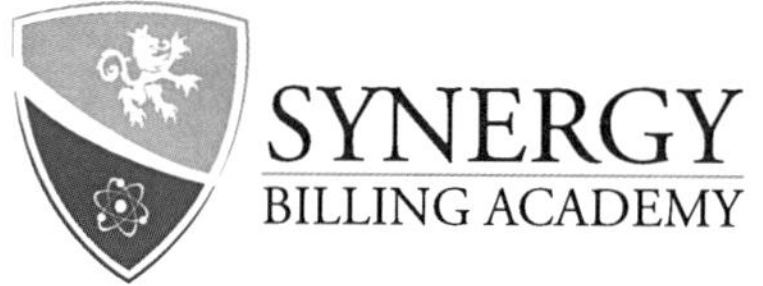

Behavioral Health Claims and Coding Manuals

DSM-V-TR

- In May 2013, DSM-V-TR (Diagnostic and Statistical Manual of Mental Disorders Fifth Text Revision) was released, marking the end of more than a decade's journey in revising the criteria for the diagnosis and classification of mental disorders.

ICD-10-CM

- On October 1, 2015, the ICD-10-CM (International Classification of Diseases 10th Revision Clinical Modification) will be released, marking the replacement of ICD-9-CM, which is what all behavioral health providers have been using to add the diagnosis to their patients' claims.

Please keep in mind that ICD-10-CM will not have any effects on Current Procedural Terminology (CPT) codes or the DMS-V-TR.

In behavioral health diagnosis, ICD-9-CM coding may use codes from the upper 200s to 300 and V Codes; however, in ICD-10-CM, we would use code range F00 and Z Codes.

ICD-9-CM Codes [4, 10]

ICD-9-CM codes have anywhere between 3 and 5 characters. The number of characters in the code will specify what type of code it is and tell you if it is a category code, a subcategory code, or a subclassification code. Below are some of the codes that we are currently using for behavioral health.

Code	Description
293.83	Mood disorder due to medical condition (e.G. Postpartum depression)
296.21	Major depressive disorder, single episode, mild
296.22	Major depressive disorder, single episode, moderate
296.30	Major depressive disorder, recurrent
296.90	Mood disorder, NOS
300.00	Anxiety disorder, NOS

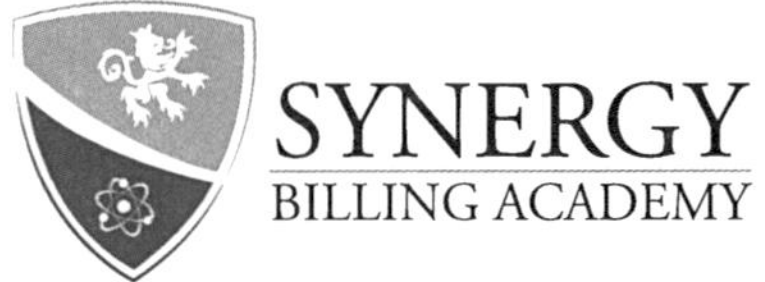

300.02	Generalized anxiety disorder
309	Adjustment disorder with depressed mood
311	Depressive disorder, not otherwise specified (NOS)
314 or 314.01	Attention Deficit/Hyperactivity Disorder (inattentive and combined types)

ICD-10-CM Chapter 5 – Mental, Behavioral, and Neurodevelopmental Disorders (F01-F99)

Transitioning to ICD-10-CM will completely change the codes used in behavioral health. Before, the code range was found in Chapter 5 and encompassed the high 200s to 300 range; now, the code range will be found in Chapter 5 and codes will start with the letter "F." Each and every one of these codes and their descriptions will be more specific to the patient's condition. Overall, ICD-9-CM codes are vague and not very descriptive, whereas ICD-10-CM codes are more descriptive.

This chapter contains more subchapters, categories, subcategories, and codes than ICD-9-CM. Consequently, when comparing ICD-10-CM to ICD-9-CM, some disorders are classified differently and we can obtain greater clinical detail.

Changes were necessary in many parts of Chapter 5 because of outdated terminology.

Given what has been discovered in the past 20 years about the effects of nicotine, ICD-10-CM contains a separate category, F17, for nicotine dependence, with subcategories to identify the specific tobacco product and nicotine-induced disorders. ICD-9-CM has a single code, 305.1, for tobacco use disorder or tobacco dependence.

There is a change in sequencing involving the intellectual disability codes (F70-F79). In ICD-9-CM, an additional code for any associated psychiatric or physical conditions should be sequenced after the intellectual disability code. In ICD-10-CM, any associated physical or developmental disorder should be coded first. [24]

Below is a breakdown of all the sections in Chapter 5:

Codes	Description
F01-F09	Mental Disorders due to known physiological conditions
F10-F19	Mental and behavioral disorders due to psychoactive substance use

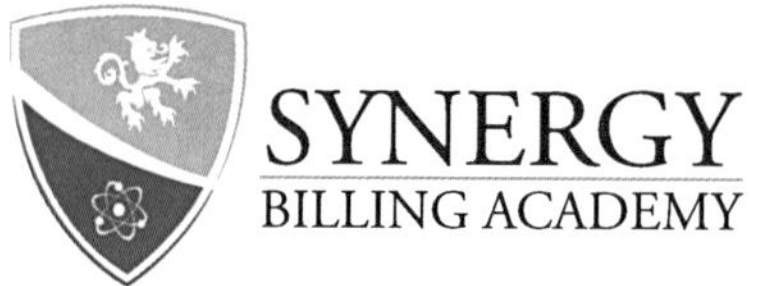

F20-F29	Schizophrenia, schizotypal, delusional, and other non-mood psychotic disorders
F30-F39	Mood [affective] disorders
F40-F48	Anxiety, dissociative, stress-related, somatoform, and other nonpsychotic mental disorders
F50-F59	Behavioral syndromes associated with physiological disturbances and physical factors
F60-F69	Disorders of adult personality and behavior
F70-F79	Intellectual disabilities
F80-F89	Pervasive and specific developmental disorders
F90-F98	Behavioral and emotional disorders with onset usually occurring in childhood and adolescence
F99	Unspecified mental disorder

ICD-10-CM Chapter Categories [24]

The codes in this chapter include disorders of psychological development but exclude symptoms, signs, and abnormal clinical laboratory findings (R00-R99). The arrangement of the codes within the various sections of ICD-10-CM is significantly different.

A number of changes to category and subcategory titles have been made.

- ICD-9-CM subcategory 296.0 is Bipolar I disorder, single manic episode, but its ICD-10-CM counterpart, category F30, is Manic episode.

There are unique codes for alcohol and drug use (not specified as abuse or dependence) and abuse and dependence, so careful review of the documentation is required. There are also changes to the codes for drug and alcohol abuse and dependence, as they no longer identify continuous or episodic use. A history of drug or alcohol dependence is coded as "in remission."

There are combination codes for drug and alcohol use and associated conditions, such as withdrawal, sleep disorders, or psychosis. There is a code for blood alcohol level (Y90.-) that can be assigned as an additional code when documentation indicates its use.

The identification of the stage of the substance use, namely continuous or episodic, is not a part of ICD-10-CM. A single ICD-10-CM code identifies not only the substance but also the

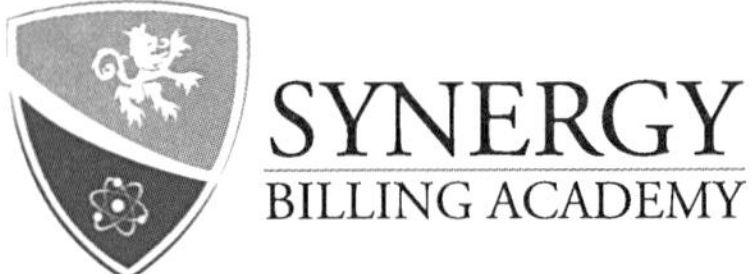

disorder the substance use induced. There continues to be a code for substance dependence "in remission."

- A fairly substantial classification change was made to codes for drug and alcohol abuse and dependence.
- The codes in this chapter are parallel to the Diagnostic and Statistical Manual of Mental Disorders – Fifth Text Revision (DSM-V TR) in most cases

Guidelines [9, 24]

Many changes were made to Chapter 5, including organization and terminology, which resulted in some guideline adjustments as well.

- In ICD-10-CM, beneath code F54, Psychological and behavioral factors associated with disorders or diseases classified elsewhere, there is a note that states to "code first the associated physical disorder."
- The equivalent ICD-9-CM code, 316, has a note to "use additional code to identify the associated physical condition."

The NCHS has published the following guidelines: [9]

A. Pain Disorders Related to Psychological Factors
B. Mental and Behavioral Disorders Due to Psychoactive Substance Use

1. In remission
2. Psychoactive substance use, abuse and dependence
3. Psychoactive substance use

A. Pain Disorders Related to Psychological Factors

- Assign code F45.41, for pain that is exclusively related to psychological disorders. As indicated by the Excludes1 note under category G89, a code from category G89 should not be assigned with code F45.41.
- Code F45.42, Pain disorders with related psychological factors, should be used with a code from category G89, Pain, not elsewhere classified, if there is documentation of a psychological component for a patient with acute or chronic pain.

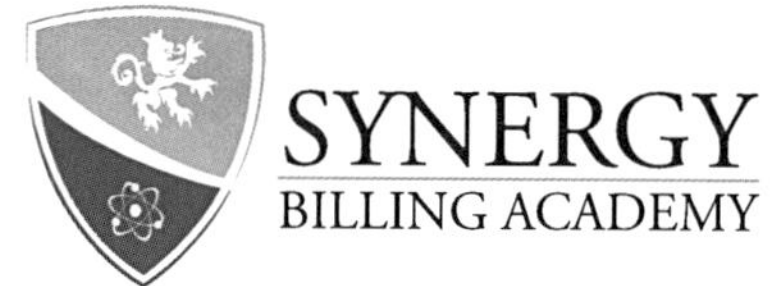

B. **Mental and Behavioral Disorders Due to Psychoactive Substance Use**

1. In remission

Selection of codes for "in remission" for categories F10-F19, Mental and behavioral disorders due to psychoactive substance use (categories F10-F19 with -.21), requires the provider's clinical judgment. The appropriate codes for "in remission" are assigned only on the basis of provider documentation (as defined in the Official Guidelines for Coding and Reporting).

2. Psychoactive substance use, abuse, and dependence

When the provider documentation refers to use, abuse, and dependence of the same substance (e.g., alcohol, opioid, cannabis, etc.), only one code should be assigned to identify the pattern of use based on the following hierarchy:

- If both use and abuse are documented, assign only the code for abuse.
- If both abuse and dependence are documented, assign only the code for dependence.
- If use, abuse, and dependence are all documented, assign only the code for dependence.
- If both use and dependence are documented, assign only the code for dependence.

3. Psychoactive substance use

As with all other diagnoses, the codes for psychoactive substance use (F10.9-, F11.9-, F12.9-, F13.9-, F14.9-, F15.9-, F16.9-) should only be assigned based on provider documentation and when they meet the definition of a reportable diagnosis (see Section III, Reporting Additional Diagnoses). The codes are to be used only when the psychoactive substance use is associated with a mental or behavioral disorder, and such a relationship is documented by the provider

Chapter 21 – Factors Influencing Health Status and Contact with Health Services

In ICD-9-CM, V Codes or health status codes are used for factors influencing health status and contact with health service. V Codes are mostly used to help explain medical history factors

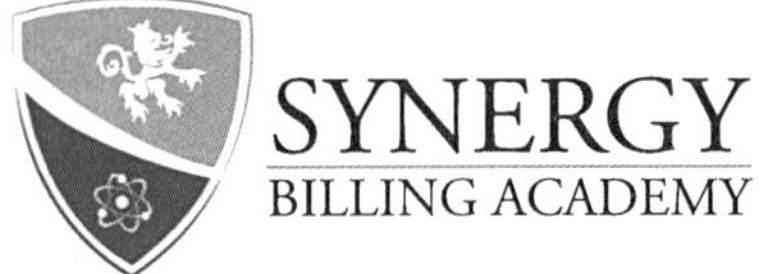

that influence treatment such as diabetes or a history of stroke, amongst others. For counseling purposes, we might need to use V Codes depending on the payer.

ICD-9-CM to ICD-10-CM

Professionals will find the listing of codes for factors influencing health status and contact with health services a little different in ICD-10-CM than what is currently found in ICD-9-CM. What were previously V Codes are now Z Codes. [24]

ICD-10-CM Chapter Categories [24]

These codes are used when a person who may or may not be sick encounters the health services for some specific purpose, such as to receive limited care or service for a current condition, or to discuss a problem which is in itself not a disease or injury.

Within in the Z Codes, some categories titles have been rephrased to better reflect the situations the codes classify. Several codes have been expanded, such as personal and family history. Codes have been added for concepts that do not exist in ICD-9-CM, and now we have instructional notes for different categories to explain how codes should be assigned. Below is a breakdown of all the sections in Chapter 21. The sections pertaining to behavioral health are:

- Z69–Z76
- Z77–Z99

CODES	DESCRIPTION
Z00-Z13	Persons encountering health services for examinations
Z14-Z15	Genetic carrier and genetic susceptibility to disease
Z16	Resistance to antimicrobial drugs
Z17	Estrogen receptor status
Z18	Retained foreign body fragment
Z20-Z28	Persons with potential health hazards related to communicable diseases
Z30-Z39	Persons encountering health services in circumstances related to reproduction
Z40-Z53	Encounters for other specific health care

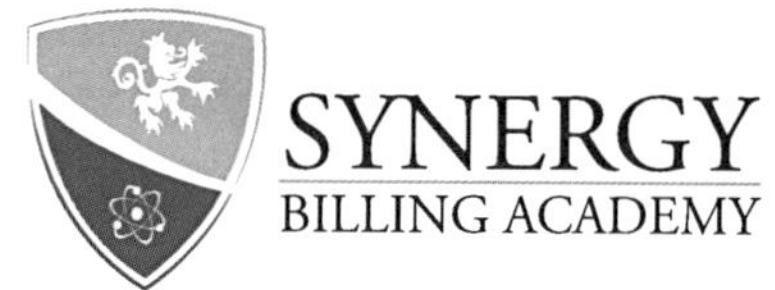

Z55-Z65	Persons with potential health hazards related to socioeconomic and psychosocial circumstances
Z66	Do not resuscitate status
Z67	Blood type
Z68	Body mass index (BMI)
Z69-Z76	***Persons encountering health services in other circumstances***
Z77-Z99	***Persons with potential health hazards related to family and personal history and certain conditions influencing health status***

Guidelines [9]

The chapter-specific guidelines provide additional information about the use of Z Codes for specified encounters.

Z Codes are for use in any health care setting. Z Codes may be used as either a first-listed (principal diagnosis code in the inpatient setting) or secondary code, depending on the circumstances of the encounter. Certain Z Codes may only be used as first-listed or principal diagnosis.

Z Codes are not procedure codes. A corresponding procedure code must accompany a Z Code to describe any procedure performed.

The NCHS has published the following guidelines: [9]

A. Use of Z Codes in Any Health Care Setting
B. Z Codes Indicate a Reason for an Encounter
C. Categories of Z Codes

1. Contact/exposure
2. Inoculations and vaccinations
3. Status
4. ***History (of)***
5. Screening
6. Observation
7. Aftercare
8. Follow-up
9. Donor
10. ***Counseling***

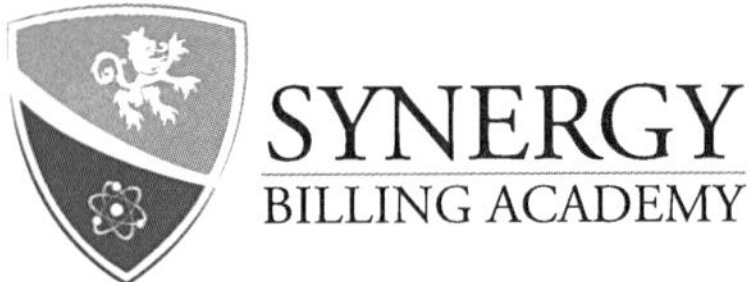

11. Encounters for obstetrical and reproductive services
12. Newborns and infants
13. Routine and administrative examinations
14. Miscellaneous Z Codes
    - Prophylactic organ removal
15. Nonspecific Z Codes
16. Z Codes that may only be principal/first-listed diagnosis

4. History (of)

There are two types of history Z Codes, personal and family. Personal history codes explain a patient's past medical condition that no longer exists and is not currently being treated, but that has the potential for recurrence and therefore may require continued monitoring.

Family history codes are for use when a patient has a family member(s) who has had a particular disease that causes the patient to be at higher risk of also developing the disease.

Personal history codes may be used in conjunction with follow-up codes and family history codes may be used in conjunction with screening codes to explain the need for a test or procedure. History codes are also acceptable on any medical record, regardless of the reason for visit. A history of an illness, even if no longer present, is important information that may alter the type of treatment ordered.

Z Code categories for history:

CODES	DESCRIPTIONS
Z80	Family history of primary malignant neoplasm
Z81	***Family history of mental and behavioral disorders***
Z82	Family history of certain disabilities and chronic diseases (leading to disablement)
Z83	Family history of other specific disorders
Z84	Family history of other conditions
Z85	Personal history of malignant neoplasm
Z86	Personal history of certain other diseases
Z87	Personal history of other diseases and conditions
Z91.4	***Personal history of psychological trauma, not elsewhere classified***

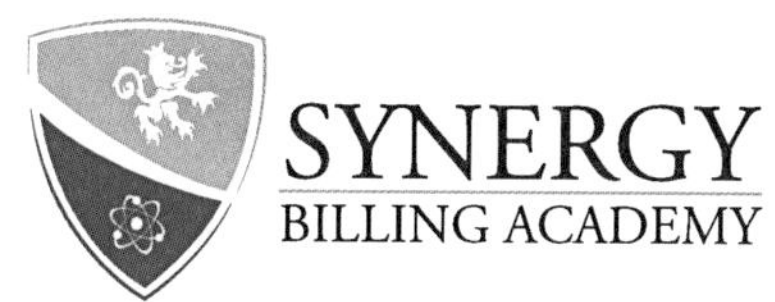

Z91.5	***Personal history of self-harm***
Z91.8	Other specified personal risk factors, not elsewhere classified Except: Z91.83, Wandering in diseases classified elsewhere
Z92	***Personal history of medical treatment*** Except: Z92.0, Personal history of contraception Except: Z92.82, Status post administration of tPA (rtPA) in a different facility within the last 24 hours prior to admission to a current facility

10. Counseling

Counseling Z Codes are used when a patient or family member receives assistance in the aftermath of an illness or injury, or when support is required in coping with family or social problems. They are not used in conjunction with a diagnosis code when the counseling component of care is considered integral to standard treatment.

Z Code categories for counseling:

CODES	DESCRIPTIONS
Z30.0	Encounter for general counseling and advice on contraception
Z31.5	Encounter for genetic counseling
Z31.6	Encounter for general counseling and advice on procreation
Z32.2	Encounter for childbirth instruction
Z32.3	Encounter for childcare instruction
Z69	Encounter for mental health services for victim and perpetrator of abuse
Z70	Counseling related to sexual attitude, behavior, and orientation
Z71	Persons encountering health services for other counseling and medical advice, not elsewhere classified
Z76.81	Expectant mother prebirth pediatrician visit

Word of Caution [12, 26]

In order to support the depth of ICD-10-CM, physician clinical documentation must, for example, contain details regarding:

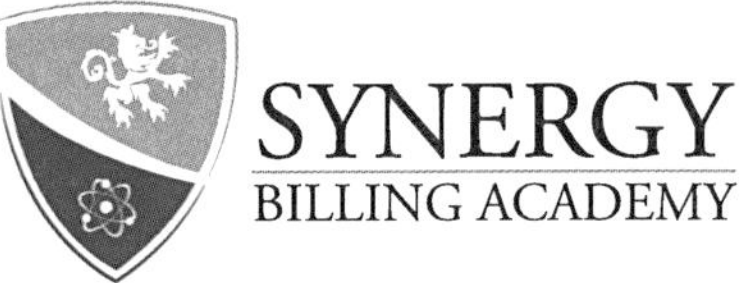

- Laterality
- Stages of healing, e.g., routine, delayed or malunion
- Trimester of pregnancy
- Episode of care, e.g., initial or subsequent encounter, sequela
- Depth, size, and cause of injuries
- Combination codes must reflect the association between conditions
- New clinical concepts such as underdosing

Helpful Tips

- Be specific in describing the patient's condition, illness, or disease.
- Distinguish between acute and chronic conditions, when appropriate.
- Identify the acute condition of an emergency situation.
  - Coma, loss of consciousness, hemorrhage, etc.
- Identify chronic complaints or secondary diagnoses.
- Identify how injuries occur.
- Be as granular as possible.
  - Acute, chronic, acute on chronic, recurrent
  - Mild, moderate, severe
  - Site or location
  - Laterality
    - Left, right, bilateral
      - Injury details
      - External cause, activity, place of occurrence

Documentation Requirements

The ICD-10 classification of mental and behavioral disorders, developed in part by the American Psychiatric Association, classifies depression by code. In typical, mild, moderate, or severe depressive episodes, the patient suffers from lowering of mood, reduction of energy, and decrease in activities. His or her capacity for enjoyment, interest, and concentration is reduced and is often marked by tiredness after even a minimum of effort. Sleep patterns are usually disturbed and appetite diminished, along with reduced self-confidence and self-esteem.

Final code selection is based on severity (mild, moderate, severe) and status. Depending on the number and severity of the symptoms, a depressive episode may be specified as mild, moderate, or severe. [35]

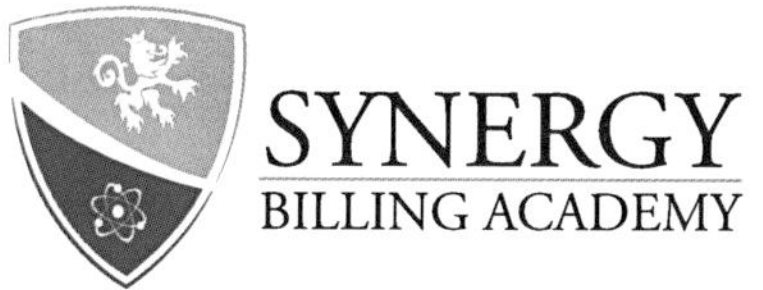

Example 1 [36]

Depression

- At a minimum, you need to identify if it is a single episode or recurrent: F32 or F33? Then there are choices:
  - Is the depression mild, moderate, or severe? 4th digit of 0, 1, or 2.
  - Are there psychotic features? F32.3 or F33.3
  - Is the depression in remission? F32.4 or F33.4

Example 2 [37]

Major Depressive Disorder F32, Major depressive disorder, single episode

According to the Fifth Edition of the Diagnostic and Statistical Manual of Mental Disorders (DSM-5), five or more of the symptoms listed below, which represent changes in functioning, must be present during the same two-weeknd time period. At least one symptom is either a depressed mood or loss of interest.

- Depressed mood most of the day, nearly every day, as indicated in the subjective report or in observation made by others
- Markedly diminished interest in pleasure in all, or almost all, activities most of the day and nearly every day
- Significant weight loss when not dieting or weight gain; for example, more than five percent of body weight gained or lost in a month or changes in appetite nearly every day
- Insomnia or hypersomnia nearly every day
- Psychomotor agitation or retardation nearly every day
- Fatigue or loss of energy nearly every day
- Feelings of worthlessness or excessive or inappropriate guilt
- Diminished ability to think or concentrate or indecisiveness nearly every day
- Recurrent thoughts of death

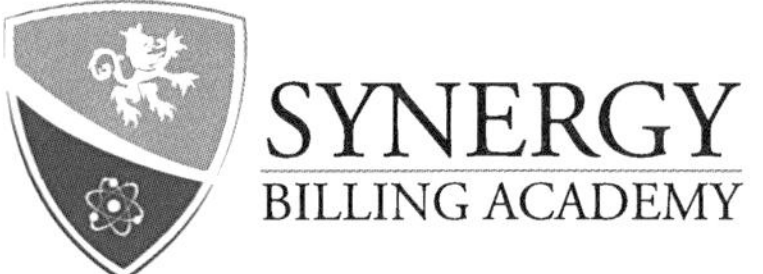

Example 3 [37]

Mild Depressive Episodes

For mild depressive episodes, two or three symptoms from the list below are usually present. The general criteria for depressive episode must be met.

At least two of the following three symptoms must be present:

- Depressed mood to a degree that is definitely abnormal to the individual, present for most of the day and almost every day, largely uninfluenced by circumstances, and sustained for at least two weeks
- Loss of interest or pleasure in activities that are normally pleasurable
- Decreased energy or increased fatigability

An additional symptom or symptoms from the following list should be present to give a total of at least four:

- Loss of confidence or self-esteem
- Unreasonable feelings of self-reproach or excessive and inappropriate guilt
- Recurrent thoughts of death or any suicidal behavior
- Complaints or evidence of diminished ability to think or concentrate, such as indecisiveness or vacillation
- Change in psychomotor activity with agitation or retardation (either subjective or objective)
- Sleep disturbance of any type
- Change in appetite (decrease or increase) with corresponding weight change

Example 4 [37]

Moderate Depressive Episodes

For moderate depressive episodes, four or more of the symptoms previously noted are usually present and the patient is likely to have great difficulty continuing with ordinary activities.

For a classification of "in remission," the patient has had two or more depressive episodes in the past but must have been free from depressive symptoms for several months. This category can still be used based on the provider's clinical determination and documentation if the patient is receiving treatment to reduce the risk of further episodes.

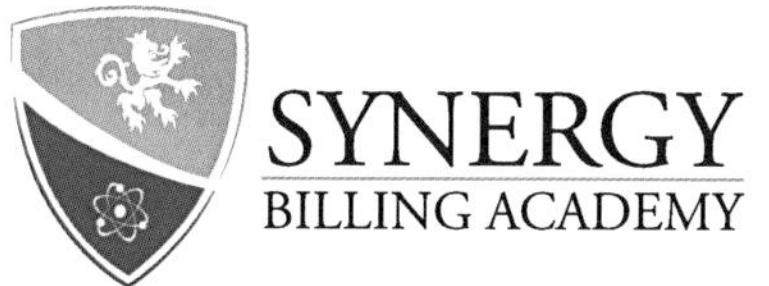

Example 5 [37]

F33, Major depressive disorder, recurrent

A recurrent depressive disorder is characterized by repeated episodes of depression without any history of independent episodes of mood elevation and increased energy or mania. There must have been at least one previous episode lasting a minimum of two weeks and separated from the current episode by at least two months. At no time in the past can there have been any hypomanic or manic episode.

Code	Description
F33.0	Major depressive disorder, recurrent, mild
F33.1	Major depressive disorder, recurrent, moderate
F33.2	Major depressive disorder, recurrent, severe without psychotic features
F33.3	Major depressive disorder, recurrent, severe with psychotic features
F33.4	Major depressive disorder, recurrent, in remission

Example 6 [37]

F33.4, Major depressive disorder, recurrent, in remission

For a classification of "in remission," the patient has had two or more depressive episodes in the past but must have been free from depressive symptoms for several months. This category can still be used based on the provider's clinical determination and documentation if the patient is receiving treatment to reduce the risk of further episodes.

Code	Description
F33.40	Major depressive disorder, recurrent, in remission, unspecified
F33.41	Major depressive disorder, recurrent, in partial remission
F33.42	Major depressive disorder, recurrent, in full remission

Notes to Remember [24]

The codes in this chapter include disorders of psychological development but exclude symptoms,

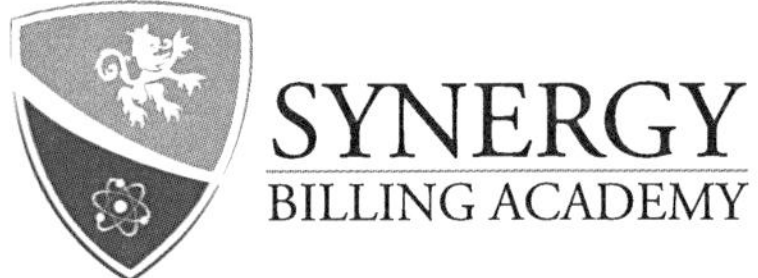

signs, and abnormal clinical laboratory findings (R00-R99). The arrangement of the codes within the various sections of ICD-10-CM is significantly different from ICD-9-CM.

A number of changes to category and subcategory titles have been made.

- Subcategory
  - In ICD-9-CM, 296.0 is bipolar 1 disorder, single manic episode.
  - In ICD-10-CM, the equivalent category is F30 for manic episode.

There are unique codes for alcohol and drug use (not specified as abuse or dependence) and abuse and dependence.

There are changes to the codes for drug and alcohol abuse and dependence, as they no longer identify continuous or episodic use. The ICD-10-CM classification system does not provide separate "history" codes for alcohol and drug abuse. These conditions are identified as "in remission" in ICD-10-CM.

A history of drug or alcohol dependence is coded as "in remission." There are combination codes for drug and alcohol use and associated conditions such as withdrawal, sleep disorders, or psychosis. There is a code for blood alcohol level (Y90.-) that can be assigned as an additional code when documentation indicates its use.

Most Used Codes by You

ICD-9-CM		ICD-10-CM	
293.81	Psychotic disorder with delusions in conditions classified elsewhere	F06.2	Psychotic disorder with delusions due to known physiological condition
293.83	Mood disorder in conditions classified elsewhere	F06.30	Mood disorder due to known physiological condition, unspecified
293.84	Anxiety disorder in conditions classified elsewhere	F06.4	Anxiety disorder due to known physiological condition
295.60	Schizophrenic disorders - residual type - unspecified	F20.5	Residual schizophrenia

Behavioral Health

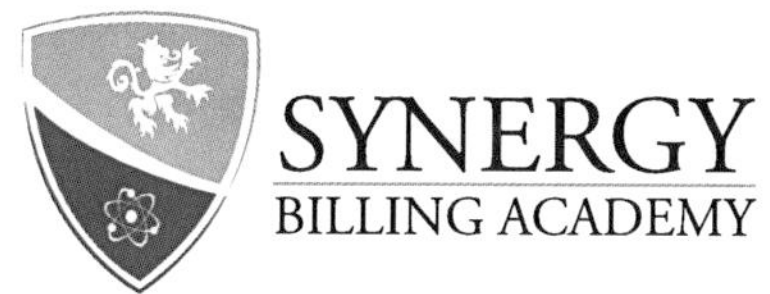

ICD-9	ICD-9 Description	ICD-10	ICD-10 Description
296.21	Majors depressive disorder, mild single episode	F32.0	Major depressive disorder, single episode, mild
296.32	Moderate recurrent major depression	F33.1	Major depressive disorder, recurrent, moderate
297.9	Unspecified paranoid state	F23	Brief psychotic disorder
300.00	Anxiety, dissociative, and somatoform disorders - anxiety state, unspecified	F41.9	Anxiety disorder, unspecified
302.70	Psychosexual dysfunction unspecified	R37	Sexual dysfunction, unspecified
302.85	Gender identity disorder in adolescents or adults	F64.1	Gender identity disorder in adolescence and adulthood
304.90	Unspecified drug dependence – unspecified	F19.20	Other psychoactive substance dependence, uncomplicated
305.1	Nondependent tobacco use disorder	F17.200	Nicotine dependence, unspecified, uncomplicated
311	Depressive disorder, not elsewhere classified	F32.9	Major depressive disorder, single episode, unspecified
314.00	Attention Deficit Disorder / ADHD unspecified	F90.9	Attention-deficit hyperactivity disorder, unspecified type
314.01	ADHD of childhood with hyperactivity	F90.0	Attention-deficit hyperactivity disorder, predominantly inattentive type
		F90.1	Attention-deficit hyperactivity disorder, predominantly hyperactive type
		F90.2	Attention-deficit hyperactivity disorder, combined type
		F90.9	Attention-deficit hyperactivity disorder, unspecified type

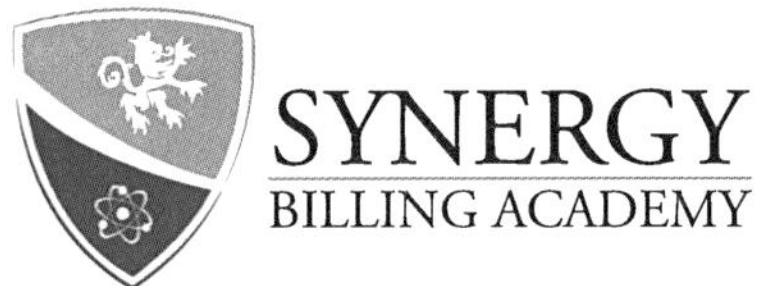

Check Your Understanding

True and False

1. Mental health and behavioral health providers use ICD-10-CM to indicate the procedures they provided for their patients.

    a. True
    b. False

2. ICD-9-CM is currently used to classify diseases.

    a. True
    b. False

3. Chapter 5 is the chapter mental and behavioral health providers will be using to document their patients' diagnoses.

    a. True
    b. False

4. Z Codes are what we knew as V Codes.

    a. True
    b. False

5. The codes we will now use start with the letter "F".

    a. True
    b. False

6. Medical claims are often rejected due to lack of documentation.

    a. True
    b. False

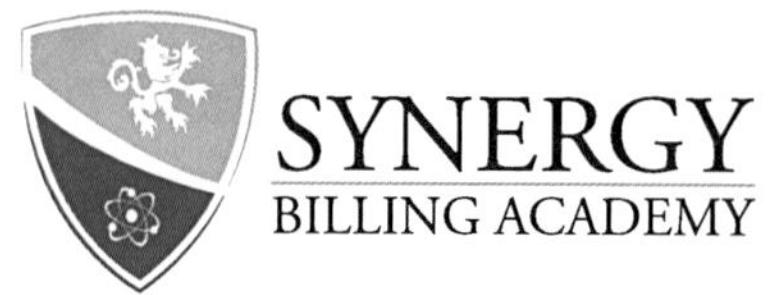

7. Complete and accurate medical records are needed to ensure proper treatment of patients.

   a. True
   b. False

8. Clinical documentation is where ICD-10-CM starts.

   a. True
   b. False

9. We now have unique codes for alcohol and drug use, abuse, and dependence.

   a. True
   b. False

10. The code for blood alcohol level is "X90."

    a. True
    b. False

ICD-10-CM International Classification of Diseases 10th Revision Clinical Modification

Dental

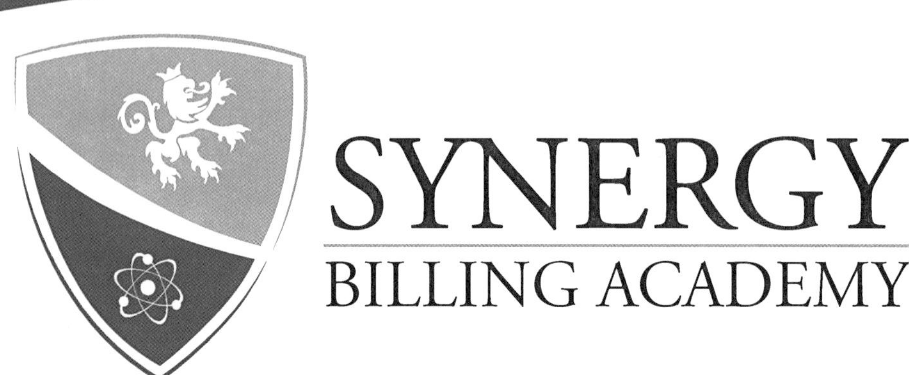

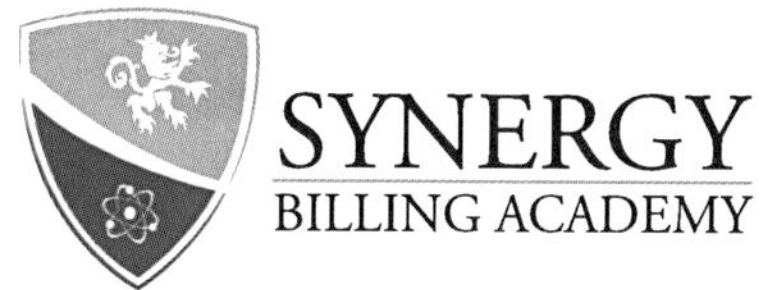

Dental Background and Practice

Dentists diagnose and treat problems with teeth, gums, and tissues in the mouth, along with giving advice and instruction on taking care of teeth and gums and administering care to help prevent future problems of patients' oral health. They provide instruction on diet, brushing, flossing, the use of fluorides, and other aspects of dental care. They remove tooth decay, fill cavities, examine X-rays, place protective plastic sealants on children's teeth, straighten teeth, and repair fractured teeth. They also perform corrective surgery on gums and supporting bones to treat gum diseases. Dentists extract teeth and make models and measurements for dentures to replace missing teeth. They also administer anesthetics and write prescriptions for antibiotics and other medications. [38, 39]

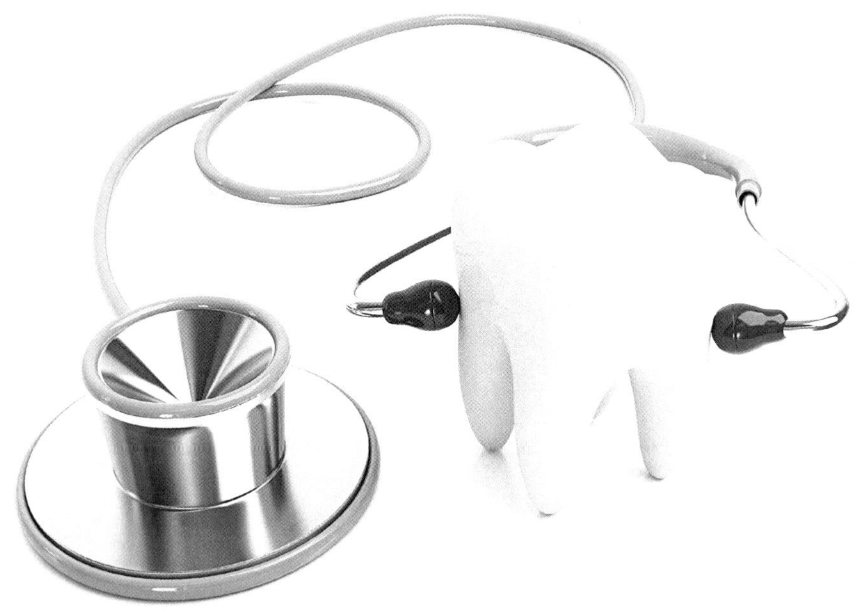

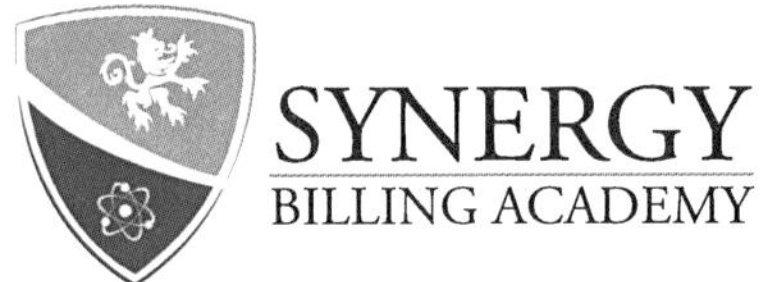

Dental Claims and Coding Manuals

On August 17, 2000, the Current Dental Terminology (CDT) was named as a HIPAA standard code set. All dental claims submitted must use a dental procedure code from the most up-to-date version based on the date of service. [40]

In 2003, it was mandated that all HIPAA-covered entities use diagnostic codes. In other words, even dentists are required to use ICD-9-CM to report a patient's diagnosis and the reason for his or her visit.

On October 1, 2015, the ICD-10-CM will be released, marking the replacement of ICD-9-CM. All dental providers have been using ICD-9-CM to add the diagnosis or reason for visit to their patients' claims for the past three decades. The change is due to the fact that ICD-9-CM codes do not have sufficient coverage, resulting in a lack of specificity for oral and dental diagnoses.

Please keep in mind that ICD-10-CM will not have any effects on Current Procedural Terminology (CPT) codes or CDT codes. CPT and CDT are used to indicate procedures and ICD-10-CM is used to indicate diagnoses.

In dentistry diagnosis coding, ICD-9-CM codes appear in code range 500 and V Codes may also be used; however, in ICD-10-CM, we would use code range K00 and Z Codes.

ICD-9-CM Code Structure

ICD-9-CM codes have anywhere from 3 to 5 characters. The number of characters in the code will specify what type of code it is and tell you if it is a category code, a subcategory code, or a subclassification code. [4, 10]

ICD-9-CM Category Codes

A three-digit category is a code that represents a single condition or disease. There are approximately 100 codes at the category level; most others require a fourth or fifth digit (subcategory and/or subclassication). [4]

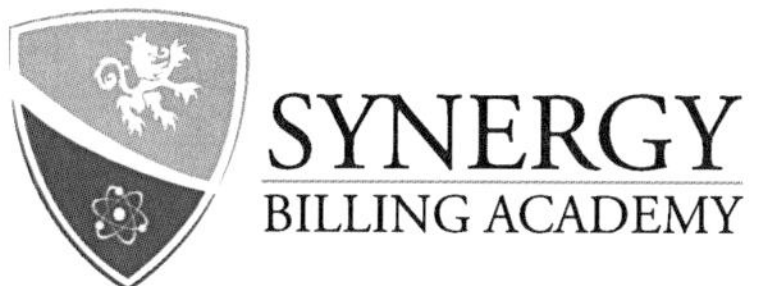

Example:

ICD-9-CM Dental Category Codes	
520	Disorders of tooth development and eruption
521	Diseases of hard tissues of teeth
522	Diseases of pulp and periapical tissues
523	Gingival and periodontal diseases
524	Dentofacial anomalies, including malocclusion
525	Other diseases and conditions of the teeth and supporting structures
526	Diseases of the jaws
527	Diseases of the salivary glands
528	Diseases of the oral soft tissues excluding lesions specific for gingiva and tongue
529	Diseases and other conditions of the tongue

ICD-9-CM Subcategory Codes

A four-digit subcategory code provides more information or specificity than the three-digit code in terms of cause, site, or manifestation of the condition. [4]

Example:

520 Disorders of Tooth Development and Eruption	
520.0	Anodontia
520.1	Supernumerary teeth
520.2	Abnormalities of size and form of teeth
520.3	Mottled teeth
520.4	Disturbances of tooth formation
520.5	Hereditary disturbances in tooth structure, not elsewhere classified
520.6	Disturbances in tooth eruption
520.7	Teething syndrome
520.8	Other specified disorders of tooth development and eruption
520.9	Unspecified disorder of tooth development and eruption

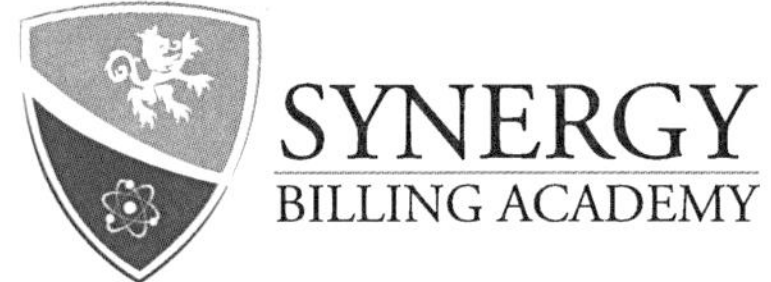

ICD-9-CM Subclassification Codes

A five-digit subclassification code adds even more information and specificity to a condition's description. You must assign the fifth digit if it is available. [4]

Example:

521 Diseases of Hard Tissues of Teeth	
521.00	Dental caries, unspecified
521.01	Dental caries limited to enamel
521.02	Dental caries extending into dentine
521.03	Dental caries extending into pulp
521.04	Arrested dental caries

ICD-10-CM Chapter 11 - Diseases of the Digestive system (K00–K95)

Transitioning to ICD-10-CM will completely change the codes used by dentists. Before, the code range was found in Chapter 9 and in the 500 range; now, in ICD-10-CM, all of our codes start with a letter designation. The section pertaining to dentists is section K00–K14. Each and every one of these codes and their descriptions will be more specific to the patient's condition. Below is the breakdown of all the sections in Chapter 11.

Code	Description
K00 - K14	***Diseases or oral cavity and salivary glands***
K20 - K31	Diseases of esophagus, stomach, and duodenum
K35 - K38	Diseases of appendix
K40 - K46	Hernia
K50 - K52	Non-infective enteritis
K55 - K64	Other diseases of intestines
K65 - K68	Diseases of peritoneum and retroperitoneum
K70 - K77	Diseases of liver
K80 - K87	Disorders of gallbladder, biliary tract, and pancreas
K90 - K95	Other diseases of digestive system

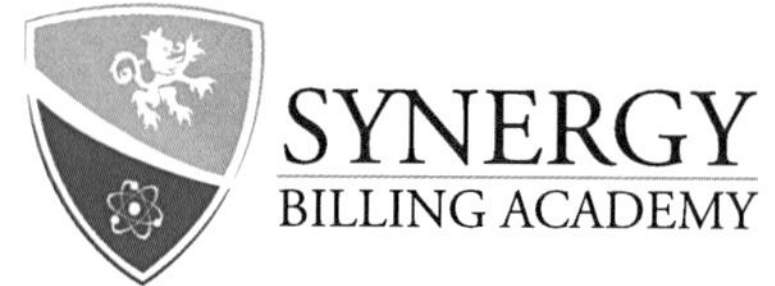

Example:

- Dental Caries, unspecified - K02.9
  - Localized destruction of calcified tissue initiated on the tooth surface by decalcification of the enamel of the teeth, followed by enzymatic lysis of organic structures, leading to cavity formation that, if left untreated, penetrates the enamel and dentin and may reach the pulp.
  - The decay of a tooth, in which it becomes softened, discolored, and/or porous.

ICD-10-CM Diseases and Disorders [24]

Some of the disease categories in this chapter have been restructured to bring together groups that are in some way related. It contains two new sections; in some cases, headings of subcategories have been changed.

Instructional notes indicating that an additional code should be assigned for associated conditions and external causes or that an underlying condition should be coded first have been expanded.

A number of new subchapters have been added to the chapter for diseases of the digestive system so that these conditions are grouped with other diseases of the digestive system. Some terminology changes and revisions to the classification of specific digestive conditions have also been made.

Guidelines [9]

Professionals must be aware of different modifications and guidelines presented in the new chapters of ICD-10-CM. ICD-10-CM requires preparation and practice due to its increased specificity. Most of the ICD-9-CM dental coding throughout Chapter 9 is directly crosswalked to an ICD-10-CM code with the exception of a few points.

Guideline modifications were made to specific codes in this chapter. No instructional notes are found at the start of the subchapter in ICD-9-CM; however, this is not the case in ICD-10-CM. At this time, there are no chapter-specific guidelines related to Chapter 11, Diseases of the Digestive System, but space has been left for future revisions.

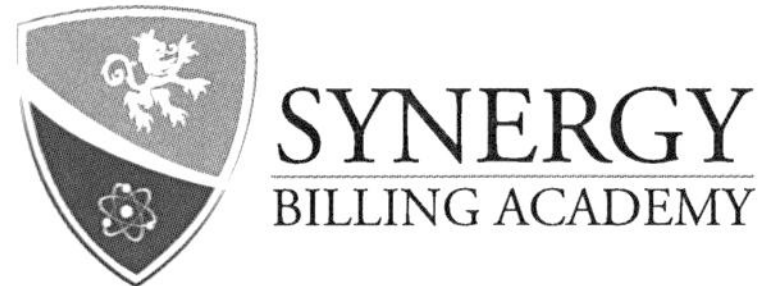

Example: [41]

- Category 521 (Dental caries): ICD-10-CM coding requires the more specific mention of whether the caries is limited to the enamel, dentin, or pulp.
- Category 525 (Edentulous - toothless): ICD-10-CM coding requires the more specific mention of the patient's class of edetulism.

Chapter 21 - Factors Influencing Health Status and Contact with Health Services

In ICD-9-CM, V Codes or health status codes are used for factors influencing health status and contact with health services. V Codes are mostly used to help explain medical history factors that influence treatment, such as diabetes or a history of stroke, amongst others. For counseling purposes, we might need to use V Codes depending on the payer.

ICD-9-CM to ICD-10-CM [24]

Professionals will find the listing of codes for factors influencing health status and contact with health services a little different in ICD-10-CM than what is currently found in ICD-9-CM. What were previously V Codes are now Z Codes. [24]

ICD-10-CM Chapter Category (Z Codes) [24]

These codes are used when a person who may or may not be sick encounters health services for some specific purpose, such as to receive limited care or service for a current condition, or to discuss a problem which is in itself not a disease or injury.

Within in the Z Codes, some category titles have been rephrased to better reflect the situations the codes classify. Several codes have been expanded, such as personal and family history. Codes have been added for concepts that do not exist in ICD-9-CM, and now we have instructional notes for different categories to explain how codes should be assigned. Below is a breakdown of all the sections in Chapter 21.

The sections pertaining to dentistry are:

- Z00 - Z13
- Z40 - Z53
- Z69 - Z96

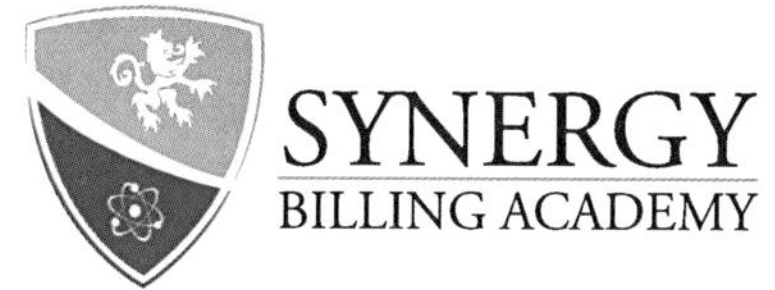

Code	Description
Z00 - Z13	***Persons encountering health services for examinations***
Z14 - Z15	Genetic carrier and genetic susceptibility to disease
Z16	Resistance to antimicrobial drugs
Z17	Estrogen receptor status
Z18	Retained foreign body fragment
Z20 - Z28	Persons with potential health hazards related to communicable diseases
Z30 - Z39	Persons encountering health services in circumstances related to reproduction
Z40 - Z53	***Encounters for other specific health care***
Z55 - Z65	Persons with potential health hazards related to socioeconomic and psychosocial circumstances
Z66	Do not resuscitate status
Z67	Blood type
Z68	Body mass index (BMI)
Z69 - Z76	***Persons encountering health services in other circumstances***
Z77 - Z99	Persons with potential health hazards related to family and personal history and certain conditions influencing health status

Chapter 21 Guidelines [9]

The chapter-specific guidelines provide additional information about the use of Z Codes for specified encounters.

Z Codes are for use in any health care setting. Z Codes may be used as either a first-listed (principal diagnosis code in the inpatient setting) or secondary code, depending on the circumstances of the encounter. Certain Z Codes may only be used as first-listed or principal diagnosis.

Z Codes are not procedure codes. A corresponding procedure code must accompany a Z Code to describe any procedure performed.

Dental Health

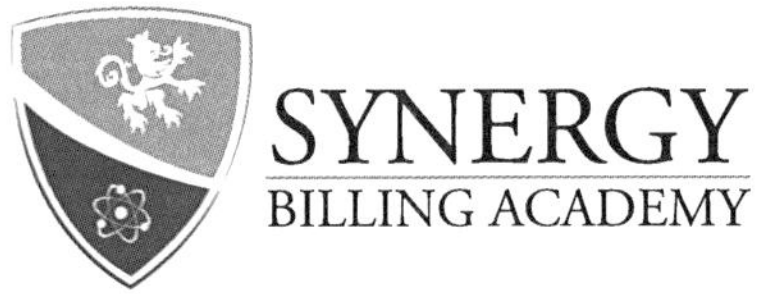

The NCHS has published the following guidelines:

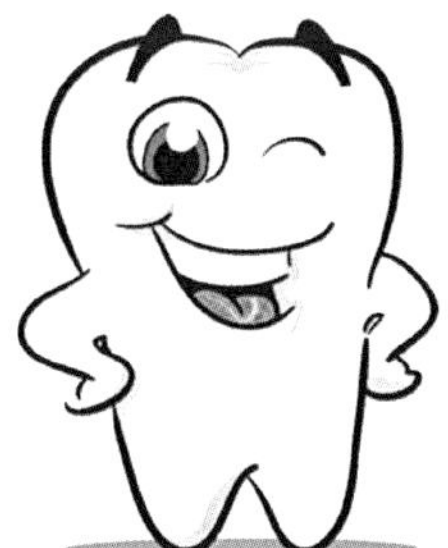

- ***Use of Z Codes in any Health Care Setting***
- ***Z Codes Indicate a Reason for an Encounter***
- Categories of Z Codes
  - Contact/Exposure
  - Inoculations and vaccinations
  - Status
  - History (of)
  - Screening
  - Observation
  - Aftercare
  - Follow-up
  - Donor
  - Counseling
  - Encounters for obstetrical and reproductive services
  - Newborns and infants
  - ***Routine and administrative examinations***
  - Miscellaneous Z Codes
    - Prophylactic organ removal
  - Nonspecific Z Codes
  - ***Z Codes that may only be principal/first-listed diagnosis***

Routine and administrative examinations

The Z Codes allow for the description of encounters for routine examinations, such as a general check-up, or examinations for administrative purposes, such as a pre-employment physical. The codes are not to be used if the examination is for diagnosis of a suspected condition or for treatment purposes. In such cases, the diagnosis code is used. Should a disease or condition be discovered during a routine exam and listed with a diagnosis, it should be coded as an additional code. Pre-existing and chronic conditions and history codes may also be included as additional codes as long as the examination is for administrative purposes and not focused on any particular condition.

Pre-operative examination and pre-procedural laboratory examination Z Codes are for use only in those situations when a patient is being cleared for a procedure or surgery and no treatment is given.

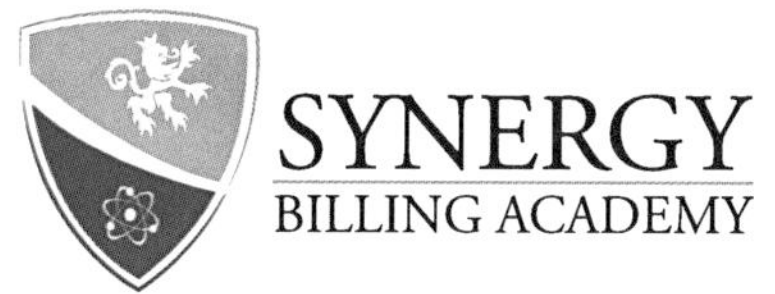

The Z Codes/Categories for Routine and Administrative Examinations	
Z00	Encounter for general examination without complaint, suspected or reported diagnosis
Z01	Encounter for other special examination without complaint, suspected or reported diagnosis
Z02	Encounter for administrative examination Except: Z02.9, Encounter for administrative examinations, unspecified

Z Codes that may only be principal/first-listed diagnosis

Code	Description
Z00	Encounter for general examination without complaint, suspected or reported diagnosis
Z01	***Encounter for other special examination without complaint, suspected or reported diagnosis***
Z02	Encounter for administrative examination
Z03	Encounter for medical observation for suspected diseases and conditions ruled out
Z04	Encounter for examination and observation for other reasons

Word of Caution [12, 26]

In order to support the depth of ICD-10-CM, physician clinical documentation must, for example, contain details regarding:

- Laterality
- Stages of healing, e.g., routine, delayed, or malunion
- Trimester of pregnancy
- Episode of care, e.g., initial or subsequent encounter, sequela
- Depth, size, and cause of injuries
- Combination codes must reflect the association between conditions
- New clinical concepts such as underdosing

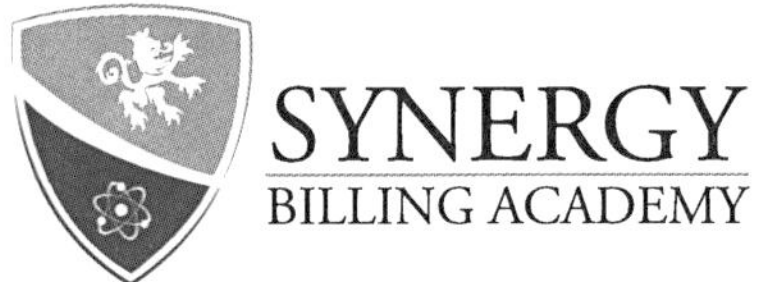

Helpful Tips

- Be specific in describing the patient's condition, illness, or disease.
- Distinguish between acute and chronic conditions, when appropriate.
- Identify the acute condition of an emergency situation.
  - Coma, loss of consciousness, hemorrhage, etc.
- Identify chronic complaints or secondary diagnoses.
- Identify how injuries occur.
- Be as granular as possible.
  - Acute, chronic, acute on chronic, recurrent
  - Mild, moderate, severe
  - Site or location
  - Laterality
    - Left, right, bilateral
      - Injury details
      - External cause, activity, place of occurrence

Documentation Requirements [41]

Example 1: [41]

Each of the characters in a code is more than just a letter or number; they all mean something. The codes help tell the complete story of why the patients were there. The documentation details are the basis of the codes. The documentation and the codes have to correlate. Incomplete medical records will result in incomplete codes.

Detail	Code	Description
What	K02	Dental caries
Where	K02.5	Dental caries on pit and fissure surface
Extent	K02.51	Dental caries on pit and fissure surface limited to enamel

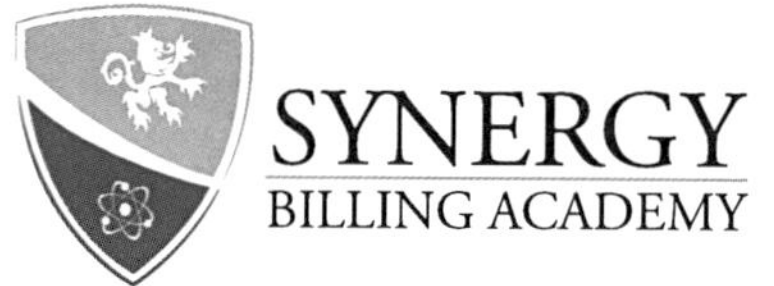

Example 2: [41]

If the patient is diabetic and is eligible for an additional prophylaxis per year, the claim may include:

- Procedure code D1110 – prophylaxis – adult
- ICD-9-CM diagnostic code – 250.0 Diabetes mellitus
- Once the ICD-10-CM codes are implemented, we would instead have to use E08.630, Diabetes due to underlying condition with periodontal disease

People who have diabetes know the disease can harm the eyes, nerves, kidneys, heart, and other important systems in the body, but patients usually do not realize that diabetes can also cause problems in their mouth. [42]

People with diabetes are at special risk for periodontal (gum) disease, an infection of the gum and bone that hold the teeth in place. Periodontal disease can lead to painful chewing difficulties and even tooth loss. Dry mouth, often a symptom of undetected diabetes, can cause soreness, ulcers, infections, and tooth decay. Smoking makes these problems worse. [42]

This is only one of the many medical conditions that can affect oral care and treatment. Others include syncope, cardiovascular disease, rheumatic heart disease, congenital health defects, coronary artery disease (CAD), myocardial infarction (MI), hypertension, heart failure, kidney disease, seizure disorder, asthma, chronic obstructive pulmonary disease (COPD); infectious diseases such as hepatitis, tuberculosis, and HIV/AIDS; blood diseases such as anemia, leukemia, and hemorrhagic disorders; and allergies such as latex allergies and drug allergies. [43]

Example 3: [41]

The following chart is an example of a patient who has dental caries. The ICD-9-CM coding of dental caries is much less specific, with just one code to describe the diagnosis. When referencing the Alphabetic Index in ICD-10-CM, a simple note of "dental caries" in the patient's chart will not be enough to select the proper diagnosis code. The example below demonstrates how ICD-10-CM forces the doctor to use much more specificity and detail within the patient's record to allow for coding the proper ICD-10-CM code.

Dental Health

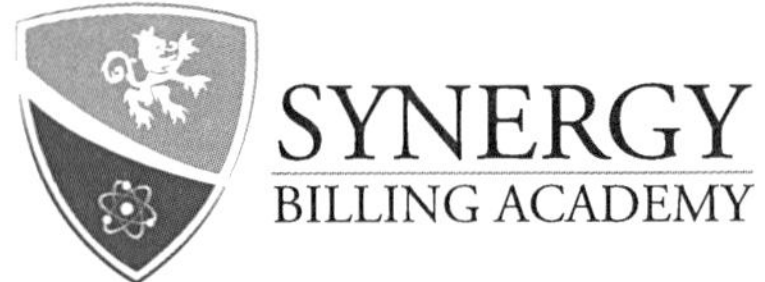

ICD-9-CM		ICD-10-CM	
521.06	Dental caries and fissure	K02.51	Dental caries on pit and fissure surface limited to enamel
		K02.52	Dental caries on pit and fissure surface penetrating into dentin
		K02.53	Dental caries on pit and fissure surface penetrating into pulp

Example 4: [41]

Many of the ICD-10-CM categories have added a note for a necessary additional code to further specify the diagnosis.

K05 (523.00) Gingivitis and periodontal diseases

- Use additional code to identify:
  - Alcohol abuse and dependence (F10-)
  - Exposure to environmental tobacco smoke (Z77.22)
  - Exposure to tobacco smoke in the prenatal period (P96.81)
  - History of tobacco use (Z87.891)
  - Occupational exposure to environmental tobacco smoke (Z57.31)
  - Tobacco dependence (F17-)
  - Tobacco use (Z72.0)

Notes to Remember [44]

Practitioners may make individual or customized plans based on the patient's health conditions. These plans are on the rise, making the selection of the appropriate codes for reimbursement a little difficult.

Many dental payers offer increased benefits for services associated with certain systemic conditions.

Some dental plans may cover specific dental procedures that may minimize the risks associated with the connection between the patient's oral and systemic health conditions. Not all plans may cover additional benefits for these conditions.

Dental Health

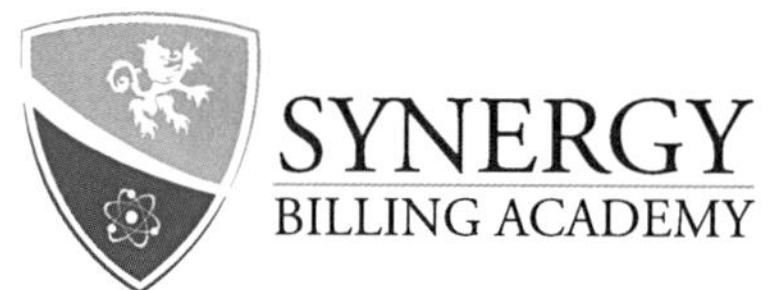

Sometimes patients are seen when they are not necessarily ill. When a patient receives preventative services such as screenings or cleanings, or to indicate history, V Codes are used. These are changing to Z Codes with ICD-10-CM.

It is important to review the guidelines and notes in each category when coding and reporting. Improved documentation is important for both reimbursement and patient care. Medical claims are often rejected and/or down-coded due to lack of documentation from providers to support the diagnosis code reported. Moreover, complete and accurate medical records are needed to ensure proper treatment of patients.

Most Used Codes

ICD-9-CM		ICD-10-CM	
520.0	Anodontia	K00.0	Anodontia
520.1	Supernumerary teeth	K00.1	Supernumerary teeth
520.2	Abnormalities of size and form of teeth	K00.2	Abnormalities of size and form of teeth
520.3	Mottled teeth	K00.3	Mottled teeth
520.4	Disturbances of tooth formation	K00.4	Disturbances of tooth formation
520.5	Hereditary disturbances in tooth structure, not elsewhere classified	K00.5	Hereditary disturbances in tooth structure, not elsewhere classified
520.6	Disturbances in tooth eruption	K00.6 K01.0 K01.1	Disturbances in tooth eruption Embedded teeth Impacted teeth
520.7	Teething syndrome	K00.7	Teething syndrome
520.8	Other specified disorders of tooth development and eruption	K00.8	Other disorders of tooth development
520.9	Unspecified disorder of tooth development and eruption	K00.9	Disorders of tooth development, unspecified
521.00	Dental caries, unspecified	K02.9	Dental caries, unspecified
521.01	Dental caries, limited enamel	K02.61	Dental caries on smooth surface limited to enamel
521.02	Dental caries extending into dentine	K02.62	Dental caries on smooth surface penetrating into dentin

Dental Health

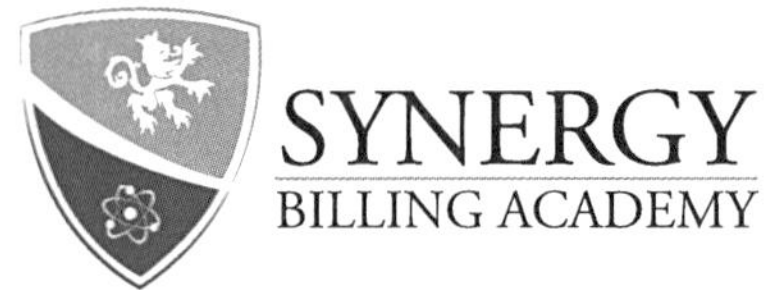

ICD-9	Description	ICD-10	Description
521.03	Dental caries extending into pulp	K02.63	Dental caries on smooth surface penetrating into pulp
521.04	Arrested dental caries	K02.3	Arrested dental caries
525.9	Dental disorder NOS	K08.9	Disorder of teeth and supporting structures, unspecified
V72.2	Dental examination	Z01.20	Encounter for dental examination and cleaning without abnormal findings
		Z01.21	Encounter for dental examination and cleaning with abnormal findings

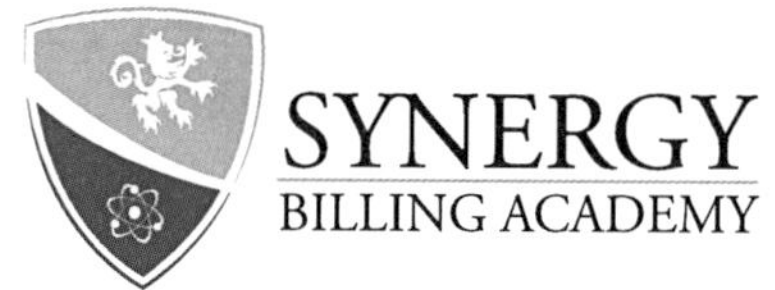

Check Your Understanding

True and False

1. ICD-10-CM is replacing the CDT.

   a. True
   b. False

2. ICD-10-CM codes are less descriptive than ICD-9-CM codes.

   a. True
   b. False

3. Diseases of oral cavity and salivary glands start with the letter "T."

   a. True
   b. False

4. Dental codes will be found in the chapter for diseases of the digestive system.

   a. True
   b. False

5. Z Codes are what we have known as V Codes.

   a. True
   b. False

6. Dentists do not need to use codes from the chapter on factors influencing health status and contact with health services.

   a. True
   b. False

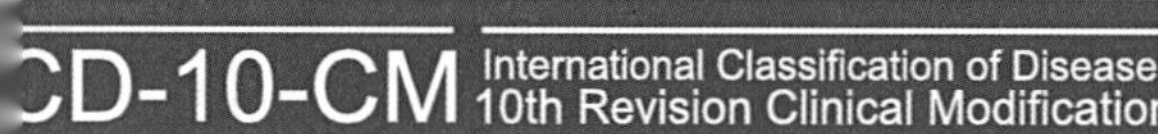

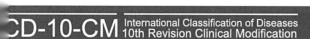

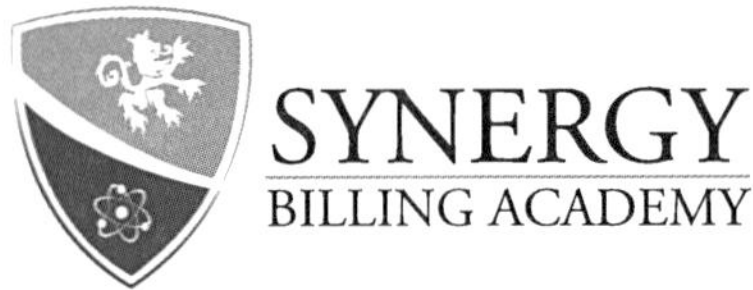

7. Medical claims are often rejected due to lack of documentation.

   a. True
   b. False

8. Complete and accurate medical records are needed to ensure proper treatment of patients.

   a. True
   b. False

9. If a diabetic patient comes in for a cleaning, we need to include a diabetes diagnosis on the patient's record.

   a. True
   b. False

10. Clinical documentation is where ICD-10-CM starts.

   a. True
   b. False

ICD-10-CM International Classification of Diseases 10th Revision Clinical Modification

Documentation Examples

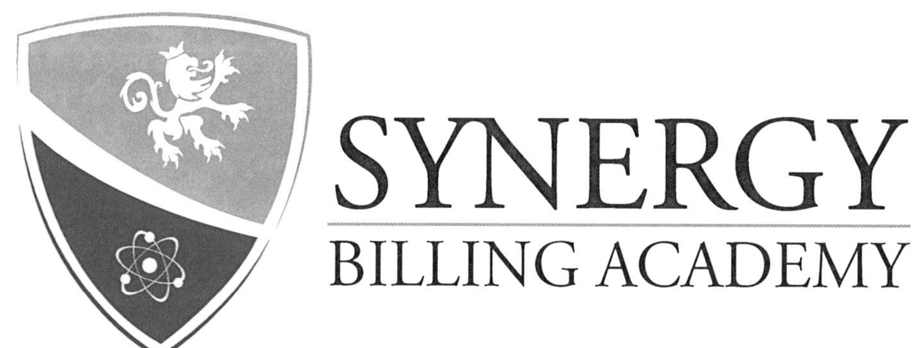

What Needs to be Documented in ICD-10-CM? [12, 26]

In order to support the depth of ICD-10-CM, physician clinical documentation must, for example, contain details regarding:

- Laterality
- Stages of healing, e.g., routine, delayed, or malunion
- Trimester of pregnancy
- Episode of care, e.g., initial or subsequent encounter, sequela
- Depth, size, and cause of injuries
- Combination codes must reflect the association between conditions
- New clinical concepts such as underdosing

Helpful Tips

- Be specific in describing the patient's condition, illness, or disease.
- Distinguish between acute and chronic conditions, when appropriate.
- Identify the acute condition of an emergency situation.
    - Coma, loss of consciousness, hemorrhage, etc.
- Identify chronic complaints or secondary diagnoses.
- Identify how injuries occur.
- Be as granular as possible.
    - Acute, chronic, acute on chronic, recurrent
    - Mild, moderate, severe
    - Site or location
    - Laterality
        - Left, right, bilateral
            - Injury details
            - External cause, activity, place of occurrence

Precision, Accuracy, and Detail

Bruxism [36]

- 27-year-old male college student is sent to the neurologist for evaluation of his sleep disorder. The patient was sent by his dentist, as he noted the ridges of his teeth had shown some wear that indicated the need for a bite guard. The physician examines

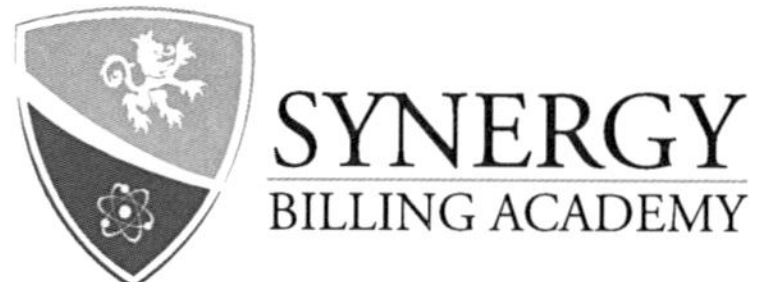

the patient and agrees with the dentist that the patient has sleep-related bruxism.

- Diagnosis code: G47.63, Sleep-related bruxism

Cholesteatoma [36]

- 40-year-old man presents to the clinic for a problem with his left ear. He states that he was trying to clean his ears but it feels like he has something growing on his left ear and it is painful. The physician examines the patient and after the exam indicates that the patient has a cholesteatoma of the left ear.
  - Diagnosis code: H60.42, Cholesteatoma of left external ear

Congenital Malformation [36]

- 5-year-old boy presents to the ENT clinic for evaluation of a deformity of his left nostril. He has had this since birth and has seen several physicians for consultation to determine what it is. He is examined by the specialist and the medical record indicates the patient has a congenital malformation of the nose unspecified. He is being referred to a children's hospital to see a world-renowned plastic surgeon.
  - Diagnosis code: Q30.9, Congenital malformation of nose, unspecified

Depression [36]

- At a minimum, you need to identify if it is a single episode or recurrent: F32 or F33? Then there are choices:
  - Is the depression mild, moderate, or severe? 4th digit of 0, 1, or 2.
  - Are there psychotic features? F32.3 or F33.3
  - Is the depression in remission?

Diabetes [36]

- 25-year-old female is seen at the diabetic clinic for evaluation of her type 1 diabetes. She is doing well, watches her diet, and exercises four days a week. She always carries snacks with her and is very aware of when her blood sugar level is low. She will return to the clinic in six months or sooner if she has any questions or concerns.

- Diagnosis code: E10.9, Type 1 diabetes mellitus without complications

- Patient presents with an ulcer on the right toe, suffers from type 2 diabetes, and has used insulin for a long time.

  - Diagnosis codes: E11.621, L97.511, Z79.4

Diabetes with CKD (Chronic Kidney Disease) [36]

- 66-year-old man presents to his physician's office for a follow-up visit for his diabetes and CKD. He has been measuring his blood sugar more consistently than in the past and states that he is "really trying." He also states that it is really hard being married to such a good baker, as he just can't leave some of those treats alone! The physician indicates that the patient has type 1 DM with diabetic CKD stage three.

  - Diagnosis codes: E10.22, Type 1 diabetes mellitus with diabetic chronic kidney disease, stage 3 (moderate); N18.3 ,Chronic kidney disease, stage 3 (moderate)

End-Stage Renal Disease [36]

- 65-year-old man with a history of kidney disease over the past couple of years has now progressed to end-stage renal disease and will be admitted in the next day or two for a procedure to insert a Hickman catheter for renal dialysis.

  - Diagnosis code: N18.6, End-stage renal disease

Fainting [36]

- 6-year-old female presents to physician's office for evaluation after fainting this morning at her home. After the study, the physician determines that there is no physiological reason for her fainting.

  - Diagnosis code: R55, Syncope and collapse

Documentation Examples

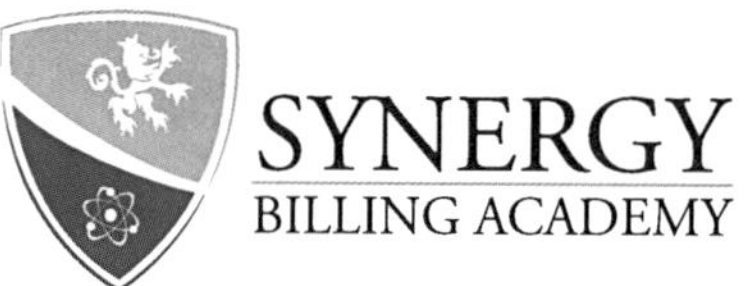

Fracture [36]

- Female with osteoporosis and pathological humerus fracture
  - ICD-9-CM: 733.01 & 733.11
  - ICD-10-CM:
    - M80.0221A, D, G, K, P, or S
    - M80.0222A, D, G, K, P, or S
  - Which side, right or left? Right = M80.021; Left = M80.22
  - What type of encounter? Initial, subsequent, or sequela?
  - What type of healing? Routine, delayed, nonunion, malunion?

Glaucoma [36]

- 58-year-old female presents to the ophthalmology clinic for evaluation of her vision. Her primary care provider referred her after she complained of having visual problems over the past few months. After careful evaluation, the ophthalmologist indicates that the patient has open-angle glaucoma.

  - Diagnosis code: H40.100, Unspecified open-angle glaucoma, stage unspecified

Headache [36]

- 46-year-old female presents to the clinic for evaluation of her headaches. She states that she gets these headaches frequently and really cannot pinpoint any specific event that brings them on. The physician examines the patient and determines that she has chronic intractable tension-type headaches.

  - Diagnosis code: G44.221, Chronic tension-type headache, intractable

Hypertension [36]

- 56-year-old male presents for follow-up for his hypertension. He has been checking his B/P at the local supermarket but thinks that he is not getting correct readings. His B/P log shows his pressures to be running between 160/90–130/60. His B/P is taken in the office and is 184/102; after 10 minutes the reading is repeated and is 180/98. The physician has decided to increase his medication and asks that he buy a B/P cuff so that he can get more accurate readings.

  - Diagnosis code: I10, Essential (primary) hypertension

Note: Even though the patient has uncontrolled B/P, it is still coded the same way.

Malignant Neoplasm [36]

- 66-year-old female with a history of severe stomach problems over the past two years presents today after studies were conducted to determine the reason for her pain. She has seen another physician who indicated that she had cancer and she wanted a second opinion. The physician indicates that the patient has cancer of the body of the stomach.
  - Diagnosis code: C16.2, Malignant neoplasm of body of stomach

Otitis Externa [36]

- 34-year-old male hairdresser presents today after trying a new dye product on his hair; after several hours, his ears became red and inflamed and are becoming progressively more painful. He has no history of any previous allergies and is otherwise healthy. After examination by the ER physician, the medical record indicates that he has bilateral acute chemical otitis externa.
  - Diagnosis code: H60.523, Acute chemical otitis externa, bilateral

Preventive Visits [36]

- 2-year-old female comes in for her 24-month check-up. She is doing well and has no complaints. She is eating well, and she continues growing in the 75% range. She will have her normal immunizations and return as needed until her next scheduled preventive service.
  - Diagnosis code: Z00.129, Encounter for routine child health examination without abnormal findings
- 10-year-old male wants to participate in sports at school but requires a physical and approval of participation. The physician does a physical as outlined on the forms that are necessary for participation and signs off with approval. The medical record indicates an examination for sports participation. Patient is scheduled for his routine preventive visit in three months.
  - Diagnosis code: Z02.5 Encounter for examination for participation in sport

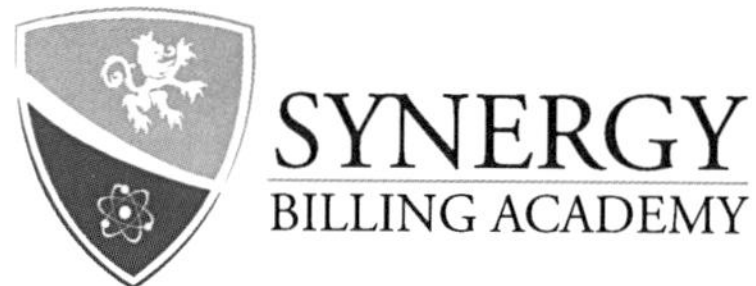

- 35-year-old male presents to the primary care provider for preoperative physical for an upcoming lung surgery. The physician indicates that the patient is doing well and has no complications or comorbidities that would limit him from having the procedure. The medical record indicates a preventive preoperative physical was performed.
  - Diagnosis code: Z01.811, Encounter for pre-procedural respiratory examination

Strep Throat [36]

- 33-year-old man presents to the physician's office with a complaint of severe sore throat. He was leaving the house to go to work this morning and went to kiss his wife. She told him he had "strep breath." His son was just diagnosed with strep throat two days ago. Physician examines the patient and does a rapid strep test which is positive.
  - Diagnosis code: J02.0, Streptococcal pharyngitis

Swimmer's Ear [36]

- 25-year-old female presents to the clinic after having pain in her right ear. She is part of the Dolphin swim team and has been practicing hard for the upcoming championships. The physician examines the patient and determines that the patient has swimmer's ear.
  - Diagnosis code: H60.331, Swimmer's ear, right ear

Easy Examples [30]

- Essential primary hypertension (401.1), I10
- Acute nasopharyngitis (460), J00
- Cough (786.2), R05
- Heartburn (787.1), R12
- Unspecified lump in breast (611.72), N63
- Laceration of scalp, initial encounter, S01.01xA
- Supervision of young primigravida, first trimester, O09.611
- Generalized abdominal tenderness, R10.817
- Adverse effect of penicillin, subsequent encounter, T36.0x5D
- Hypothermia, initial encounter,T36.xxxA

Documentation Examples

SYNERGY
BILLING ACADEMY

Pre-Procedural Consultations [30]

- Encounter for pre-op cardiovascular exam, Z01.810
- Encounter for pre-op respiratory exam, Z01.811
- Encounter for pre-op lab (blood/urine) exam, Z01.812
- Encounter for other pre-op exam, Z01.818

Routine Pediatric Encounters [30]

- Healthy, newborn exam, < 8 days old, Z00.110
- Healthy, newborn exam, 8–28 days old, Z00.111
- Routine child health exam with abnormality, Z00.121
- Routine child health exam without abnormality, Z00.129

Routine GYN Encounters [30]

- General, routine, GYN exam with abnormality, Z01.411
- General, routine, GYN exam without abnormality, Z01.419
- Supervision normal 1st pregnancy, 1st trimester, Z34.01
- Supervision normal 1st pregnancy, 2nd trimester, Z34.02
- Supervision normal 1st pregnancy, 3rd trimester, Z34.03

ICD-10-CM International Classification of Diseases 10th Revision Clinical Modification

Guideline Examples

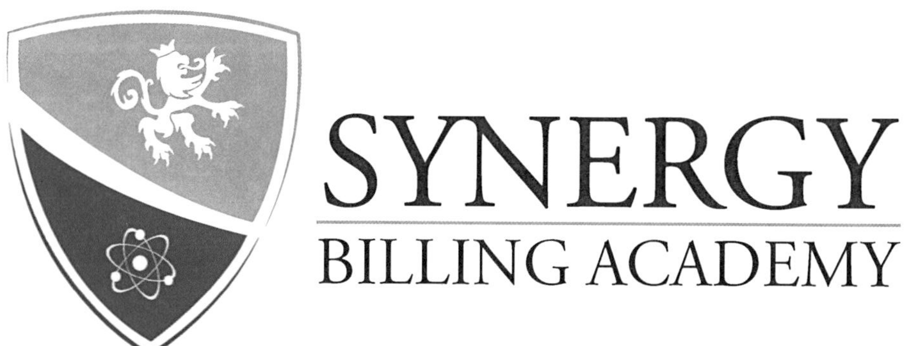

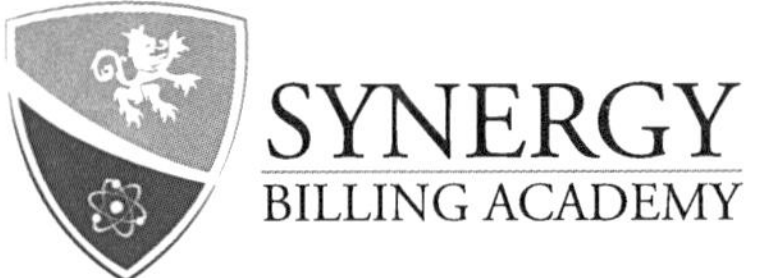

Bronchitis Guideline [9, 10, 31]

To code bronchitis to the correct level of specificity, the documentation should indicate whether the condition is acute or chronic and any associated conditions such as asthma, COPD, emphysema, and whether this is an exacerbation of the condition. The guidance also states to use additional code(s) to identify: exposure to environmental tobacco smoke, exposure to tobacco smoke in the perinatal period, history of tobacco use, occupational exposure to environmental tobacco smoke, tobacco dependence, or tobacco use.

Code: J40 Bronchitis, not specified as acute or chronic

Otitis Media Guideline [9, 10, 31]

Otitis media is classified as either nonsuppurative or suppurative in ICD-10-CM and the documentation should also include whether the condition is acute or chronic. In order to code otitis media to the correct level of specificity, documentation should indicate the type (acute, chronic, suppurative, etc.) and whether the condition is recurrent.

Laterality is also a component of the code and the documentation should specify if the condition is unilateral or bilateral. There are instructional notes to use additional code(s) for any associated perforated tympanic membrane (H72-). There are also instructional notes to use additional code(s) to identify exposure to environmental tobacco smoke (Z77.22), exposure to tobacco smoke in the perinatal period (P96.81), history of tobacco use (Z87.891), occupational exposure to environmental tobacco smoke (Z57.31), or tobacco use (Z72.0).

Code: H66.93 Otitis media, unspecified, bilateral

Ovarian Cysts Guideline [9, 10, 31]

In order to code ovarian cysts to the correct level of specificity, documentation should indicate the type of cyst (follicular, corpus luteum, etc.).

Codes: Z01.411 Encounter for gynecological examination (general) (routine) with abnormal findings
N83.20 Ovarian cyst; unspecified
Z12.72 Encounter for screening for malignant neoplasm of vagina

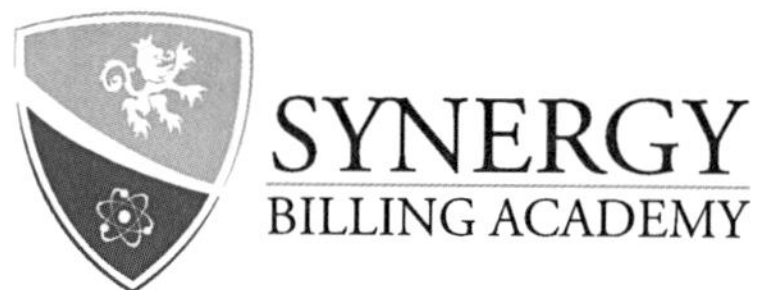

Pregnancy Guideline [9, 10, 31]

In order to code pregnancy supervision, the documentation should indicate the trimester of the patient. The trimester in ICD-10-CM has been defined in Chapter 15, Pregnancy, Childbirth, and the Puerperium as follows: 1st trimester – less than 14 weeks 0 days, 2nd trimester – 14 weeks 0 days to less than 28 weeks 0 days, 3rd trimester – 28 weeks 0 days until delivery. Trimesters are counted from the first day of the last menstrual period.

Pregnancy has many code selections for the supervision of pregnancy. Normal first pregnancy, other pregnancy, unspecified pregnancy, high risk pregnancy are some of the options. Each code set also has a code for first, second, and third or unspecified trimester. With pregnancy, you will also have to use a secondary code that specifies the weeks of pregnancy.

Code: Z34.90 Supervision of normal pregnancy, unspecified, unspecified trimester

ICD-10-CM International Classification of Diseases 10th Revision Clinical Modification

Documentation Requirements

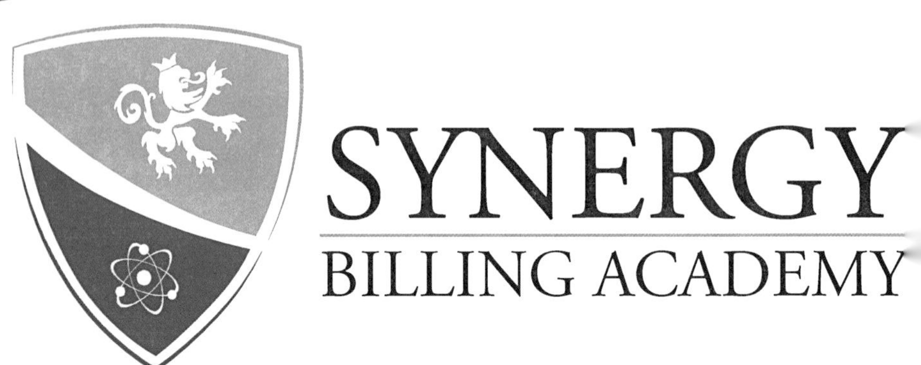

Documentation Requirements

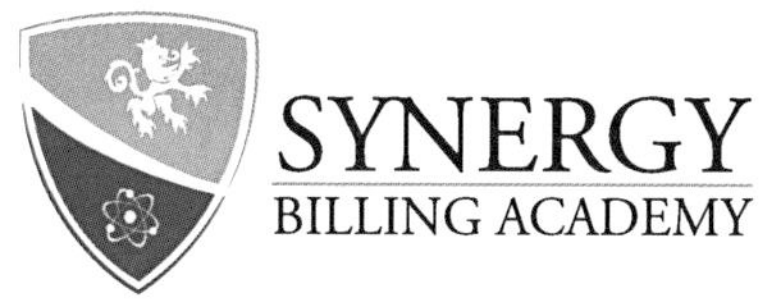

Alzheimer's Disease [32]

It is important for providers to understand the elements necessary for the documentation of Alzheimer's disease in ICD-10-CM. Please make sure to document the following key pieces of information:

- Type
  - Early onset
    - Presenile dementia
  - Late onset
    - Senile dementia
  - Other
  - Unspecified
- If applicable, also document:
  - Delirium
  - Dementia
    - With behavioral disturbance
    - Without behavioral disturbance

Anemia [46]

It is important for providers to understand the elements necessary for the documentation of anemia in ICD-10-CM. Please make sure to document the following key pieces of information:

- Cause of anemia:
  - Chronic anemia secondary to malignancy
  - Chronic anemia secondary to chronic kidney disease (CKD)
  - Acute blood loss anemia secondary to acute gastrointestinal (GI) bleed
  - Acute post-operative blood loss anemia (if greater than expected blood loss during surgery)
  - Chronic idiopathic anemia
- Type of anemia:
  - Iron Deficiency
  - Pernicious
  - Aplastic
  - Sickle Cell
  - Blood Loss Anemia

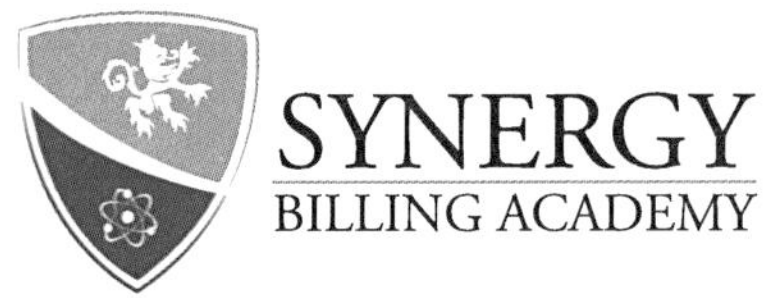

- Acuity
  - Acute
  - Chronic
  - Acute on chronic

Appendicitis [32]

It is important for providers to understand the elements necessary for the documentation of appendicitis in ICD-10-CM. Please make sure to document the following key pieces of information:

- Acute
  - With generalized peritonitis
    - Ruptured appendix
  - **With localized peritonitis**
    - **Peritoneal abscess**
    - **With or without rupture of appendix**
      - **Other**
      - **Unspecified**
    - Without peritonitis
- Other
  - Chronic
  - Recurrent
- Unspecified

Asthma [32]

In ICD-10-CM, the provider will be required to grade asthma by its severity and whether it is intermittent or persistent.

There are three severity categories: mild, moderate, and severe. The "mild" category is further classified as mild intermittent or mild persistent.

- Asthma types
  - Mild intermittent
    - Mild intermittent, uncomplicated
    - Mild intermittent with acute exacerbation
    - Mild intermittent with status asthmaticus

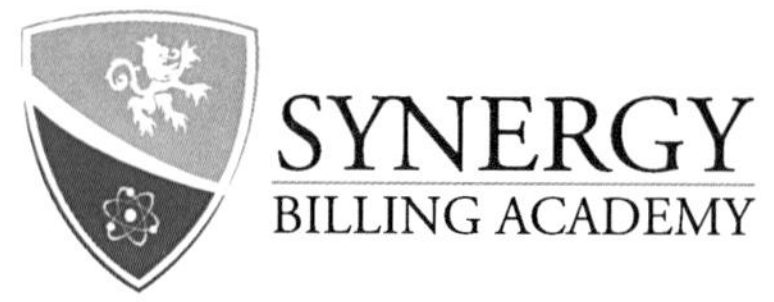

- Mild persistent
    - Mild persistent, uncomplicated
    - Mild persistent with acute exacerbation
    - Mild persistent with status asthmaticus
- Moderate persistent
    - Moderate persistent, uncomplicated
    - Moderate persistent with acute exacerbation
    - Moderate persistent with status asthmaticus
- Severe persistent
    - Severe persistent, uncomplicated
    - Severe persistent with acute exacerbation
    - Severe persistent with status asthmaticus

ICD-10-CM change: Documentation of a history of tobacco use, tobacco dependence, or exposure to environmental tobacco smoke is also important.

Congestive Heart Failure [32]

The documentation concepts necessary to describe congestive heart failure in ICD-9-CM will not change in ICD-10-CM.

The two important concepts to remember when documenting congestive heart failure are acuity and type.

In certain cases, the type may not be known. Therefore, it is acceptable to document what you know and update your documentation as test results become available, e.g., echocardiogram results, ejection fraction, etc.

- Acuity
    - Acute
    - Chronic
    - Acute on chronic
- Type
    - Systolic
    - Diastolic
    - Combined systolic and diastolic

Document associated conditions such as aortic valve disease, coronary artery disease (CAD), cardiomyopathy (type), or mitral valve disease (stenosis, insufficiency).

Documentation Requirements

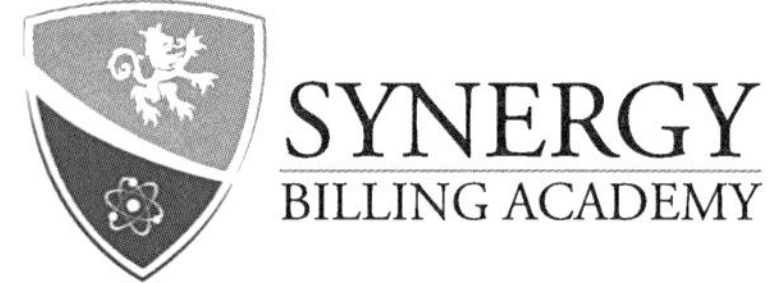

Debridement [32]

It is important for providers to understand the elements necessary for the documentation of excisional vs. non-excisional debridement.

- Excisional debridement involves the cutting away of tissue/necrosis/slough and falls under the "Excision" definition in ICD-10-CM.
- Non-excisional debridement is defined as the non-operative brushing, irrigating, scrubbing, or washing away of devitalized tissue. It falls under the "Extraction" definition in ICD-10-CM. Either can be performed at the bedside, in the ER, or in the OR.

Key documentation concepts:

- Location of the debridement (e.g., right ankle, left wrist)
- Condition requiring debridement (e.g., ulcer, necrosis, abscess)
- Instrument used (e.g., scissors, scalpel, curette, water jet, etc. If blade is used, please note size)
- Method used (e.g., irrigating, brushing, cutting)
- Depth of the debridement noting the deepest layer: skin, subcutaneous, fascia, muscle, bone
- Description of the tissue removed
- Descriptor: incisional or excisional

Dermatitis [32]

It is important for providers to understand the elements necessary for the documentation of dermatitis in ICD-10-CM. Please make sure to document the following key pieces of information:

- **Allergic contact dermatitis, due to:**
  - Metals
  - Adhesives
  - Dyes
  - Animal dander
- **Irritant contact dermatitis, due to:**
  - Detergents
  - Oils and greases
  - Solvents
  - Metals

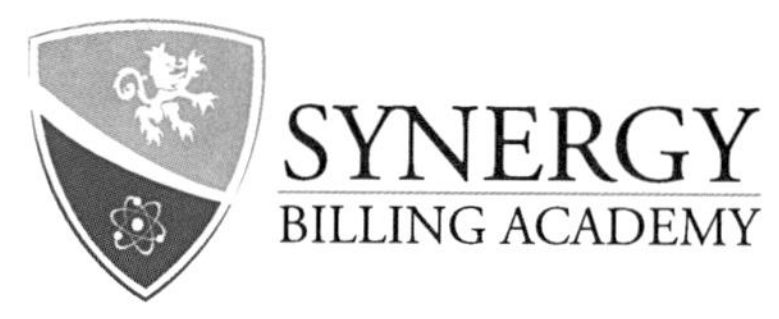

- **Unspecified contact dermatitis, due to:**
  - Dyes
- **Causative agents for all types**
  - **Cement**
  - Cosmetics
  - Drugs in contact with skin
  - Food in contact with skin
  - Insecticide
  - Plants (except food)
  - Plastic or rubber
  - **Other agents**
  - Unspecified cause

Diabetes Mellitus [32]

It is important for providers to understand the elements necessary for the documentation of diabetes mellitus in ICD-10-CM. Please make sure to document the following key pieces of information:

- Type
  - Type 1
  - Type 2
  - **Drug/chemical induced**
  - **Due to underlying condition**
  - **Specified type**
- **Control**
  - **Inadequately controlled**
  - **Out of control**
  - **Poorly controlled**
  - Hypoglycemia
  - **Hyperglycemia**
- **Manifestation/Complication**
  - **Arthropathy**
  - Circulatory complications
  - Hyperosmolarity
    - With or without coma
  - Hypoglycemia
    - With or without coma

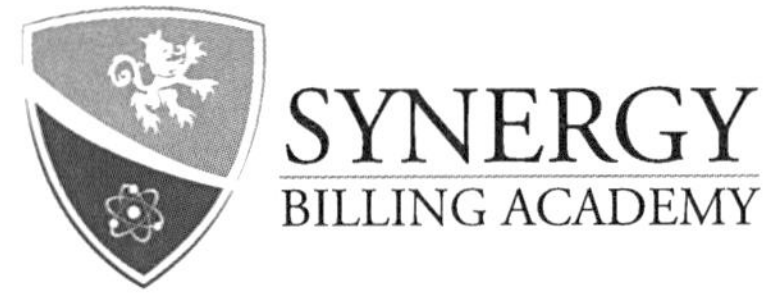

  - Ketoacidosis
    - With or without coma
  - Kidney complications
  - Neurological complications
  - Ophthalmic complications
  - **Oral complications**
  - **Skin complications**
  - Without complications
- Insulin use
  - No longer required for Type 1

Edema [32]

It is important for providers to understand the elements necessary for the documentation of edema in ICD-10-CM. Please make sure to document the following key pieces of information:

- **Localized**
- **Generalized**
- **Unspecified**
  - **Fluid retention**
- Site specific
- As a manifestation

Feeding Problems of Newborn [32]

It is important for providers to understand the elements necessary for the documentation of feeding problems of newborn in ICD-10-CM. Please make sure to document the following key pieces of information:

- Difficulty feeding at breast
- Failure to thrive
- Overfeeding
- Regurgitation and rumination
- Slow feeding
- Underfeeding
- Vomiting
  - Bilious
  - Other

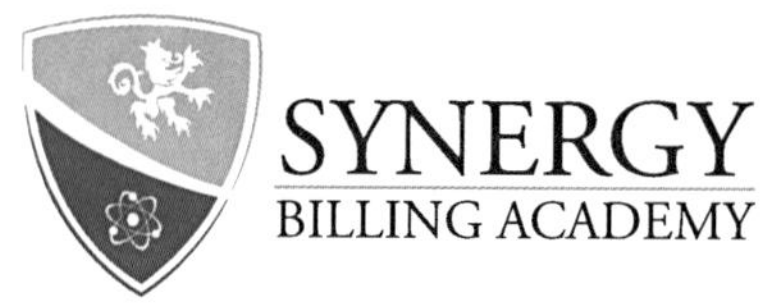

- **Other**
- **Unspecified**
- "Newborn" is defined as the first 28 days of life
  - If condition first presents after 28 days, it is not considered a newborn condition. These codes can be used throughout the life of the patient, if the condition is still present after 28 days.

Fractures [46]

It is important for providers to understand the elements necessary for the documentation of fractures in ICD-10-CM. Please make sure to document the following key pieces of information:

- Laterality
- Mechanism of injury
- Etiology of fracture
  - Traumatic, pathologic, osteoporosis, neoplastic disease
- Site
  - Name of the bone
  - Medial, lateral, midshaft, epiphysis, etc.
- Displaced vs. non-displaced
- Closed or open
  - Gustilo Anderson classification for open fractures
- Type of fracture
  - Comminuted, greenstick, oblique, segmental, spiral, transverse, compression, burst, etc.
- Note injury to surrounding tissue
- Encounter type
  - Initial encounter for fracture (type)
  - Subsequent encounter for fracture with routine healing
  - Subsequent encounter for fracture with delayed healing
  - Subsequent encounter for fracture with nonunion
  - Subsequent encounter for fracture with malunion
  - Sequela

Example: Instead of documenting "Fractured R arm," you will now document "Fell while running, traumatic, acute, closed, transverse right distal radial fracture with surrounding soft tissue hematoma and swelling."

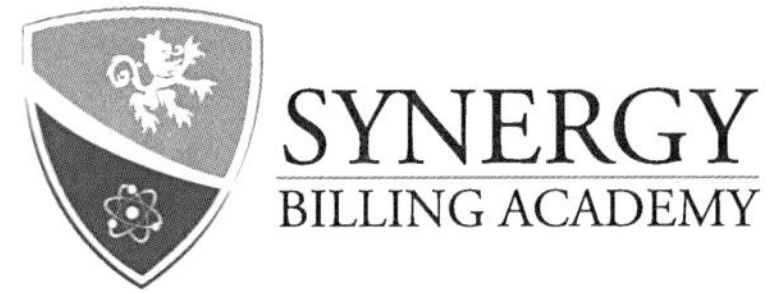

Glaucoma [32]

It is important for providers to understand the elements necessary for the documentation of glaucoma in ICD-10-CM. Please make sure to document the following key pieces of information:

- Type
  - Glaucoma suspect
  - Open-angle
  - Primary angle-closure
  - Secondary to:
    - Eye trauma
    - Eye inflammation
    - Other eye disorders
    - Drugs
  - Other glaucoma
  - Unspecified glaucoma
  - Glaucoma in diseases classified elsewhere
- Stage
  - Mild
  - Moderate
  - Severe
  - Indeterminate
  - Unspecified
- **Laterality**
  - **Right**
  - **Left**
  - **Bilateral**
  - **Unspecified**

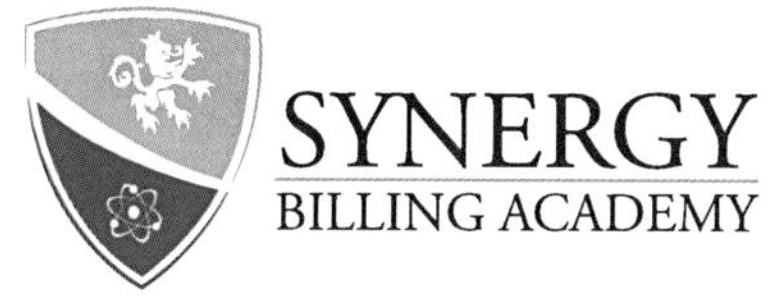

Gout [32]

It is important for providers to understand the elements necessary for the documentation of gout in ICD-10-CM. Please make sure to document the following key pieces of information:

- Type
  - Acute
  - Chronic
    - With or without tophus
  - Unspecified
- **Cause**
  - **Drug-induced**
  - **Idiopathic**
  - **Primary**
  - **Lead-induced**
  - **Saturnine**
  - **Renal impairment**
  - **Other secondary**
  - **Unspecified**
- **Site**
  - **Ankle and foot**
  - **Hip**
  - **Knee**
  - **Elbow**
  - **Hand**
  - **Shoulder**
  - **Wrist**
  - **Vertebrae**
  - **Multiple**
  - **Unspecified**
- **Laterality of extremities**
  - **Right**
  - **Left**
  - **Unspecified**

Documentation Requirements

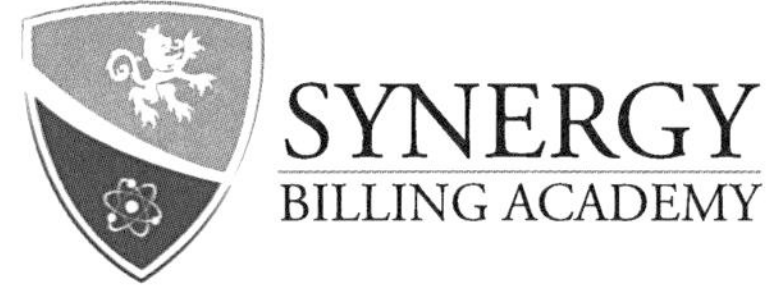

Myocardial Infarctions [46]

It is important for providers to understand the elements necessary for the documentation of myocardial infarctions in ICD-10-CM. Document the following:

- Type of MI
  - ST elevation MI (STEMI)
  - Non-ST elevation MI (NSTEMI)
- Site of MI (including wall and vessel)
- Episode of care
  - Initial: within four-week time frame (28 days)
  - Subsequent: care for a subsequent, new MI occurring within four-week (28 days) time frame of the initial MI
- Complications
  - List all complications related to the MI
- Site for initial episode of STEMI
  - Anterior wall
    - Left main coronary artery
    - Left anterior descending artery
    - Other coronary artery of anterior wall
  - Inferior wall
    - Right coronary artery
    - Other coronary artery of inferior wall
  - Other
    - Left circumflex coronary artery
    - Other specified
  - Unspecified
- **Site for subsequent episode STEMI**
  - **Anterior wall**
  - **Inferior wall**
  - **Other**
- **NSTEMI – initial/subsequent**
  - **No site required**
  - **Episode of care reporting only**
- **Episode of care**
  - **Initial (four-week time frame)**
  - **Subsequent (care for a subsequent, new MI occurring within the four-week time frame of the initial MI)**

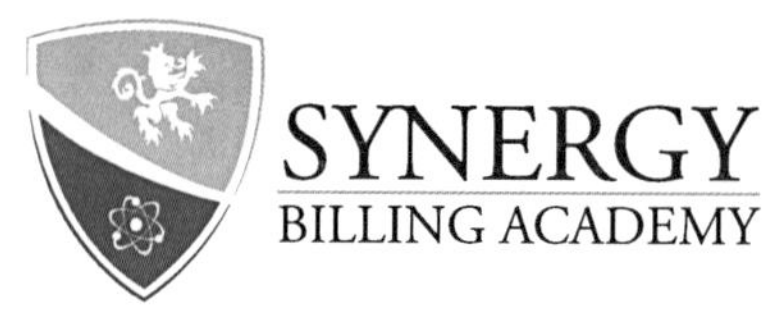

- Complications
  - Same as ICD-9-CM
- **Type**
  - **ST elevation MI (STEMI)**
  - **Non-ST elevation MI (NSTEMI)**

Obesity [32]

It is important for providers to understand the elements necessary for the documentation of obesity in ICD-10-CM. Please make sure to document the following key pieces of information:

- **Obesity**
  - **Drug-induced**
  - Morbid
    - **Due to excess calories**
    - **With alveolar hypoventilation**
  - **Other**
    - **Due to excess calories**
  - **Constitutional**
- Overweight
- Body Mass Index (BMI)

Pneumonia [32]

It is important for providers to understand the elements necessary for the documentation of pneumonia in ICD-10-CM. Please make sure to document the following key pieces of information:

- Acuity
  - Acute
  - Chronic
- Laterality
  - Left
  - Right
  - Bilateral
- Location
  - Upper lobe
  - Middle lobe
  - Lower lobe

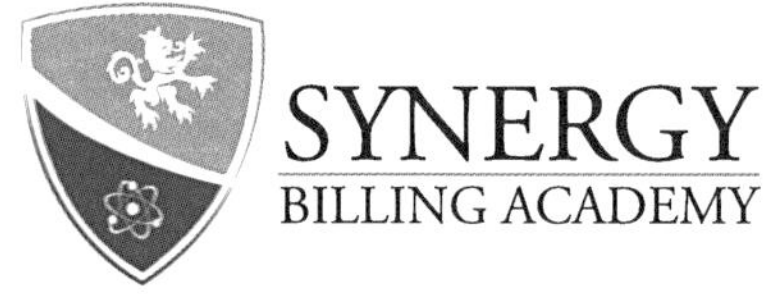

- Cause (if known)
  - Community acquired, hospital acquired, aspiration, ventilator-associated, chemical, bacterial, viral, associated with HIV/AIDS, etc.
- Organism (if known)
  - A positive sputum culture is not required to document the type of pneumonia you "suspect" is being treated, for example: "suspect gram neg. pneumonia."
- Document associated issues
  - Abscess, cavitation, empyeme, sepsis, respiratory failure (acute, chronic, or acute on chronic, hypoxic/hypercapnic)

Poor Fetal Growth – Maternal Record [32]

It is important for providers to understand the elements necessary for the documentation of poor fetal growth for the maternal record in ICD-10-CM. Please make sure to document the following key pieces of information:

- **Maternal care for known or suspected poor fetal growth**
  - **Due to known or suspected**
    - **Placental insufficiency**
    - **Other poor fetal growth**
      - **Light-for-dates NOS**
      - **Small-for-dates NOS**
- **Trimester**
  - **First (less than 14 weeks 0 days)**
  - **Second (14 weeks 0 days to less than 28 weeks 0 days)**
  - **Third (28 weeks 0 days until delivery)**
  - Unspecified
- **Fetus affected by complication**
  - **Multiple gestation pregnancy**
    - **Fetus 1**
    - **Fetus 2**
    - **Fetus 3**
    - **Fetus 4**
    - **Fetus 5**
    - **Other**
  - **Unspecified or not applicable (e.g., single fetus)**

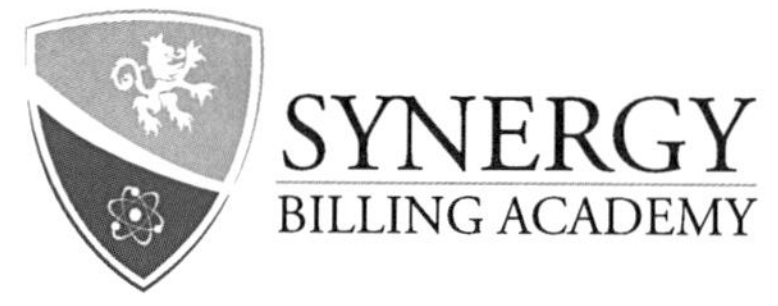

Poor Fetal Growth – Perinatal Record [32]

It is important for providers to understand the elements necessary for the documentation of poor fetal growth for the perinatal record in ICD-10-CM. Please make sure to document the following key pieces of information:

- Light-for-dates
- Small-for-dates
- **Small-and-light-for-dates**
- **Fetal (intrauterine) malnutrition <u>not</u> light or small for gestational age**
- **Newborn affected by slow intrauterine growth, unspecified birthweight in grams**
  - **Unspecified to 2,499g**

Regional Enteritis – Crohn's Disease [32]

It is important for providers to understand the elements necessary for the documentation of regional enteritis – Crohn's disease in ICD-10-CM. Please make sure to document the following key pieces of information:

- Site
  - Small intestine
  - Large intestine
  - Both small and large intestine
  - Unspecified site
- **With complication**
  - **Abscess**
  - **Fistula**
  - **Intestinal obstruction**
  - **Rectal bleeding**
  - **Other**
  - **Unspecified**
- **Without complication**

Respiratory Failure [32]

It is important for providers to understand the elements necessary for the documentation of respiratory failure in ICD-10-CM. Please make sure to document the following key pieces of information:

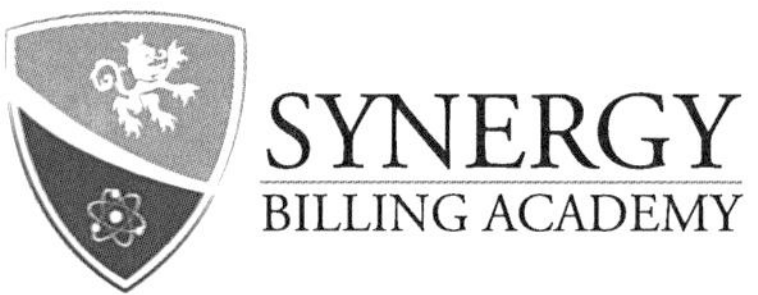

- Status
  - Acute
  - Chronic
  - Acute and/on chronic
  - **Unspecified**
- **With**
  - **Hypercapnia**
  - **Hypoxia**
  - **Unspecified whether with hypoxia or hypercapnia**

Scoliosis [32]

It is important for providers to understand the elements necessary for the documentation of scoliosis in ICD-10-CM. Please make sure to document the following key pieces of information:

- **Type**
  - Idiopathic
    - Infantile
    - **Juvenile**
    - **Adolescent**
    - **Other idiopathic**
  - **Neuromuscular**
    - **Identify underlying condition**
  - **Other secondary**
  - Thoracogenic
  - Other forms of scoliosis
  - Unspecified scoliosis
- **Region**
  - **Occipito-atlanto-axial** (only applicable to neuromuscular scoliosis)
  - **Cervical**
  - **Cervicothoracic**
  - **Thoracic**
  - **Thoracolumbar**
  - **Lumbar**
  - **Lumbosacral**
  - **Sacral/sacrococcygeal** (only applicable to infantile idiopathic scoliosis)
  - **Unspecified**

Documentation Requirements

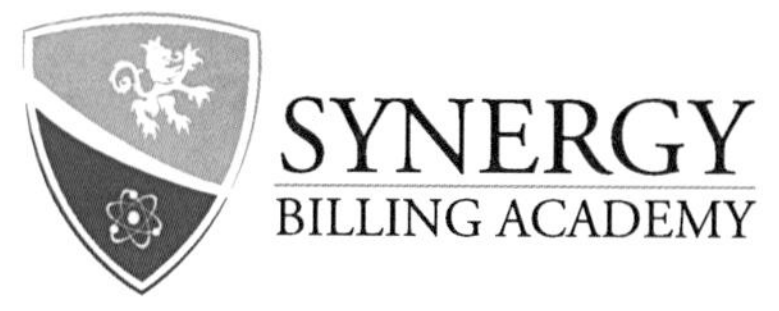

Sepsis [32]

It is important for providers to understand the elements necessary for the documentation of sepsis in ICD-10-CM. Please make sure to document the following key pieces of information:

- Was the sepsis present on admission?
- Is the sepsis with or without shock?
- The causal agent or presence of underlying systemic infection, if known (e.g., bacterial, fungal, candida)
    - Sepsis due to MRSA pneumonia or MRSA pneumonia with sepsis
- Sepsis due to a post-procedural infection
    - If unknown agent or source, document "sepsis, unknown source"
- Associated organ dysfunction when documenting severe sepsis
    - Severe sepsis due to MRSA pneumonia with resulting acute respiratory failure
    - If more than one organ is affected, document individually

Document underlying local infection; specify causal relationship to local infection and/or procedure. Identify:

- Causative organism
    - Staphylococcus
        - MSSA
        - MRSA
        - Other specified
        - Unspecified
    - **Streptococcus**
        - **Group A**
        - **Group B**
        - Pneumoniae
        - **Other**
        - **Unspecified**
    - Other gram negative
    - Anaerobes
- Any associated
    - Organ dysfunction or failure
    - Severe sepsis
    - Septic shock
- **SIRS is only applicable for non-infectious process**

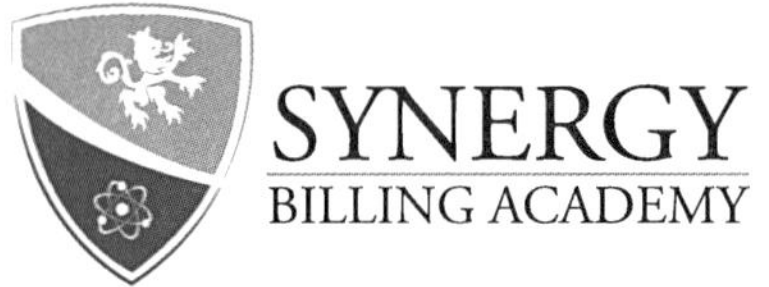

ICD-10-CM change: There is no longer a code for SIRS due to an infectious process. There are two categories for SIRS of a noninfectious origin, one without acute organ dysfunction and one with acute organ dysfunction. In ICD-10-CM, there is no such thing as urosepsis.

Specificity in documentation clearly defines your patient's severity of illness and risk of mortality. Accurate documentation is the key!

Traumatic Fracture [32]

It is important for providers to understand the elements necessary for the documentation of traumatic fracture in ICD-10-CM. Please make sure to document the following key pieces of information:

- **Site**
  - **Neer classification proximal end of humerus**
  - **Salter-Harris classification for physeal fractures**
- **Open**
  - **Gustilo Anderson classification for long bone fractures**
- Closed
- **Episode of care**
  - **Initial (active phase of treatment)**
  - **Subsequent (after active phase)**
    - **With delayed healing**
    - **With malunion**
    - **With nonunion**
    - **With routine healing or aftercare**
  - **Sequela/Late Effect**

Ulcer – Chronic Skin Ulcer – Non-Pressure [32]

It is important for providers to understand the elements necessary for the documentation of ulcers – chronic skin ulcer – non-pressure in ICD-10-CM. Please make sure to document the following key pieces of information:

- **Site**
  - **Back**
  - **Buttock**
  - Lower limb

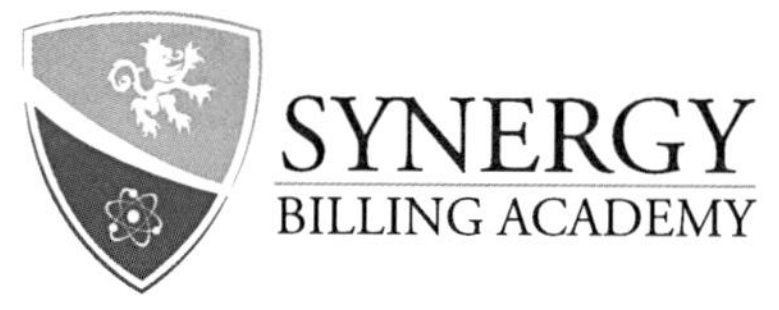

    - Ankle
    - Calf
    - Heel and midfoot
      - Plantar surface
    - Other part of foot
      - Toes
    - Thigh
    - **Other part of lower leg**
    - **Unspecified part of lower leg**
  - **Skin of other sites**
- **Ulcer depth**
  - **Limited to skin breakdown**
  - **With fat layer exposed**
  - **With muscle necrosis**
  - **With bone necrosis**
  - **Unspecified severity**
- **Laterality of lower limb**
  - **Right**
  - **Left**
- **Causal condition of lower limb ulcer**
  - Atherosclerosis of lower extremity
  - Chronic venous hypertension
  - Diabetic ulcers
  - Postphlebitic syndrome
  - **Postthrombotic syndrome**
  - **Varicose ulcer**
- **Gangrene**

Ulcer – Pressure Ulcer [32]

It is important for providers to understand the elements necessary for the documentation of ulcer – pressure ulcer in ICD-10-CM. Please make sure to document the following key pieces of information:

- Site
  - Ankle
  - Back
    - Lower

Documentation Requirements

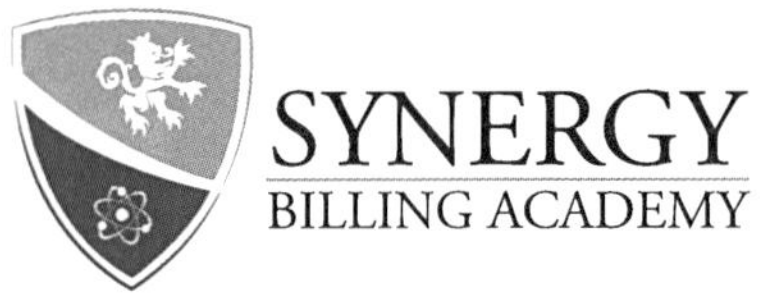

        - Upper
            - Shoulder blade
        - Unspecified part
    - Buttock
    - **Contiguous sites of back, buttock, hip**
    - Elbow
    - Head
        - **Face**
    - Heel
    - Hip
    - **Sacral region**
        - Coccyx, **tailbone**
    - Other
    - Unspecified
- **Stage**
    - **Stage 1**
    - **Stage 2**
    - **Stage 3**
    - **Stage 4**
    - Unstageable
    - Unspecified
- **Laterality of limbs and trunk**
    - **Right**
    - **Left**
    - **Unspecified**

ICD-10-CM International Classification of Diseases 10th Revision Clinical Modification

Code Conversion Guide

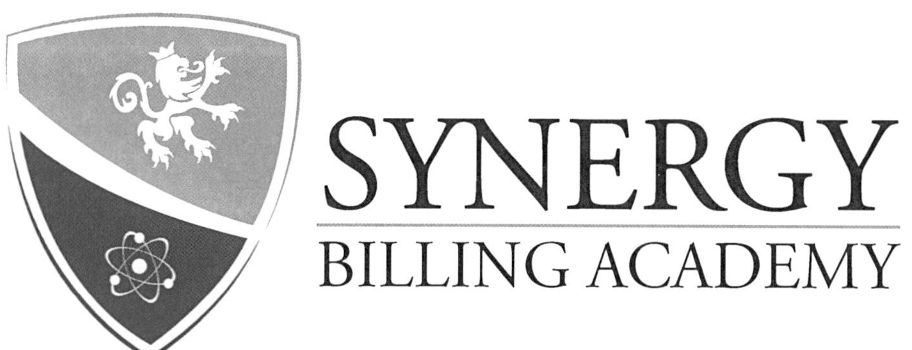

Code Conversion Guide

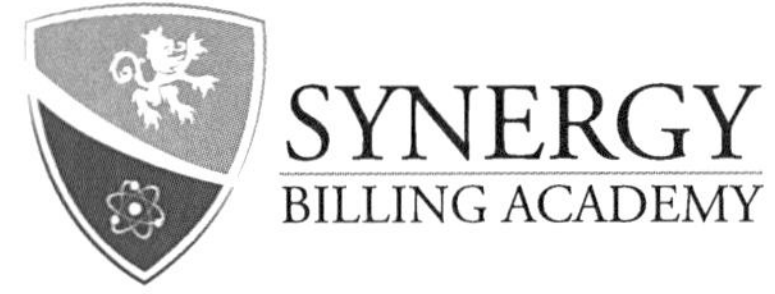

Chapter 1: Infectious and Parasitic Diseases

ICD-9-CM		ICD-10-CM	
034.0	Streptococcal sore throat	J02.0 J03.00	Streptococcal pharyngitis Acute streptococcal tonsillitis, unspecified
041.00	Streptococcus, unspecified	B95.5	Unspecified streptococcus as the cause of diseases classified elsewhere
042	HIV disease	B20	Human immunodeficiency virus [HIV] disease
052.9	Varicella without mention of complication	B01.9	Varicella without complication
054.10	Genital herpes, unspecified	A60.9	Anogenital herpesviral infection, unspecified
070.53	Hepatitis E without mention of hepatic coma	B17.2	Acute hepatitis E
078.10	Viral warts, unspecified	B07.9	Viral wart, unspecified
079.4	Human papillomavirus	B97.7	Papillomavirus as the cause of diseases classified elsewhere
099.41	Chlamydia trachomatis	N34.1	Nonspecific urethritis
110.1	Dermatophytosis of nail	B35.1	Tinea unguium
112.1	Candidiasis of vulva and vagina	B37.3	Candidiasis of vulva and vagina

Chapter 2: Neoplasms

ICD-9-CM	ICD-10-CM
Neoplasms (140-239)	Neoplasms (C00-D49) – C = Cancer

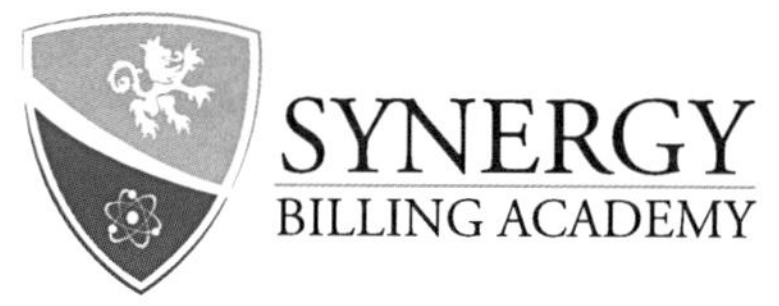

Chapter 3: Endocrine, Nutritional and Metabolic Diseases, and Immunity Disorders

ICD-9-CM		ICD-10-CM	
244.9	Unspecified hypothyroidism	E03.9	Hypothyroidism, unspecified
250.00	Diabetes mellitus without mention of complication, Type II or unspecified type, not stated as uncontrolled	E11.9	Type 2 diabetes mellitus without complications
250.01	Diabetes mellitus without mention of complication, Type I [juvenile type], not stated as uncontrolled	E10.9	Type 1 diabetes mellitus without complications
250.02	Diabetes mellitus without mention of complication,Type II or unspecified type, uncontrolled	E11.65	Type 2 diabetes mellitus with hyperglycemia
250.21	Diabetes w/hyperosmolarity Type I	E10.69	Type 1 diabetes mellitus with other specified complication
250.62	Diabetes Type II, uncontrolled with neurological manifestations	E11.40 E11.65	Type 2 diabetes mellitus with diabetic neuropathy, unspecified Type 2 diabetes mellitus with hyperglycemia
257.2	Other testicular hypofunction	E29.1	Testicular hypofunction
266.2	Other B-complex deficiencies	E53.8	Deficiency of other specified B group vitamins
272.0	Pure hypercholesterolemia	E78.0	Pure hypercholesterolemia
272.2	Mixed hyperlipidemia	E78.2	Mixed hyperlipidemia
272.4	Other and unspecified hyperlipidemia	E78.4 E78.5	Other hyperlipidemia Hyperlipidemia, unspecified
274.10	Gouty arthropathy, unspecified	M10.30	Gout due to renal impairment, unspecified site
277.7	Dysmetabolic Syndrome X	E88.81	Metabolic syndrome
278.00	Obesity, unspecified	E66.9	Obesity, unspecified
278.01	Morbid obesity	E66.01	Morbid (severe) obesity due to excess calories

Code Conversion Guide

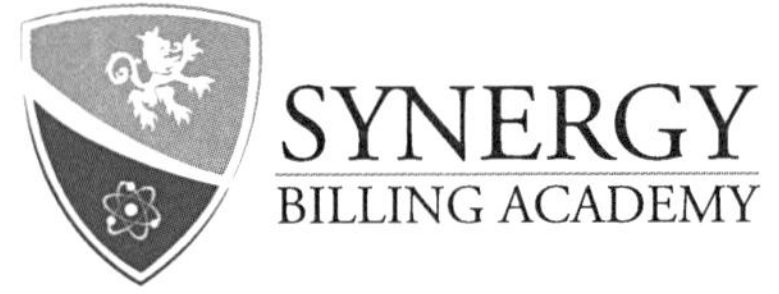

Chapter 4: Diseases of Blood and Blood-Forming Organs

ICD-9-CM		ICD-10-CM	
285.9	Unspecified anemia	D64.9	Anemia, unspecified

Chapter 5: Mental, Behavioral, and Neurodevelopmental Disorders

ICD-9-CM		ICD-10-CM	
293.81	Psychotic disorder with delusions in conditions classified elsewhere	F06.2	Psychotic disorder with delusions due to known physiological condition
293.83	Mood disorder in conditions classified elsewhere	F06.30	Mood disorder due to known physiological condition, unspecified
293.84	Anxiety disorder in conditions classified elsewhere	F06.4	Anxiety disorder due to known physiological condition
295.60	Schizophrenic disorders – residual type – unspecified	F20.5	Residual schizophrenia
296.21	Major depressive disorder, mild single episode	F32.0	Major depressive disorder, single episode, mild
296.32	Moderate recurrent major depression	F33.1	Major depressive disorder, recurrent, moderate
297.9	Unspecified paranoid state	F23	Brief psychotic disorder
300.00	Anxiety, dissociative and somatoform disorders – anxiety state, unspecified	F41.9	Anxiety disorder, unspecified
302.70	Psychosexual dysfunction unspecified	R37	Sexual dysfunction, unspecified
302.85	Gender identity disorder in adolescents or adults	F64.1	Gender identity disorder in adolescence and adulthood
304.90	Unspecified drug dependence – unspecified	F19.20	Other psychoactive substance dependence, uncomplicated
305.1	Nondependent tobacco use disorder	F17.200	Nicotine dependence, unspecified, uncomplicated

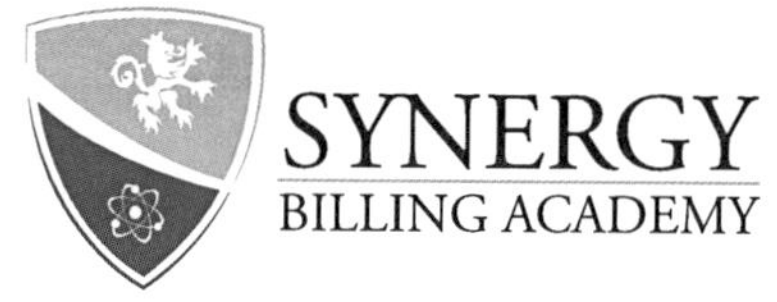

Chapter 6: Diseases of Nervous System and Sense Organs

ICD-9-CM		ICD-10-CM	
338.4	Chronic pain syndrome	G89.4	Chronic pain syndrome
367.1	Myopia	H52.13	Myopia, bilateral
372.00	Acute disorders of conjunctiva unspecified	H10.33	Unspecified acute conjunctivitis, bilateral
381.02	Acute mucoid otitis media	H65.119	Acute and subacute allergic otitis media (mucoid) (sanguinous) (serous), unspecified ear
382.9	Unspecified otitis media	H66.90	Otitis media, unspecified, unspecified ear

Chapter 7: Diseases of Circulatory System

ICD-9-CM		ICD-10-CM	
401.0	Essential hypertension, malignant	I10	Essential (primary) hypertension
401.1	Essential hypertension, benign	I10	Essential (primary) hypertension
401.9	Essential hypertension, unspecified	I10	Essential (primary) hypertension
415.19	Pulmonary embolism and infarction, other	I26.99	Other pulmonary embolism without acute cor pulmonale
428.0	Congestive heart failure, unspecified	I50.9	Heart failure, unspecified
429.2	Unspecified cardiovascular disease	I25.10	Atherosclerotic heart disease of native coronary artery without angina pectoris

Code Conversion Guide

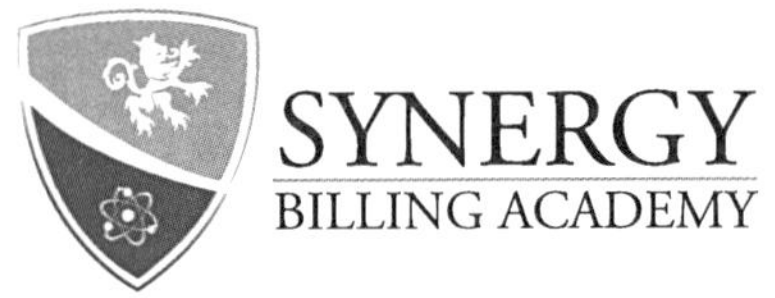

Chapter 8: Diseases of Respiratory System

ICD-9-CM		ICD-10-CM	
460	Acute nasopharyngitis	J00	Acute nasopharyngitis [common cold]
461.9	Acute sinusitis, unspecified	J01.90	Acute sinusitis, unspecified
462	Acute pharyngitis	J02.9	Acute pharyngitis, unspecified
465.9	Acute upper respiratory infection, unspecified site NOS	J06.9	Acute upper respiratory infection, unspecified
466.0	Acute bronchitis	J20.9	Acute bronchitis, unspecified
466.19	Acute bronchiolitis due other infections organisms	J21.8	Acute bronchiolitis due to other specified organisms
472.0	Chronic rhinitis	J31.0	Chronic rhinitis
472.1	Chronic pharyngitis	J31.2	Chronic pharyngitis
472.2	Chronic nasopharyngitis	J31.1	Chronic nasopharyngitis
473.9	Unspecified sinusitis	J32.9	Chronic sinusitis, unspecified
477.0	Allergic rhinitis due to pollen	J30.1	Allergic rhinitis due to pollen
477.9	Allergic rhinitis, cause unspecified	J30.0 J30.9	Vasomotor rhinitis Allergic rhinitis, unspecified
486	Pneumonia, organism unspecified	J18.9	Pneumonia, unspecified organism
490	Bronchitis, not specified as acute or chronic	J40	Bronchitis, not specified as acute or chronic
491.20	Obstructive chronic bronchitis, without exacerbation	J44.9	Chronic obstructive pulmonary disease, unspecified
493.00	Extrinsic asthma, unspecified	J45.20	Mild intermittent asthma, uncomplicated
493.90	Asthma NOS	J45.909 J45.998	Unspecified asthma, uncomplicated Other asthma
496	(Chronic airway obstruction, not elsewhere classified)	J44.9	Chronic obstructive pulmonary disease, unspecified

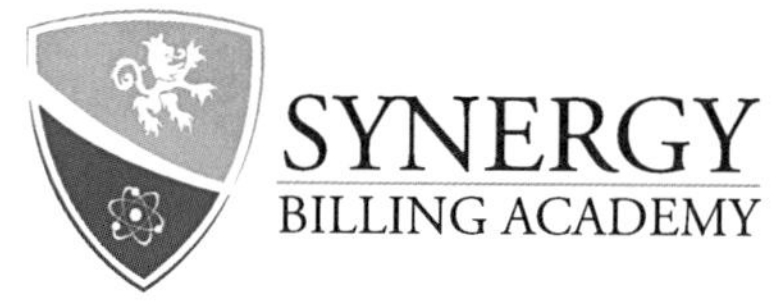

Chapter 9: Diseases of Digestive System

ICD-9-CM		ICD-10-CM	
521.00	Unspecified dental caries	K02.9	Dental caries, unspecified
525.9	Toothache	K08.9	Disorder of teeth and supporting structures, unspecified
530.11	Reflux esophagitis	K21.0	Gastro-esophageal reflux disease with esophagitis
530.81	Esophageal reflux	K21.9	Gastro-esophageal reflux disease without esophagitis
564.00	Unspecified constipation	K59.00	Constipation, unspecified

Chapter 10: Diseases of Genitourinary System

ICD-9-CM		ICD-10-CM	
599.0	Urinary tract infection, site not specified	N39.0	Urinary tract infection, site not specified
616.10	Vaginitis	N76.0 N76.1 N76.2 N76.3	Acute vaginitis Subacute and chronic vaginitis Acute vulvitis Subacute and chronic vulvitis
616.11	Vaginitis and vulvovaginitis in diseases classified elsewhere	N77.1	Vaginitis, vulvitis and vulvovaginitis in diseases classified elsewhere
623.5	Vaginal discharge (unspecified)	N89.8	Other specified noninflammatory disorders of vagina
626.2	Excessive or frequent menstruation	N92.0	Excessive and frequent menstruation with regular cycle

Code Conversion Guide

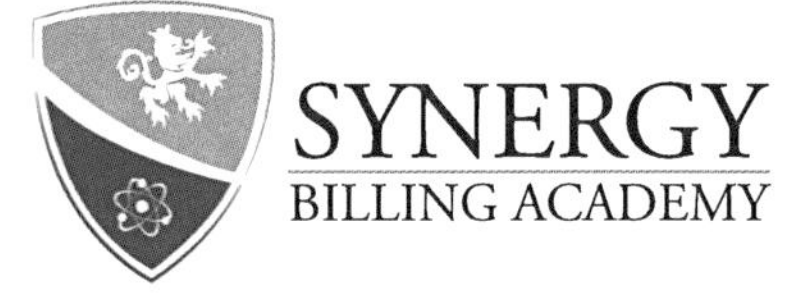

Chapter 11: Complications of Pregnancy, Childbirth, and the Puerperium

ICD-9-CM		ICD-10-CM	
654.23	Previous c-section delivery antepartum condition	O34.21	Maternal care for scar from previous cesarean delivery

Chapter 12: Diseases of the Skin and Subcutaneous Tissue

ICD-9-CM	ICD-10-CM
Diseases of the Skin and Subcutaneous Tissue (680–709)	Diseases of the Skin and Subcutaneous Tissue (L00–L99)

Chapter 13: Diseases of Musculoskeletal System and Connective Tissue

ICD-9-CM		ICD-10-CM	
714.0	Rheumatoid arthritis	M06.9	Rheumatoid arthritis, unspecified
715.90	Osteoarthritis unspecified, site unspecified	M15.9 M19.90	Polyosteoarthritis, unspecified Unspecified osteoarthritis, unspecified site
716.90	Unspecified arthropathy, site unspecified	M12.9	Arthropathy
719.41	Pain in joint, shoulder region	M25.519	Pain in unspecified shoulder
719.44	Pain in joint, hand	M79.643 M79.646	Pain in unspecified hand Pain in unspecified finger(s)
719.46	Pain in joint, lower leg	M25.569	Pain in unspecified knee
719.47	Pain in joint, ankle and foot	M25.579	Pain in unspecified ankle and joints of unspecified foot
719.48	Pain in joint, other specified sites	M25.50	Pain in unspecified joint
719.49	Pain in joint, multiple sites	M25.50	Pain in unspecified joint

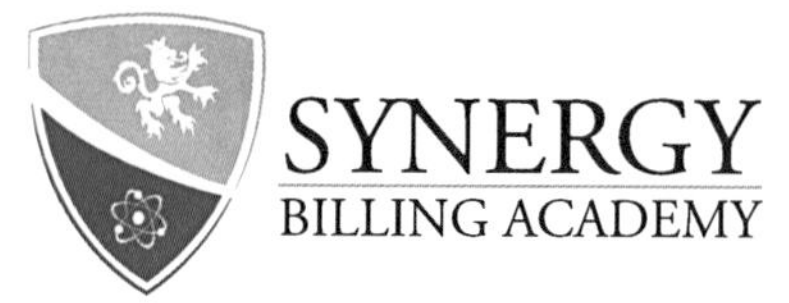

723.1	Cervicalgia	M54.2	Cervicalgia
724.2	Lumbago	M54.5	Low back pain
724.4	Thoracic or lumbosacral neuritis or radiculitis, unspecified	M54.14 M54.15 M54.16 M54.17	Radiculopathy, thoracic region Radiculopathy, thoracolumbar region Radiculopathy, lumbar region Radiculopathy, lumbosacral region
724.5	Back pain	M54.89 M54.9	Other dorsalgia Dorsalgia, unspecified
728.85	Spasm of muscle	M62.40 M62.838	Contracture of muscle, unspecified site Other muscle spasm
729.1	Unspecified myalgia and myositis	M60.9 M79.1 M79.7	Myositis, unspecified Myalgia Fibromyalgia

Chapter 14: Congenital Anomalies

ICD-9-CM	ICD-10-CM
Congenital Anomalies (740–759)	Congenital Malformations, Deformations, and Chromosomal Abnormalities (Q00–Q99)

Chapter 15: Certain Conditions Originating in Perinatal

ICD-9-CM	ICD-10-CM
Certain Conditions Originating in the Perinatal Period (760–779)	Certain Conditions Originating in the Perinatal Period (P00–P96)

Code Conversion Guide

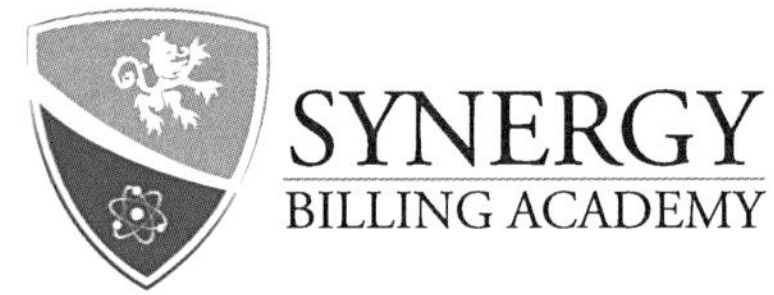

Chapter 16: Symptoms, Signs, and Ill-Defined Conditions

ICD-9-CM		ICD-10-CM	
780.52	Insomnia, unspecified	G47.00	Insomnia, unspecified
780.60	Fever, unspecified	R50.2 R50.9	Drug-induced fever Fever, unspecified
780.79	Other malaise and fatigue	G93.3 R53.1 R53.81 R53.83	Postviral fatigue syndrome Weakness Other malaise Other fatigue
782.1	Rash and other nonspecific skin eruption	R21	Rash and other nonspecific skin eruption
782.3	Edema	R60.0 R60.1 R60.9	Localized edema Generalized edema Edema, unspecified
784.0	Headache	G44.1 R51	Vascular headache, not elsewhere classified Headache
786.05	Shortness of breath	R06.02	Shortness of breath
786.2	Cough	R05	Cough
786.50	Chest pain, unspecified	R07.9	Chest pain, unspecified
788.1	Dysuria	R30.0 R30.9	Dysuria Painful micturition, unspecified
789.00	Abdominal pain, unspecified site	R10.9	Unspecified abdominal pain
789.01	Abdominal pain, right upper quadrant	R10.11	Right upper quadrant pain

Chapter 17: Injury and Poisoning

ICD-9-CM	ICD-10-CM
Injury and Poisoning (800–999)	Injury, Poisoning, and Certain Other Consequences of External Causes (S00–T88) T = Toxicity

Code Conversion Guide

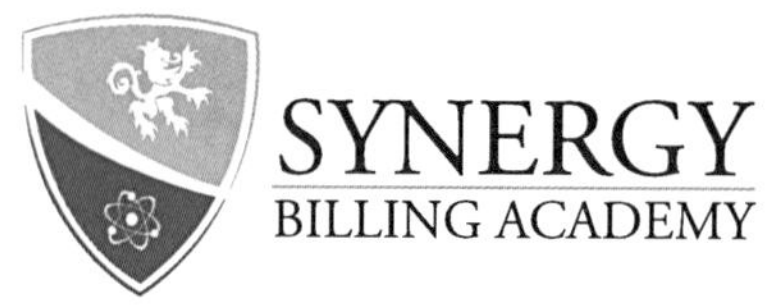

V Codes

ICD-9-CM		ICD-10-CM	
V01.6	Contact with or exposure to venereal	Z20.2	Contact with and (suspected) exposure to infections with a predominantly sexual mode of transmission
V03.81	Hemophilus influenza, type B vaccine	Z23	Encounter for immunization
V03.82	Pneumococcal vaccine	Z23	Encounter for immunization
V03.89	Other specified vaccination	Z23	Encounter for immunization
V03.9	Vaccine for bacterial disease	Z23	Encounter for immunization
V04.81	Need for prophylactic vaccination and inoculation, influenza	Z23	Encounter for immunization
V04.89	Vaccine for viral disease	Z23	Encounter for immunization
V05.3	Viral hepatitis	Z23	Encounter for immunization
V05.8	Need for prophylactic vaccine and inoculation against other specified	Z23	Encounter for immunization
V05.9	Need for prophylactic vaccine and inoculation against unspecified	Z23	Encounter for immunization
V06.1	Diphtheria-tetanus-pertussis	Z23	Encounter for immunization
V06.4	Measles-mumps-rubella	Z23	Encounter for immunization
V06.8	Other combination	Z23	Encounter for immunization
V06.9	Unspecified combination vaccine	Z23	Encounter for immunization
V07.8	Need for other specified prophylactic or treatment	Z41.8	Encounter for other procedures for purposes other than remedying health state
V15.81	Noncompliance with medical treatment	Z91.19	Patient's noncompliance with other medical treatment and regimen
V15.82	Personal history of tobacco use, presenting hazards to health	Z87.891	Personal history of nicotine dependence
V20.0	Health supervision of infant or child – foundling	Z76.1	Encounter for health supervision and care of foundling

Code Conversion Guide

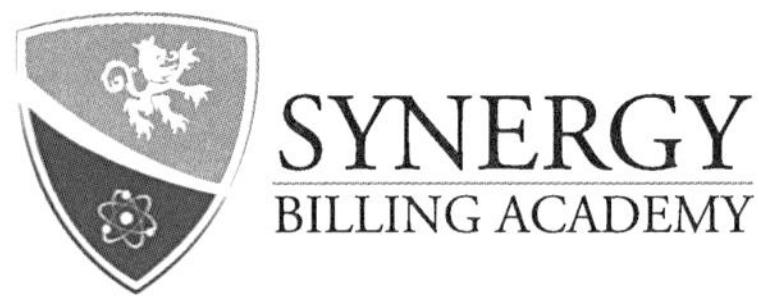

V20.1	Health supervision – other healthy infant/child receiving care	Z76.2	Encounter for health supervision and care of other healthy infant and child
V20.2	Routine infant/child check-up	Z00.129	Encounter for routine child health examination without abnormal findings
V22.0	Supervision of normal first pregnancy	Z34.00	Encounter for supervision of normal first pregnancy, unspecified trimester
V22.1	Supervision of other normal pregnancy	Z34.80 Z34.90	Encounter for supervision of other normal pregnancy, unspecified trimester Encounter for supervision of normal pregnancy, unspecified, unspecified trimester
V22.2	Pregnant state, incidental	Z33.1	Pregnant state, incidental
V24.2	Routine postpartum follow-up	Z39.2	Encounter for routine postpartum follow-up
V25.02	General counseling for initiation of other contraceptive measures	Z30.018	Encounter for initial prescription of other contraceptives
V25.09	Other general counseling and advice on contraceptive management	Z30.09	Encounter for other general counseling and advice on contraception
V25.40	Contraception maintenance	Z30.40	Encounter for surveillance of contraceptives, unspecified
V25.49	Surveillance other previous contraceptive method	Z30.49	Encounter for surveillance of other contraceptives
V27.0	Outcome of delivery single live born	Z37.0	Single live birth
V29.0	Observation and evaluation of newborns and infants suspected infectious condition	P00.2	Newborn (suspected to be) affected by maternal infectious and parasitic diseases
V52.3	Fitting and adjustment of dental prosthetic device	Z46.3	Encounter for fitting and adjustment of dental prosthetic device
V62.3	Educational circumstance	Z55.9	Problems related to education and literacy, unspecified

Code Conversion Guide

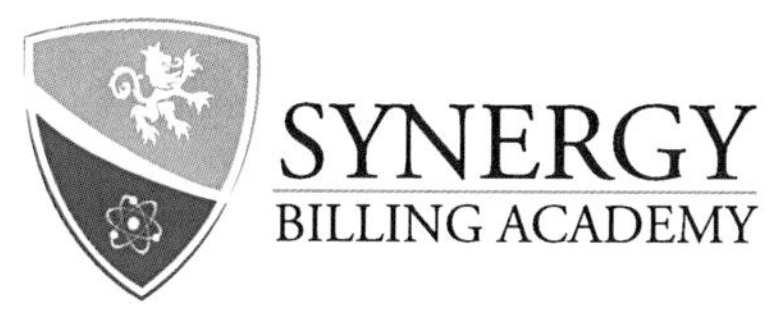

V65.40	Counseling NOS	Z71.9	Counseling, unspecified
V65.49	Other specified counseling	Z71.89	Other specified counseling
V68.01	Disability examination	Z02.71	Encounter for disability determination
V68.1	Issue of repeat prescriptions	Z76.0	Encounter for issue of repeat prescription
V69.2	Problems related to high-risk sexual behavior	Z72.51	High-risk heterosexual behavior
V70.0	Exam, general adult medical	Z00.00	Encounter for general adult medical examination without abnormal findings
V70.3	Exam, marriage/camp/school/ sports	Z02.89	Encounter for other administrative examinations
V70.5	Health examination of defined subpopulation	Z02.1 Z02.3 Z02.89	Encounter for pre-employment examination Encounter for examination for recruitment to armed forces Encounter for other administrative examinations
V72.2	Dental examination	Z01.20 Z01.21	Encounter for dental examination and cleaning without abnormal findings Encounter for dental examination and cleaning with abnormal findings
V72.31	Exam, gynecological	Z01.411 Z01.419	Encounter for gynecological examination (general) (routine) with abnormal findings Encounter for gynecological examination (general) (routine) without abnormal findings
V72.32	Encounter for pap cervical smear to confirm findings of recent normal smear following initial abnormal smear	Z01.42	Encounter for cervical smear to confirm findings of recent normal smear following initial abnormal smear

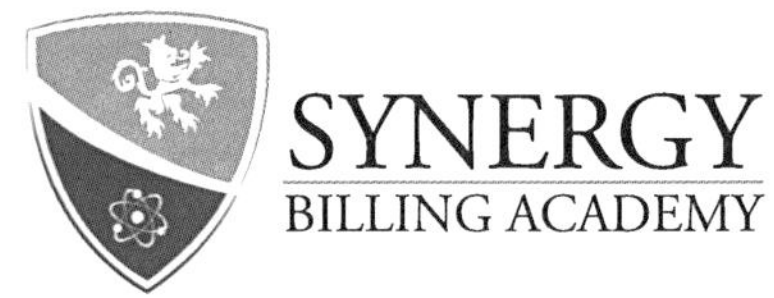

V72.41	Pregnancy examination or test negative	Z32.02	Encounter for pregnancy test, result negative
V72.85	Other specified examination	Z01.89	Encounter for other specified special examinations
V74.1	Screening examination for pulmonary tuberculosis	Z11.1	Encounter for screening for respiratory tuberculosis
V74.5	Screening for venereal disease STI	Z11.3	Encounter for screening for infections with a predominantly sexual mode of transmission
V76.2	Screening for malignant neoplasm, cervix	Z12.4	Encounter for screening for malignant neoplasm of cervix
V76.44	Special screening for malignant neoplasm of prostate	Z12.5	Encounter for screening for malignant neoplasm of prostate
V77.91	Screening for lipoid disorders	Z13.220	Encounter for screening for lipoid disorders
V78.0	Screening for iron deficiency – anemia	Z13.0	Encounter for screening for diseases of the blood and blood-forming organs and certain disorders involving the immune mechanism

E Codes: External Causes of Injury and Poisoning

ICD-9-CM	ICD-10-CM
Supplemental Classification of External Causes of Injury and Poisoning (E800-E99)	Injury, Poisoning, and Certain Other Conse quences of External Causes (S00-T88) T = Toxicity; External Causes of Morbidity (V01-Y99); Y = Why did it happen?

ICD-10-CM International Classification of Diseases 10th Revision Clinical Modification

Frequently Asked Questions

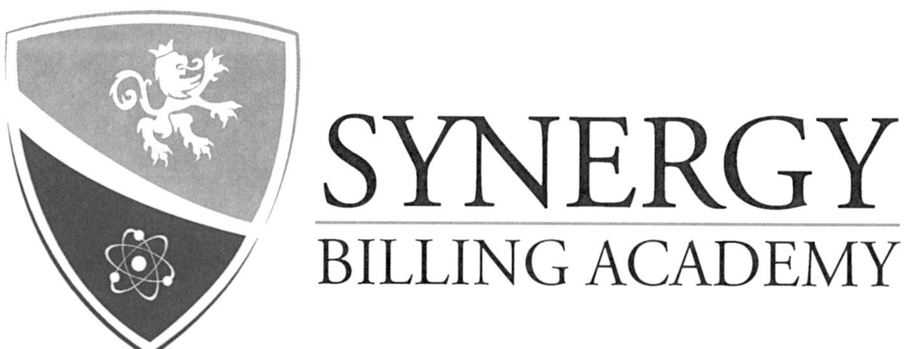

Frequently Asked Questions

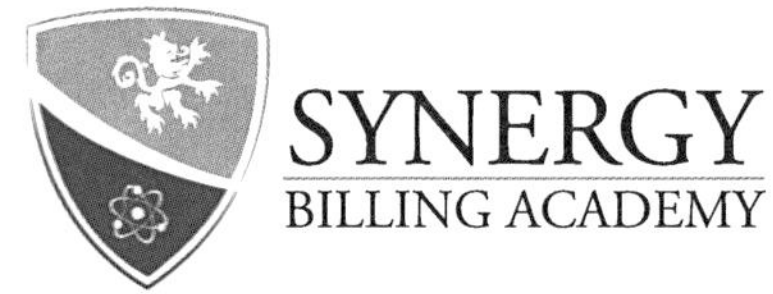

What is ICD-10? [47]

ICD-10 is a diagnostic coding system implemented by the World Health Organization (WHO) in 1993 to replace ICD-9, which was developed by WHO in the 1970s. ICD-10 is used in almost every country in the world, except the United States.

When we hear "ICD-10-CM" in the United States, it usually refers to the U.S. clinical modification of ICD-10: ICD-10-CM. This code set is scheduled to replace ICD-9-CM, our current U.S. diagnostic code set, on October 1, 2015.

Another designation, ICD-10-PCS, for "procedural coding system," will also be adopted in the United States. ICD-10-PCS will replace Volume 3 of ICD-9-CM as the inpatient procedural coding system. The final rule stated that CPT would remain the coding system for physician services.

Why is the United States moving to ICD-10-CM?

The ICD-9-CM code set is more than 30 years old and has become outdated. It is no longer considered usable for today's treatment, reporting, and payment processes. It does not reflect advances in medical technology and knowledge. In addition, the format limits our ability to expand the code set and add new codes.

ICD-9-CM has several problems. Foremost, it is out of room. Because the classification is organized scientifically, each three-digit category can have only 10 subcategories. Most numbers in most categories have been assigned diagnoses. Medical science keeps making new discoveries, yet there are no numbers to assign these diagnoses.

Computer science, combined with the new, more detailed codes in ICD-10-CM, will allow for better analysis of disease patterns and treatment outcomes that can advance medical care. These same details will streamline claims submissions, as these details will make the initial claim much easier for payers to understand.

The ICD-10-CM code set reflects advances in medicine and uses current medical terminology. The code format is expanded, which means that it can include greater detail within the code. This greater detail means that the code can provide more specific information about the diagnosis. The ICD-10-CM code set is also more flexible, allowing future expansion and encompassing new technologies and diagnoses. However, we expect the transition period to be disruptive for physicians; you are urged to begin preparing now.

Frequently Asked Questions

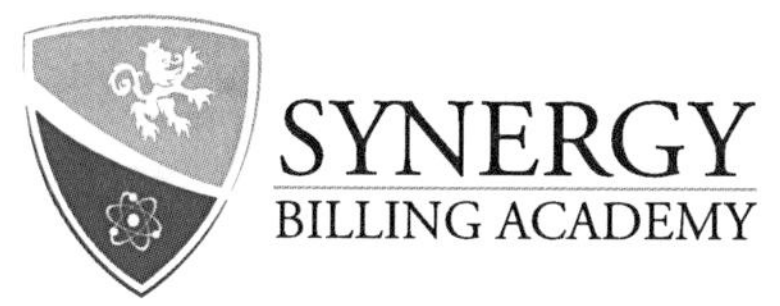

How is ICD-10-CM different from our current system?

In many ways, ICD-10-CM is much like ICD-9-CM. The guidelines, conventions, and rules are very similar. The organization of the codes is very similar. Anyone who is qualified to code ICD-9-CM should be able to make the transition to coding ICD-10-CM.

Many improvements have been made to coding in ICD-10-CM. For example, a single code can report a disease and its current manifestation (e.g., type 2 diabetes with diabetic retinopathy). In fracture care, the code differentiates an encounter for an initial fracture; follow-up of fracture healing normally; follow-up with fracture in malunion or nonunion; or follow-up for late effects of a fracture. Obstetrical codes now designate the trimester, adding specificity.

While much has been said about the huge increase in the number of codes under ICD-10-CM, some of this growth is due to laterality. While an ICD-9-CM code may identify a condition of, for example, the ovary, the parallel ICD-10-CM code identifies four codes: unspecified ovary, right ovary, left ovary, or bilateral condition of the ovaries.

The major differences between the two systems are differences that will affect information technology and software at your practice. Here's a chart showing the differences:

Issue	ICD-9-CM	ICD-10-CM
Volume of codes	Approximately 13,600	Approximately 69,000
Composition of codes	Mostly numeric, with E and V codes being alphanumeric. Valid codes have three, four, or five digits.	All codes are alphanumeric, beginning with a letter and with a mix of numbers and letters thereafter. Valid codes may have three, four, five, six, or seven digits.
Duplication of code sets	Currently, only ICD-9-CM codes are required. No mapping is necessary.	For a period of two years or more, systems will need to access both ICD-9-CM codes and ICD-10-CM codes as the country transitions between code sets. Mapping will be necessary so that equivalent codes can be found for issues of disease tracking, medical necessity edits and outcomes studies.

Frequently Asked Questions

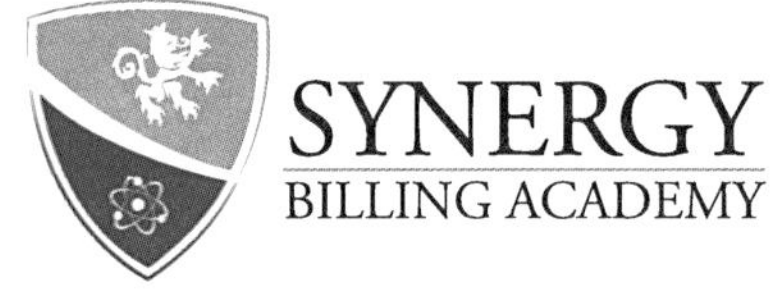

Because ICD-10-CM has more codes, is it more difficult to use than ICD-9-CM?

Just as the size of a dictionary or phone book doesn't make it more difficult to use, a higher number of codes doesn't necessarily increase the complexity of the coding system—in fact, it makes it easier to find the right code. Greater specificity and clinical accuracy make ICD-10-CM easier to use than ICD-9-CM. Because ICD-10-CM is much more specific, is more clinically accurate, and uses a more logical structure, it is much easier to use than ICD-9-CM. The Alphabetic Index and electronic coding tools will continue to facilitate proper code selection.

Explain the difference between ICD-10-CM and ICD-10-PCS.

ICD-10-CM is the diagnosis code set that will be replacing ICD-9-CM Volumes 1 and 2. ICD-10-CM will be used to report diagnoses in all clinical settings. ICD-10-PCS is the procedure code set that will be replacing ICD-9-CM Volume 3. ICD-10-PCS will be used to report hospital inpatient procedures only.

What is ICD-10-PCS?

ICD-10-PCS is a code set designed to replace Volume 3 of ICD-9-CM for inpatient procedure reporting. It will be used by hospitals and by payers. ICD-10-PCS is significantly different from Volume 3 and from CPT codes and will require significant training for users.

ICD-10-PCS will not affect coding of physician services in practice offices. However, physicians should be aware that documentation requirements under ICD-10-PCS are quite different, so their inpatient medical record documentation will be affected by this change.

ICD-10-PCS has nearly 79,000 seven-digit alphanumeric codes. Codes are selected from complex grids based on the type of procedure performed, approach, body part, and other characteristics. The code system does not use medical terminology based on Latin or eponyms.

Will ICD-10-PCS replace CPT?

No. ICD-10-PCS will be used to report hospital inpatient procedures only. The Current Procedural Terminology (CPT) and Healthcare Common Procedure Coding System (HCPCS) will continue to be used to report services and procedures in outpatient and office settings.

Frequently Asked Questions

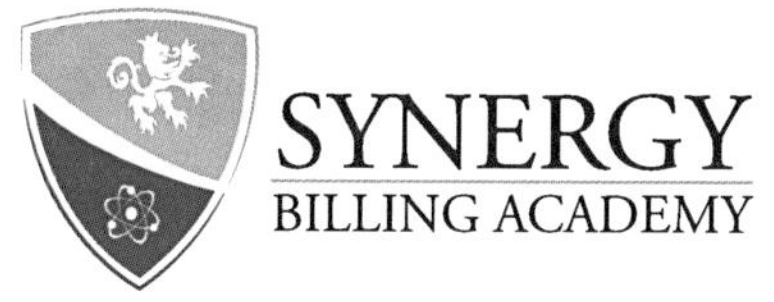

When will ICD-10-CM and ICD-10-PCS be implemented?

The Centers for Medicare and Medicaid Services (CMS) announced in January of 2009 that ICD-10-CM and ICD-10-PCS will be implemented into the HIPAA-mandated code set on October 1, 2015. Additionally, effective January 1, 2012, you must be ready to submit your claims electronically using the X12 Version 5010 and NCPDP Version D.0 standards. This is also a prerequisite for implementing the new ICD-10-CM/PCS codes. All services and discharges performed on or after October 1, 2015, must be coded using the ICD-10-CM/PCS code set. The necessary system and workflow changes need to be in place by the compliance date in order for you to send and receive the ICD-10-CM/PCS codes.

Do I have to upgrade to ICD-10-CM/PCS?

Yes. The conversion to ICD-10-CM/PCS is a HIPAA code set requirement. Providers, including physicians, are HIPAA "covered entities," which means that you must comply with the HIPAA requirements.

Who else has to upgrade to ICD-10-CM/PCS?

Health care clearinghouses and payers are also HIPAA-covered entities, so they are required to convert to ICD-10-CM/PCS as well.

I thought HIPAA code set standards only applied to the HIPAA electronic transactions. What if I don't use the HIPAA electronic transactions?

It is correct that HIPAA code set requirements apply only to the HIPAA electronic transactions. But it would be much too burdensome on the industry to use ICD-10-CM/PCS in electronic transactions and ICD-9-CM in manual transactions. Payers are expected to require that ICD-10-CM/PCS codes be used in other transactions, such as on paper, through a dedicated fax machine, or via the phone.

What if I'm not ready by the compliance deadline?

Any ICD-9-CM codes used in transactions for services or discharges on or after October 1, 2015, will be rejected as non-compliant and the transactions will not be processed. You will have disruptions in the processing of your transactions and receipt of your payments. Physicians are urged to set up a line of credit to mitigate any cash flow interruptions that may occur.

Frequently Asked Questions

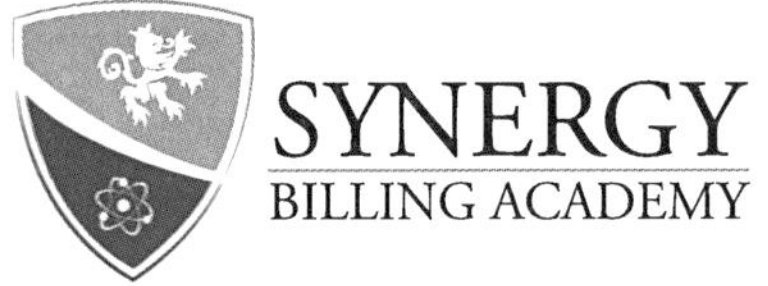

Deadlines for other HIPAA requirements have been delayed. Will the compliance date for ICD-10-CM/PCS be delayed?

Do not expect there to be a delay in the ICD-10-CM/PCS compliance deadline. The Centers for Medicare and Medicaid Services (CMS) is responsible for oversight of compliance with the HIPAA code set requirements. CMS has made it clear that there will be no extension of the deadline for ICD-10-CM/PCS. Work within Medicare to upgrade to the ICD-10-CM/PCS transactions is on schedule and they expect to be ready on time.

What is the grace period for the use of ICD-9-CM codes submitted after implementation of the new ICD-10-CM/PCS codes?

CMS has indicated that there will be no delay in implementation of ICD-10. The following are excerpts from the CMS website:

Remember: ICD-10-CM/PCS compliance date for implementation

- October 1, 2015 – Compliance date for implementation of ICD-10-CM (diagnoses) and ICD-10-PCS (procedures)
  - No delays
  - No grace period
- Implementation planning should be undertaken with the assumption that the Department of Health and Human Services (HHS) will not grant an extension beyond the October 1, 2015, compliance date.

HHS has no plans to extend the compliance date for implementation of ICD-10-CM/PCS; therefore, covered entities should plan to complete the steps required in order to implement ICD-10-CM/PCS by October 1, 2015.

Who is affected by the transition to ICD-10-CM/PMS? If I don't deal with Medicare claims, will I have to transition?

Everyone covered by HIPAA must use ICD-10-CM/PCS starting October 1, 2015. This includes health care providers and payers who do not deal with Medicare claims. Organizations that are not covered by HIPAA but use ICD-9-CM codes should be aware that their coding may become obsolete if they do not transition to ICD-10-CM/PCS.

Frequently Asked Questions

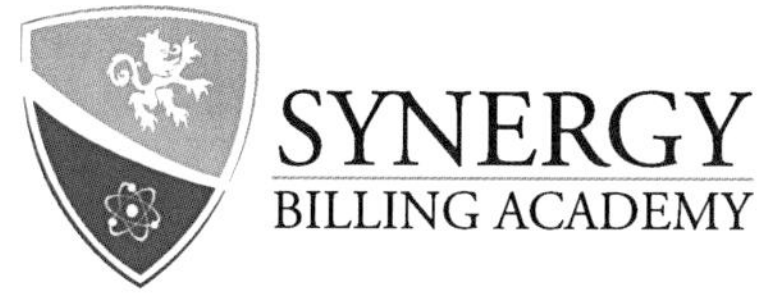

Do state Medicaid programs need to transition to ICD-10-CM/PCS?

Yes. Like everyone else covered by HIPAA, state Medicaid programs must use ICD-10-CM/PCS for services provided on or after October 1, 2015.

What happens if I do not switch to ICD-10-CM/PCS?

Claims for all health care services and hospital inpatient procedures performed on or after October 1, 2015, must use ICD-10-CM/PCS diagnosis and inpatient procedure codes. (This does not apply to CPT coding for outpatient procedures.) Claims that do not use ICD-10-CM/PCS diagnosis and inpatient procedure codes cannot be processed. It is important to note, however, that claims for services provided before October 1, 2015, must use ICD-9-CM diagnosis and inpatient procedure codes.

Codes change every year, so why is the transition to ICD-10-CM/PCS any different from the annual code changes?

ICD-10-CM/PCS codes are completely different from ICD-9-CM codes. Currently, ICD-9-CM codes are mostly numeric and have three to five digits. ICD-10-CM/PCS codes are alphanumeric and contain three to seven characters. ICD-10-CM/PCS is more robust and descriptive with "one-to-many" matches to ICD-9-CM in some instances. As with ICD-9-CM codes, ICD-10-CM/PCS codes will be updated every year. ICD-9-CM codes will not continue to be updated after October 1, 2015.

What should providers do to prepare for the transition to ICD-10-CM/PCS?

For providers who have not yet started to transition to ICD-10-CM/PCS, we have provided some action steps to take now. Some of these activities, such as establishing a transition team and communicating to internal staff, might not be necessary for small practices where one or two people would be handling the transition activities.

- Establish a transition team or ICD-10CM/PCS project coordinator, depending on the size of your organization, to lead your transition to ICD-10-CM/PCS. Develop a plan for making the transition to ICD-10-CM/PCS; include a timeline that identifies tasks to be completed and crucial milestones/relationships, task owners, resources needed, and estimated start and end dates.

Frequently Asked Questions

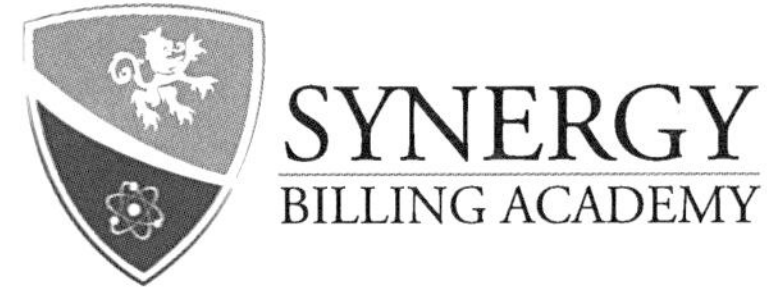

- Determine how ICD-10-CM/PCS will affect your organization. Start by reviewing how and where you currently use ICD-9-CM codes. Make sure you have accounted for the use of ICD-9-CM in authorizations/pre-certifications, physician orders, medical records, superbills/ encounter forms, practice management and billing systems, and coding manuals.
- Review how ICD-10-CM/PCS will affect clinical documentation requirements and electronic health record (EHR) templates.
- Communicate the plan, timeline, and new system changes and processes to your organization, and ensure that leadership and staff understand the extent of the effort the ICD-10-CM/PCS transition requires.
- Secure a budget that accounts for software upgrades/software license costs, hardware procurement, staff training costs, revision of forms, workflow changes during and after implementation, and risk mitigation.
- Talk with your payers, billing and IT staff, and practice management system and/or EHR vendors about their preparations and readiness.
- Coordinate your ICD-10-CM/PCS transition plans among your trading partners and evaluate contracts with payers and vendors for policy revisions, testing timelines, and costs related to the ICD-10-CM/PCS transition.

Why should I prepare now for the ICD-10-CM/PCS transition?

The transition from ICD-9-CM to ICD-10-CM/PCS will change how you do business. Health care organizations, from large national plans to small provider offices, laboratories, medical testing centers, hospitals, and more will need to devote staff time and financial resources for transition activities.

What does ICD-10-CM/PCS compliance mean?

All HIPAA-covered entities must be able to successfully conduct health care transactions using the ICD-10-CM/PCS diagnosis and procedure codes. ICD-9-CM diagnosis and procedure codes can no longer be used for services provided on or after the October 1, 2015, implementation date.

Frequently Asked Questions

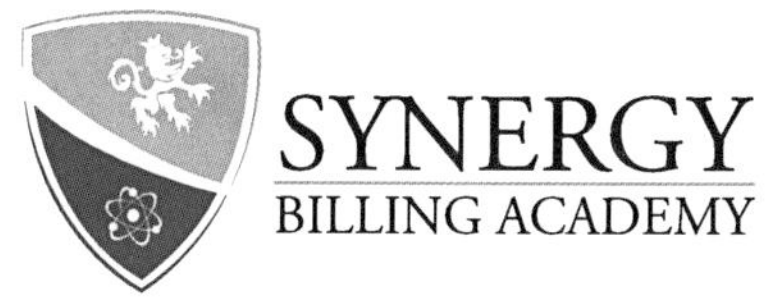

What is the primary purpose of this change?

The primary purpose of the change to ICD-10-CM/PCS is to improve clinical communication. It allows for the capture of more data about signs, symptoms, risk factors, and comorbidities and better describes the clinical issues overall. It will also enable the United States to exchange information across international borders.

What is the deciding factor on when to use ICD-10-CM/PCS codes?

For outpatient services, ICD-10-CM codes are required for dates of service on or after the compliance date. For inpatient services, ICD-10-PCS codes are required on the date of discharge after the compliance date.

Will there be a period of time when both codes will be required on the same claim?

No. Per CMS guidance, ICD-9-CM codes will no longer be accepted on institutional, professional or supplier claims (including electronic and paper) with FROM date of service or date of discharge through dates on or after October 1, 2015. A claim cannot contain both ICD-9-CM codes and ICD-10-CM/PCS codes. Institutional claims will be returned to the health care provider. Professional and supplier claims will be returned as not able to process.

Will ICD-10-CM/PCS codes be required for authorization of services that occur after October 1, 2015?

Yes. ICD-10-CM/PCS codes will be required for dates of service after the implementation date.

What changes in payment will there be with the change to ICD-10-CM/PCS?

There should be no change to the way a claim is paid from ICD-9-CM to ICD-10-CM/PCS codes, unless a diagnosis-related group (DRG) change has taken place or a contract has been rewritten to incorporate a change of reimbursement.

What do you offer for implementation training and when should our office begin?

Synergy has custom-made services for you!

Frequently Asked Questions

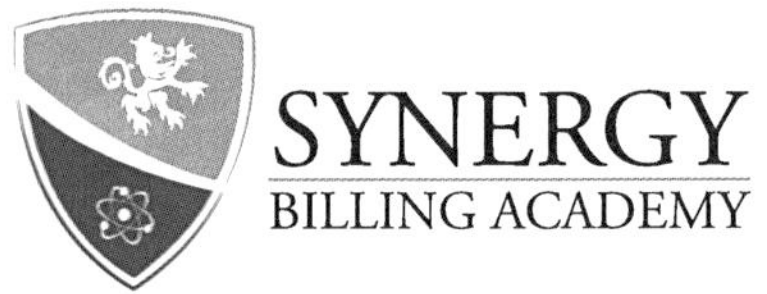

- **Taskforce**

  Thanks to our proactive approach, we have a highly knowledgeable team to help you navigate through this transition without impacting your cash flow. You can rely on us, the FQHC billing experts, to ensure that your cash flow is not interrupted.

- **Internal Training**

  As one of the top companies in the nation, all of our employees and team members go through a series of in-house training sessions to stay abreast of all the new changes in billing and the new ICD-10-CM code set.

- **Online Webinars**

  We offer online training webinars covering a range of topics, from an introduction to ICD-10-CM to training on coding each body system.. Because we understand the work load, these webinars will be offered at a time of your convenience. Once these are completed, you will have access to unlimited recordings for refreshers.

- **On-Site Training**

  Training is the only step that will ensure a smooth transition to the ICD-10-CM code set. Along with the webinars, we also offer on-site training programs which will help to make the transition successful. The on-site training programs are designed to fit your needs and are based on your timetable.

- **Quick Guide**

  As we move from having about 14,000 codes to having about 68,000 codes, Synergy will provide you with a crosswalk of the top 150 used by FQHCs, moving from ICD-9-CM codes to ICD-10-CM.

Frequently Asked Questions

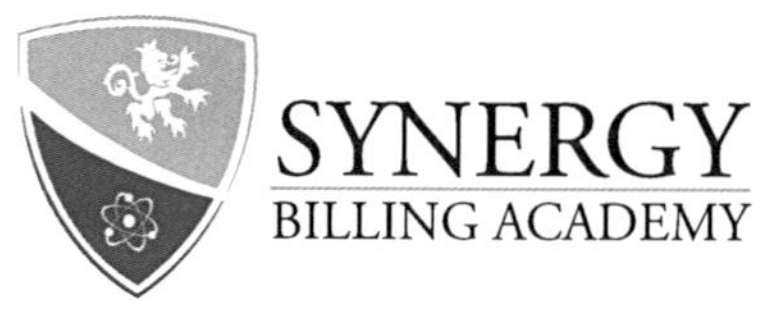

- **FAQ Bulletins**

  There are a lot of assumptions and questions regarding the new code set. Here at Synergy, we understand your concerns and will provide you with answers to all of your ICD-10-CM questions.

- **Open Forum**

  As our partner, you will have the ability to join our blog to discuss questions, answers, and solutions in real time.

- **ICD-10-CM Support**

  Here at Synergy Billing Academy, we have taken a proactive approach to ensure that the necessary steps are in place to keep your practice running smoothly with no interruption in your revenue cycle. With Synergy by your side, you have nothing to worry about; we will make sure that you are prepared for October 1, 2015.

ICD-10-CM International Classification of Diseases 10th Revision Clinical Modification

Myths Versus Facts

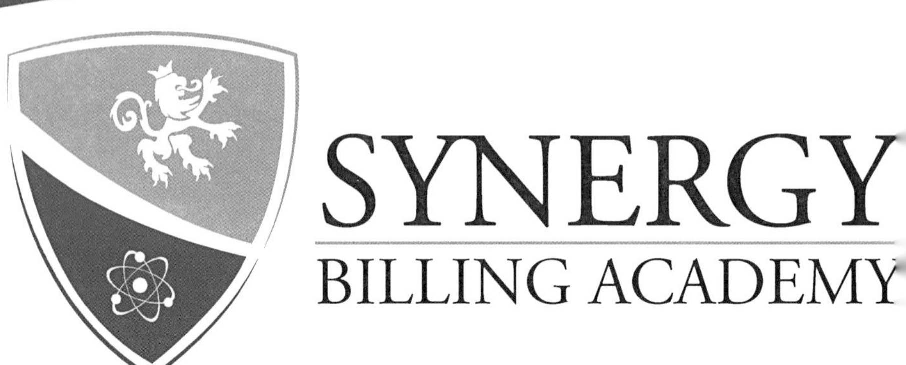

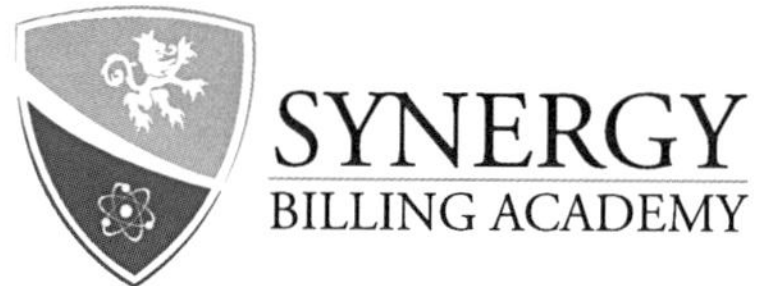

There will be another delay to the ICD-10-CM/PCS implementation deadline. [49, 50]

CMS has confirmed that there will be no more delays, but it's understandable that so many people expect one. We already received an extension from the original deadline in 2013 and much of the industry is still behind in preparation. Despite this, October 1, 2015, is still the official deadline. It is important that health care organizations are prepared to submit claims with ICD-10-CM/PCS codes by this date. Pat Brooks, senior technical advisor at CMS, confirms that "the ICD-10 CM/PCS implementation date will not be delayed further."

CMS and HHS currently have no plans to move the date or extend the conversion process. Any provider who is not ready to use ICD-10-CM/PCS codes starting on October 1, 2015, will not be reimbursed for services performed on or after that date if they are coded in ICD-9-CM. The two-year delay from 2013 to 2015 has already caused significant disruptions in the planning process.

All Health Insurance Portability and Accountability Act (HIPAA)-covered entities must implement the new code sets with dates of service, or date of discharge for inpatients, that occur on or after October 1, 2015. Covered entities should plan to complete the steps required to implement ICD-10-CM/PCS on October 1, 2015.

With less than a year left to prepare, it's essential that you plan well to be ready for the transition. As you are preparing, think about everywhere you currently use an ICD-9-CM code and create a gap analysis so these areas can be modified for ICD-10-CM/PCS.

Training your staff for ICD-10-CM/PCS will also need to be a major focus, as billers and coders will need to code in the new system. Remember to include time to train your physicians and clinical staff, because they will need to know what type of documentation to provide in patient charts to help the coders identify the appropriate ICD-10-CM/PCS code.

Even with thorough planning in place, you may still experience payment delays once ICD-10-CM/PCS takes effect. It is strongly recommended that you establish a loan or line of credit to help tide your organization over if you experience delays in reimbursement during the transition.

Implementation of ICD-10-CM/PCS can wait until after electronic health records and other health care initiatives have been established.

Implementation of ICD-10-CM/PCS cannot wait for the implementation of other health care initiatives. As management of health information becomes increasingly electronic, the cost of

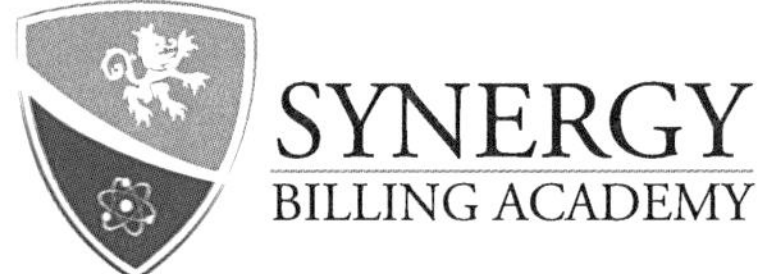

implementing a new coding system will increase due to required systems and applications upgrades.

Non-covered entities that are not covered by HIPAA, such as worker's compensation and auto insurance companies that use International Classification of Diseases, 9th Edition, Clinical Modification (ICD-9-CM), may choose not to implement ICD-10-CM/PCS.

Because ICD-9-CM will no longer be maintained after ICD-10-CM/PCS is implemented, it is in non-covered entities' best interest to use the new coding system. The increased detail in ICD-10-CM/PCS is of significant value to non-covered entities. The Centers for Medicare and Medicaid Services (CMS) will work with non-covered entities to encourage their use of ICD-10-CM/PCS.

All HIPAA-covered entities, including physicians and hospitals, are mandated to switch to ICD-10CM/PCS in 2015. But that doesn't include every single type of organization that currently uses ICD-9-CM. Worker's compensation and auto insurance companies, for example, use ICD-9-CM codes but are not required to make the leap to ICD-10-CM/PCS. But it's in their best interests to do so, according to CMS, because physicians and hospitals will be using the newer codes. The increased detail and specificity will be just as useful for worker's comp as it is for the emergency department. CMS will work with non-covered entities to help them make the transition. State Medicaid Programs will also receive CMS help to ensure that they will meet the deadline.

State Medicaid plans are not required to transition to ICD-10-CM/PCS.

All entities coved by HIPAA will need to transition to ICD-10-CM/PCS, and this includes all state Medicaid plans. Major industry changes like this are challenging for state Medicaid plans due to their limited funding, so CMS is providing special assistance to help them with this massive transition. However, it is possible that some state Medicaid plans will not be ready by the October 1, 2015, deadline.

Other payers that are not covered by HIPAA, such as property and casualty insurance, worker's compensation, and auto insurance, are encouraged, but not required, to become ICD-10-CM/PCS compliant. While some states are requiring these payers to transition to ICD-10-CM/PCS, others will not switch to ICD-10-CM/PCS.

You will likely continue to use ICD-9-CM codes for at least some payers after October 1, 2015, such as those not covered by HIPAA and state Medicaid plans still in transition. It will be important to talk with your practice, revenue cycle management vendors, and clearinghouse to make sure

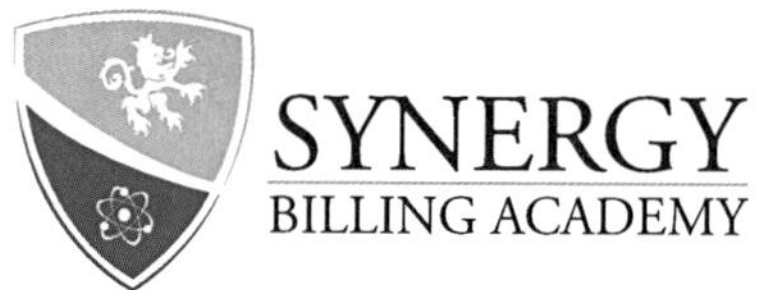

your system can accommodate both the ICD-9-CM and the ICD-10-CM/PCS code sets. This will help keep your revenue from being at risk from these payers.

Everything is going to get more complicated—prohibitively so.

ICD-10-CM/PCS has a lot of codes, 140,000 of them, to be exact; but just as increasing the number of words in a dictionary doesn't make it harder to use, the greater number of ICD-10-CM/PCS codes won't significantly affect the complexity of coding, CMS explains. Electronic decision support tools and organized code books will make finding the right code easy, and the new logical structure of ICD-10-CM/PCS will help coders find exactly what they're looking for.

Nonspecific codes are still available for use if supported by clinical documentation, and much of the detail necessary for ICD-10-CM/PCS coding is already present. Providers do not need to perform unnecessary diagnostic tests just to get to the most specific code that exists in the code book. Superbills based on ICD-10-CM/PCS won't necessarily be any longer or more complicated than ICD-9 superbills and codes can be crosswalked to help the conversion process.

The increased number of codes in ICD-10-CM/PCS will make the new coding system impossible to use.

Just as an increase in the number of words in a dictionary doesn't make it more difficult to use, the greater number of codes in ICD-10-CM/PCS doesn't necessarily make it more complex to use. In fact, the greater number of codes in ICD-10-CM/PCS makes it easier for you to find the right code. In addition, just as you don't have to search the entire list of ICD-9-CM codes for the proper code, you also don't have to conduct searches of the entire list of ICD-10-CM/PCS codes. The Alphabetic Index and electronic coding tools are available to help you select the proper code. It is anticipated that the improved structure and specificity of ICD-10-CM/PCS will assist in developing increasingly sophisticated electronic coding tools, helping you to select the codes more quickly. Because ICD-10-CM/PCS is much more specific, is more clinically accurate, and uses a more logical structure, it is much easier to use than ICD-9-CM. Most physician practices use a relatively small number of diagnosis codes that are generally related to a specific type of specialty.

Unnecessarily detailed medical record documentation will be required when ICD-10-CM/PCS is implemented.

As with ICD-9-CM, ICD-10-CM/PCS codes should be based on medical record documentation.

Myths Versus Facts

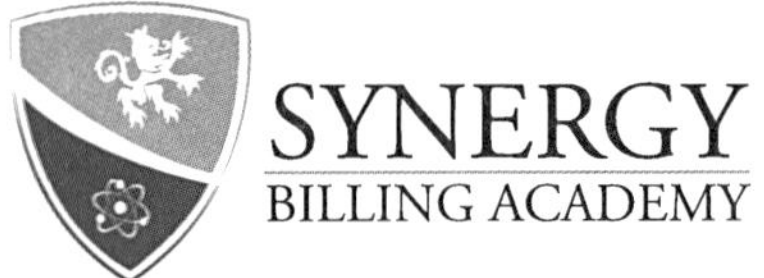

While documentation supporting accurate and specific codes will result in higher quality data, nonspecific codes are still available for use when documentation doesn't support a higher level of specificity.

As demonstrated by the American Hospital Association/American Health Information Management Association field testing study, much of the detail contained in ICD-10-CM is already in medical record documentation, but is not currently needed for ICD-9-CM coding.

Medically unnecessary diagnostic tests will need to be performed to assign an ICD-10-CM code.

As with ICD-9-CM, ICD-10-CM codes are derived from documentation in the medical record. Therefore, if a diagnosis has not yet been established, you should code the condition to its highest degree of certainty (which may be a sign or symptom) when using both coding systems. In fact, ICD-10-CM contains many more codes for signs and symptoms than ICD-9-CM, and it is better designed for use in ambulatory encounters when definitive diagnoses are often not yet known. Nonspecific codes are still available in ICD-10-CM/PCS for use when more detailed clinical information is not known.

My electronic medical records system will automate the conversion of ICD-10-CM/PCS for me.

The use of an electronic medical record (EMR) will not automate the conversion of ICD-9-CM to ICD-10-CM/PCS. Many organizations and physicians are implementing electronic medical records with the belief that the EMR will take care of their transition to ICD-10-CM/PCS. Although the implementation or use of an EMR can help with the documentation challenges providers will confront in the new ICD-10-CM/PCS world, the use of an EMR alone is not a magic bullet.

Implementing ICD-10-CM/PCS won't change my current workflow.

Some experts predict ICD-10-CM/PCS could increase physician documentation time by 15 percent. Challenges will exist for physicians when assigning and ranking of diagnoses for the patient's encounter.

In the current EMR environment, many providers are completing data elements and selecting diagnosis codes from drop-down lists. In many cases, the number of codes from which to select a diagnosis will increase exponentially. Medicare also has indicated it may no longer reimburse for claims submitted using "unspecified" codes.

Myths Versus Facts

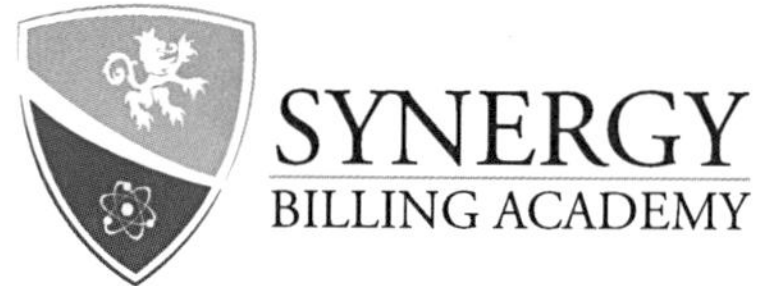

ICD-10-CM/PCS was developed without clinical input.

The development of ICD-10-CM/PCS involved significant clinical input. A number of medical specialty societies contributed to the development of the coding systems.

ICD-10-CM/PCS was developed a number of years ago, so it is probably already out of date.

Prior to the implementation of the partial code freeze, ICD-10-CM/PCS codes had been updated annually since their original development to keep pace with advances in medicine and technology and changes in the health care environment. The ICD-9-CM Coordination and Maintenance Committee implemented a partial freeze during which only codes capturing new technologies and new diseases would be added to ICD-9-CM and ICD-10-CM/PCS. The code freeze resulted in the following updates:

- On October 1, 2011, the last regular, annual updates were made to both code sets.
- On October 1, 2012, and October 1, 2013, only limited code updates for new technologies and new diseases were made to both code sets as required by Section 503(a) of Public Law 108-173.
- On October 1, 2014, only limited code updates for new technologies and new diseases were made to the ICD-10-CM/PCS code sets to capture new technologies and diseases. No further updates will be made to ICD-9-CM on or after October 1, 2015, as it will no longer be used for reporting.
- On October 1, 2015, regular updates to ICD-10-CM/PCS will resume.

Current Procedural Terminology (CPT) will be replaced by ICD-10-PCS.

ICD-10-PCS will only be used for facility reporting of hospital inpatient procedures and will not affect the use of CPT.

ICD-10-CM-based superbills will be too long or too complex to be of much use.

Practices may continue to create superbills that contain the most common diagnosis codes used in their practice. ICD-10-CM-based superbills will not necessarily be longer or more complex than ICD-9-CM-based superbills. Neither current superbills nor ICD-10-CM-based superbills provide all possible code options for many conditions. The superbill conversion process includes conducting a review that includes removing rarely used codes and crosswalking common codes from ICD-9-CM to ICD-10-CM, which can be accomplished by looking up codes in the ICD-10-CM code book or using the General Equivalence Mappings (GEMs).

Myths Versus Facts

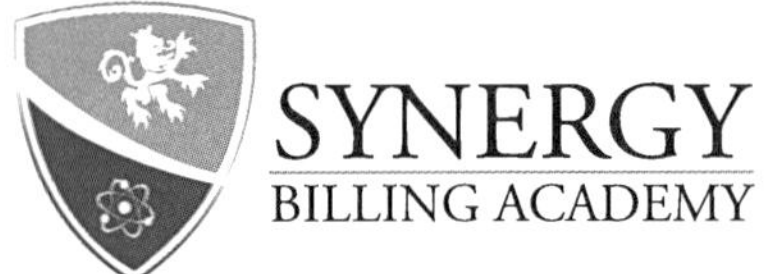

The GEMs were developed to provide help in coding medical records.

CMS developed the GEMs, or General Equivalence Mappings, to help guide the industry as we convert payment systems, coverage edits, and other databases from ICD-9-CM to ICD-10-CM/PCS.

While the GEMs are helpful to show which ICD-10-CM/PCS codes may correspond to your existing ICD-9-CM codes, they are not intended to be used to code ICD-10-CM/PCS claims because they do not include all the necessary information for the coding process. When providers code claims, they need to refer to clinical documentation in the patient's medical record to identify the most appropriate ICD-10-CM/PCS code. The ICD-10-CM/PCS code set has more than five times the amount of codes as ICD-9-CM, so the detail in the patient record will provide the specificity coders need to choose the correct code.

The GEMs are a handy tool intended to help update payment systems, risk adjustment logic, quality measures, and research databases by mapping one code set to the other. They are not a one-to-one solution for coding an individual clinical chart. Mapping is not the same as coding, CMS warns, because the GEMs do not allow for the selection of the most accurate and applicable ICD-10-CM/PCS code.

Mapping is not the same as coding:

- Mapping links concepts in two code sets without considering patient medical record information.
- Coding involves the assignment of the most appropriate code based on medical record documentation and applicable coding rules/guidelines.
- The GEMs can be used to convert the following databases from ICD-9-CM to ICD-10-CM/PCS:
  - Payment systems
  - Quality measures
  - Payment and coverage edits
  - A variety of research applications involving trend data
  - Risk adjustment logic

The GEMs are free of charge and available to any provider who wishes to use them. Code books, which are available in physical hard copies and electronic editions, should be used to deal with individual patient charts.

ICD-10-CM International Classification of Diseases 10th Revision Clinical Modification

Unusual New Codes

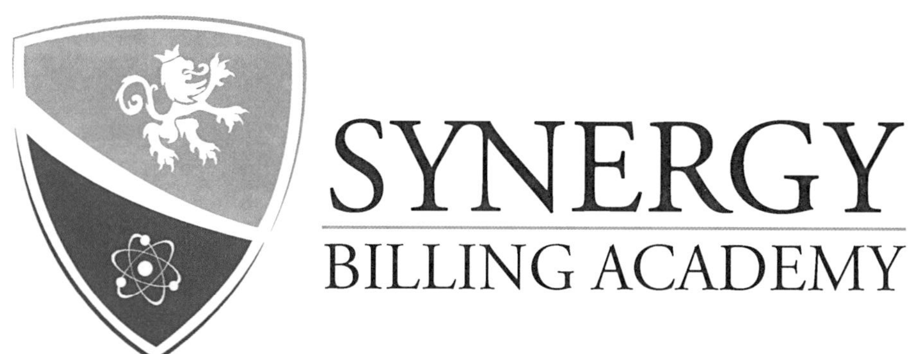

Unusual New Codes

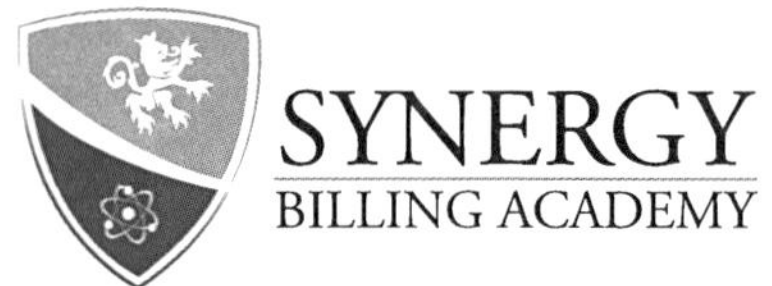

Unusual New Codes [10]

1. F40.243 Fear of flying
2. R42 Dizziness and giddiness
3. R46.0 Very low level of personal hygiene
4. R46.1 Bizarre personal appearance
5. R46.4 Slowness and poor responsiveness
6. T15.91XA Foreign body on external eye, part unspecified, right eye, initial encounter
7. T50.5X6A Underdosing of appetite depressants, initial encounter
8. T63.442S Toxic effect of venom of bees, intentional self-harm, sequela
9. T71.231D Asphyxiation due to being trapped in a discarded refrigerator, accidental
10. V61.6XXD Passenger in heavy transport vehicle injured in collision with pedal cycle in traffic accident, subsequent encounter
11. V80.730A Animal-rider injured in collision with trolley
12. V90.37XA Submersion due to falling or jumping from crushed water skis
13. V91.07XA Burn due to water skis on fire, initial encounter
14. V91.07XD Burn due to water skis on fire, subsequent encounter
15. V91.30XA Hit or struck by falling object due to accident on merchant ship, initial encounter
16. V91.35XA Hit or struck by falling object due to accident in canoe or kayak
17. V94.810 Civilian watercraft involved in water transport accident with military watercraft
18. V95.42XA Forced landing of spacecraft injuring occupant, initial encounter
19. V96.00XS Unspecified balloon accident injuring occupant, sequela
20. V97.33XD Sucked into jet engine, subsequent encounter

Have you suffered a burn due to your flaming water-skis?
Your doctor will soon have a code for that.

Unusual New Codes

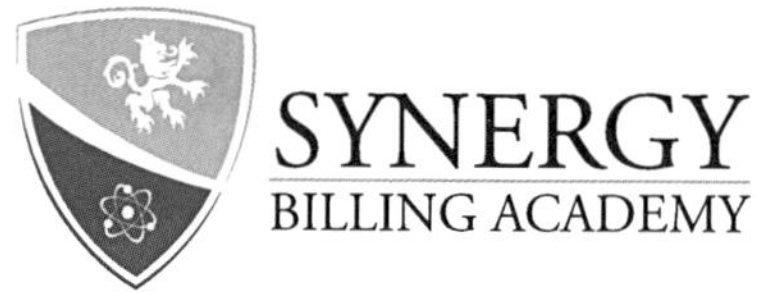

21. W16.221 Fall into bucket of water, causing drowning and submersion
22. W21.00XA Struck by hit or thrown ball, unspecified type, initial encounter
23. W22.02XA Walked into lamppost, initial encounter
24. W22.02XD Walked into a lamppost, subsequent encounter
25. W25 Contact with sharp glass
26. W29.0 Contact with powered kitchen appliance, subsequent encounter
27. W34.110 Accidental malfunction of BB gun
28. W45.1 Paper entering through skin
29. W49.01XA Hair causing external constriction
30. W50.1XXS Accidental kick by another person, sequela
31. W56.11XD Bitten by sea lion
32. W56.21XA Bitten by orca, initial encounter
33. W56.22XA Struck by orca, initial encounter
34. W56.49 Other contact with shark
35. W59.21XS Bitten by turtle
36. W59.22XS Struck by turtle, sequela
37. W61.12XA Struck by macaw – (Pesky, talking birds)
38. W61.42XD Struck by turkey, subsequent encounter
39. W61.62 Struck by duck
40. X52 Prolonged stay in weightless environment
41. Y34 Unspecified event, undetermined intent
42. Y92.146 Hurt at swimming pool of prison as the place of occurrence
43. Y92.241 Hurt at the library
44. Y92.253 Hurt at the opera – opera house as the place of occurrence of the external cause
45. Y93.D Contact with scissors; activities involving arts and handcrafts
46. Y93.D1 Stabbed while crocheting; activity, knitting and crocheting
47. Z37.54 Sextuplets, all liveborn
48. Z62.1 Parental overprotection
49. Z62.891 Sibling rivalry
50. Z63.1 Problems in relationship with the in-laws
51. Z73.1 Type A behavior pattern
52. Z73.4 Inadequate social skills, not elsewhere classified
53. Z89.419 Acquired absence of unspecified great toe

ICD-10-CM International Classification of Diseases 10th Revision Clinical Modification

References

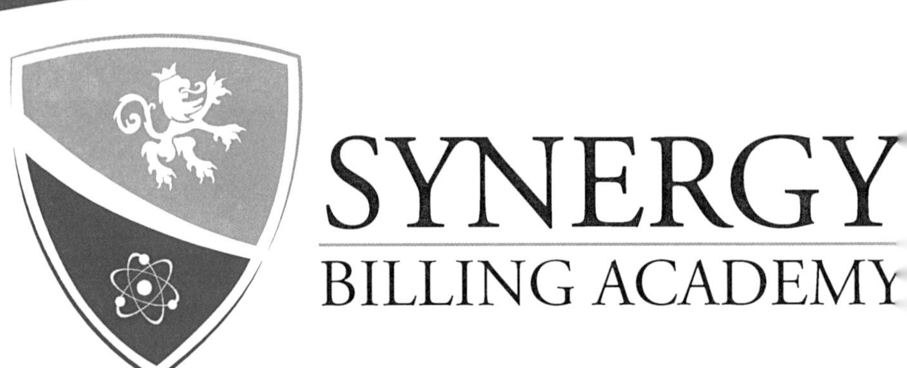

References

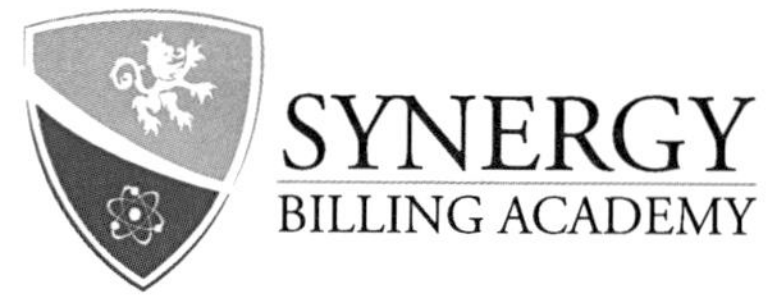

1. American Academy of Professional Coders. (n.d.). What is Medical Coding? Retrieved from http://www.aapc.com/medical-coding/medical-coding.aspx

2. World Health Organization (WHO). (2001, July 6). History of the development of the ICD. Retrieved from http://www.who.int/classifications/icd/en/HistoryOfICD.pdf

3. Harrison, C. (2010). ICD-9-CM Basics. In Medical Office Handbook. Boston, MA: McGraw Hill Higher Education.

4. Buck, C. J. (2013). Step-by-Step Medical Coding (2013 ed.). St. Louis, MO: Elsevier/Saunders.

5. Buck, C. J., & Netter, F. H. (2013). 2013 ICD-9-CM for Hospitals, Volumes 1, 2, & 3 (Professional ed.). St. Louis, Mo.: Elsevier.

6. Centers for Disease Control and Prevention. (2011). ICD-9-CM Official Guidelines for Coding and Reporting. Retrieved from http://www.cdc.gov/nchs/data/icd/icd9cm_guidelines_2011.pdf

7. Centers for Medicare and Medicaid Services. (2013, June 4). ICD-10 Small-MedPractice Handbook. Retrieved from http://www.cms.gov/Medicare/Coding/ICD10/Downloads/ICD-10_Small-MedPractice_Handbook_060413[1].pdf

8. Centers for Medicare and Medicaid Services. (2015, June 1). ICD-10-CM Classification Enhancements. Retrieved from http://www.cms.gov/Medicare/Coding/ICD10/downloads/ICD-10QuickRefer.pdf

9. Centers for Disease Control and Prevention. (2015). ICD-10-CM Official Guidelines for Coding and Reporting. Retrieved from http://www.cdc.gov/nchs/data/icd/icd10cm_guidelines_2015.pdf

10. Buck, C. J., & Buck, C. J. (2013). 2013 ICD-10-CM Draft (2013 ed.). St. Louis, Mo.: Elsevier.

11. Centers for Medicare and Medicaid Services. (2015, June 1). ICD-10-CM/PCS The Next Generation Of Coding. Retrieved from http://www.cms.gov/Medicare/Coding/ICD10/downloads/ICD-10Overview.pdf

12. ADP AdvancedMD. (n.d.). My ICD-10. Retrieved from http://myicd10.advancedmd.com/assets/uploads/ADP_AdvancedMD_Chart_Audit_Webinar_AAPC_2013.pdf

13. Centers for Medicare and Medicaid Services. (2013, March 19). 2013 Webinar Series #1 – Pathway through the ICD-10 Maze. Retrieved from http://www.cms.org/uploads/first-step-slides_3-19.ppt

References

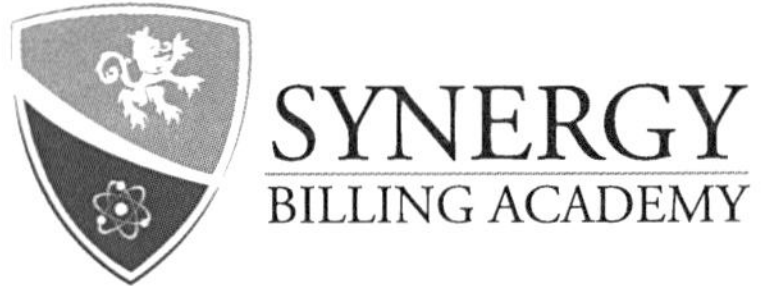

14. Nichols, J. (2011, March 1). Applications and Technologies Collaborative - ICD-10 – Physician Impacts. Retrieved from http://www.christianacare.org/workfiles/medicaldentalstaff/icd10/ICD-10-Physician-Impacts-3-7-11.pdf

15. Zeisset, Ann. "Coding Injuries in ICD-10-CM." Journal of AHIMA 82, no.1 (January 2011): 52-54. Retrieved from http://library.ahima.org/xpedio/groups/public/documents/ahima/bok1_048533.hcsp?dDocName=bok1_048533

16. Cruz, A., & Shebala, S. (2013, April 8). ICD-10-CM: Training. Retrieved from http://www.nmhima.org/wp-content/uploads/ICD-10-CM-AHIMA.pdf

17. American Academy of Professional Coders. (n.d.). ICD-10 Documentation Example. Retrieved from http://www.aapc.com/icd-10/icd-10-documentation-example.aspx

18. Leppert, M. (2014, January 10). Beware the Boiling Water Toss | ICD-10 Trainer. Retrieved from http://blogs.hcpro.com/icd-10/2014/01/beware-the-boiling-water-toss/

19. American Academy of Professional Coders. (2011, July 13). ICD-10 Clinical Documentation Improvement. Retrieved from http://news.aapc.com/index.php/2011/07/icd-10-clinical-documentation-improvement/

20. Ormondroyd, T., Scott, B., & Oliver, C. (2013, March 20). Helping Physicians Succeed in an ICD-10 World. Retrieved from http://icd10.dignityhealthmember.org/Media/documents/Helping_Physicians_Succeed.pdf

21. Medex Diagnostic & Treatment Center. (n.d.). Family Physicians Education and Training. Retrieved from http://www.medexwellness.com/37-health-database/family-practice.html?layout=blog&Itemid=110

22. ICARE Clinics. (n.d.). ICARE-CLINICS. Retrieved from http://www.icare-clinics.com/blog-detail/MQ==

23. 23. Shah Associates. (n.d.). Internal Medicine. Retrieved from http://www.shah-associates.com/specialties/Internal-Medicine/10

24. Devault, K., Barta, A., & Endicott, M. (2013). ICD-10-CM Coder Training Manual 2013. S.l.: Amer Health Info Mgmt Asc.

25. American Congress of Obstetricians and Gynecologists. (2005, February 6). Women's Health Care Physicians. Retrieved from https://www.acog.org/About_ACOG/Scope_of_Practice

26. Brown, M., & Stilley, P. (2013, May 1). Documentation and the Government. Retrieved from http://static.aapc.com/a3c7c3fe-6fa1-4d67-8534-a3c9c8315fa0/e0bdf19e-6a7c-4179-9300-8acc467f224e/3e149886-7ad5-4868-99a8-7784fc95b8a5.pdf

References

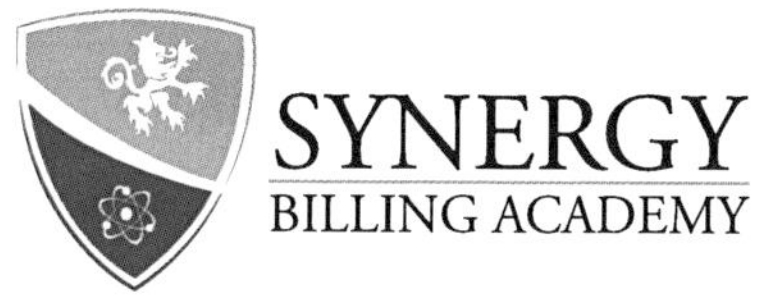

27. Eramo, L. (2014, January 23). 6 ICD-10 Tips for OB/GYN Specialists. Retrieved from http://gettingpaid.kareo.com/gettingpaid/2014/01/6-icd-10-tips-for-obgyn-specialists/

28. Dr. Lockwood, C. (2013, September 1). ICD-10 and the OB/GYN. Retrieved from http://contemporaryobgyn.modernmedicine.com/contemporary-obgyn/news/icd-10-and-obgyn?page=full

29. American Academy of Professional Coders. (2013, February 15). OB/GYN Quick Reference for ICD-10-CM. Retrieved from http://cloud.aapc.com/documents/OB-GYN-Quick-Reference_ICD-10-CM.pdf

30. Enos, N. (2014, January 29). 2014 CPT Code Update and ICD-10 Changes for OB/GYN. Retrieved from http://chmbinc.com/wp-content/uploads/2014/01/PowerPoint-Slides.pdf

31. American Academy of Professional Coders. (2012, May 25). ICD-10 Assessment Summary. Retrieved from http://cloud.aapc.com/pdf/Sample-I-10-Report.pdf

32. Munson Healthcare. (2015). ICD-10 Quick Reference Cards - For Physicians - Munson Healthcare. Retrieved from http://www.munsonhealthcare.org/icd10/quick

33. Association of American Medical Colleges. (2011, November 1). Behavioral and Social Science Foundations for Future Physicians. Retrieved from https://www.aamc.org/download/271020/data/behavioralandsocialsciencefoundationsforfuturephysicians.pdf

34. Renz, L. (2013, November 10). How does ICD-10 affect Mental Health!? Revised June 19, 2015, Retrieved from http://pimsyehr.com/resources/icd-10/189-icd-com-pmh-phc-cdb-how-does-icd-10-affect-mental-health

35. World Health Organization (WHO). (2004, July 13). The ICD-10 Classification of Mental and Behavioural Disorders. Retrieved from http://www.who.int/classifications/icd/en/bluebook.pdf

36. Cain, C., & Bredemeyer, B. (2013, March 12). ICD-10-CM Coding for Internal Medicine including Primary Care, Pediatrics and OB/GYN. Retrieved from http://betterhealth.mckesson.com/wp-content/uploads/MED3000-ICD-10-slide-deck-3-14-13.pdf

37. American Academy of Professional Coders. (2013, October 29). ICD-10 Resource: Coding for Major Depressive Disorder. Retrieved from http://cloud.aapc.com/documents/Depressive-Disorder-ICD-10-BH.pdf

38. U.S. Bureau of Labor Statistics. (n.d.). Dentists. from http://www.bls.gov/ooh/healthcare/dentists.htm

39. Career Cornerstone Center: Careers in Science, Technology, Engineering, Math and Medicine. (n.d.). Retrieved from http://www.careercornerstone.org/dentist/dentist.htm

References

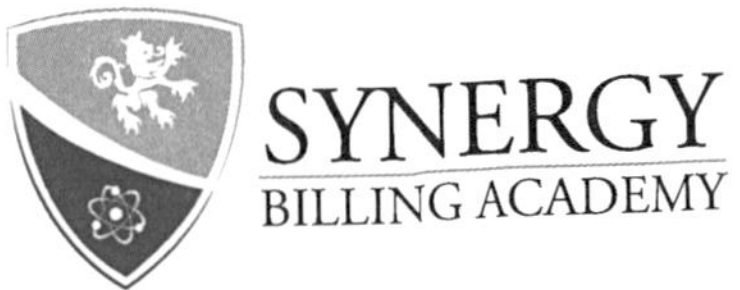

40. American Dental Association. (n.d.). Code on Dental Procedures and Nomenclature (CDT). Retrieved from http://www.ada.org/3827.aspx

41. American Association of Oral and Maxillofacial Surgeons. (n.d.). Difference in Coding Dentoalveolar Codes in ICD-10-CM. Retrieved from http://www.aaoms.org/members/resources/practice-management-and-allied-staff/practice-management-and-allied-staff-news-and-materials/difference-in-coding-dentoalveolar-codes-in-icd-10-cm

42. National Institute of Dental and Craniofacial Research. (2014, October 8). Diabetes and Oral Health. Retrieved from http://www.nidcr.nih.gov/OralHealth/Topics/Diabetes/

43. Govoni, M., & Leeuw, W. (2005, November 15). Dental Care - Medical Conditions that Affect Dental Treatment. Revised January 20, 2015, Retrieved from http://www.dentalcare.com/en-US/dental-education/continuing-education/ce76/ce76.aspx?ModuleName=coursecontent&PartID=6&SectionID=-1

44. Workgroup for Electronic Data Interchange. (2013, January 14). ICD-10-CM Training Module for Dental Practitioners. Retrieved from https://www.wedi.org/forms/uploadFiles/2303D00000045.toc.Jan.14DentalWebinar.pdf

45. American Health Information Management Association. (n.d.). Choose Your Path to ICD-10. Retrieved from http://www.ahima.org/topics/icd10

46. Crozer-Keystone Health System. (n.d.). ICD-10 Tips for All Specialties. Retrieved from http://www.crozerkeystone.org/healthcare-professionals/icd-10-update/updates-on-icd-10-clinical-documentation-improvement/

47. Centers for Medicare and Medicaid Services. (n.d.). The Small Physician Practice's Route to ICD-10. Retrieved from http://www.roadto10.org/

48. Eramo, L. (2013, October 28). 6 Key ICD-10 Changes for Primary Care. Retrieved from http://gettingpaid.kareo.com/gettingpaid/2013/10/6-key-icd-10-changes-for-primary-care/

49. Centers for Medicare and Medicaid Services. (2015, June 1). ICD-10-CM/PCS Myths and Facts. Retrieved from https://www.cms.gov/Medicare/Coding/ICD10/downloads/ICD-10MythsandFacts.pdf

50. Centers for Medicare and Medicaid Services. (n.d.). ICD-10-CM/PCS Myths and Facts - Centers for Medicare & Medicaid Services. Retrieved from https://www.cms.gov/Outreach-and-Education/Medicare-Learning-Network-MLN/MLNProducts/MLN-Publications-Items/ICN902143.html